P9-DVL-177

Publisher's Note

on is designed to provide accurate and authoritative information in regard to the
covered. It is sold with the understanding that the publisher is not engaged in
hological, financial, legal, or other professional services. If expert assistance or
eeded, the services of a competent professional should be sought.

the U.S.A. by Publishers Group West; in Canada by Raincoast Books; in Great
ft Book Company, Ltd.; in South Africa by Real Books, Ltd.; in Australia by
n New Zealand by Tandem Press.

94 Aphrodite Matsakis
    New Harbinger Publications, Inc.
    5674 Shattuck Avenue
    Oakland, CA 94609

Susan Sanford
ayle Zanca

ss Catalog Card Number: 93-087082
7 Hardcover

d.

ited States of America on recycled paper.

blications Web address: www.newharbinger.com

1   10   9   8   7   6

Post-Trau
Stress Dis

A COMPLETE TREAT

This publicati
subject matter
rendering psy
counseling is

Distributed in
Britain by Airl
Boobook; and i

Copyright © 19

Cover design by
Text Design by

Library of Congr
ISBN 1-879237-68

All rights reserve

Printed in the Un

New Harbinger P

00   99   98

15   14   13   12

Aphrodite M

Edited by

NEW HARBINGE

This book is dedicated to all who suffer and all who will suffer in our trauma-ridden world. Hopefully, aside from offering specific techniques and theories, this book will help teach respect and compassion for trauma survivors and their pain.

Contents

List of Handouts

Acknowledgments

I would like to gratefully acknowledge Ms. Leslie Tilley for her careful editing of this book and Dr. Matthew McKay for his guidance and support. I would also like to gratefully acknowledge the many scholars and clinicians, most of whom I have never met, but whose works have inspired me and taught me about trauma and its effects. These individuals include Jonathan Shay, Ph.D., M.D.; Judith Herman, M.D.; Christine Courtois, Ph.D.; Judeit Sprei-Ott, Ph.D.; Judith Peterson, Ph.D.; Richard Kluft, M.D.; Frank Putnam; Richard Lowenstein, M.D.; Besssel van der Kolk, M.D.; Lenore Walker, Ph.D.; Eric Gerdemen, Ph.D.; Irene Frieze, Ph.D.; and Irwin Parsons, Ph.D.

I also want to thank my colleagues Peter Valerio, M.A.C.P.C.; Carole Rayburn, Ph.D.; Wayne Miller, M.A., M.S.W.; Edward Jordan, Ph.D.; and William Washington, M.S.W., for sharing their expertise in working with trauma survivors.

My daughters, Theodora and Magdalena, deserve special recognition for their patience and support, and the staff at New Harbinger needs to be commended for its timely and careful efforts on behalf of this book.

Introduction

In your career as a therapist, you are bound to be confronted with trauma survivors, many of whom suffer from post-traumatic stress disorder, or PTSD. But, because PTSD was only officially recognized by the American Psychiatric Association in 1980 (in the *Diagnostic and Statistical Manual of Mental Disorders*, Third Edition, *DSM-III*), many mental health professionals are still in the process of learning about it. To date, PTSD is one of the least known and least appreciated of the anxiety disorders. As a result, many individuals who suffer from PTSD have not been properly diagnosed and thus have not received adequate help. You may be the first therapist to recognize the symptoms of PTSD or to create a therapeutic setting that permits the trauma to reveal itself or be discussed so that the wounds caused by the trauma can begin to heal.

Not every individual who is traumatized develops PTSD. However, as of this writing PTSD symptoms are estimated to affect, at minimum, some 8 percent of our population (Wolfe 1989). This 8-percent figure does not consist only of combat veterans but includes victims of domestic violence, natural disasters, stranger crime, and vehicular, technological, and occupational accidents. Given the escalation of crime in our country and the continued prevalence of other forms of trauma, this figure can only be expected to increase.

For example, according to Justice Department figures there was an estimated 59 percent increase in rapes and attempted rapes in the United States between 1991 and 1992. In a parallel manner, there was an 8 percent rise in violent crimes (*Washington Post* 20 April 1992). Statistics also indicate a rise in child abuse (*Washington Post* 29 Sept. 1992). Whether these increases are artifacts of increased public awareness of the problem, improved reporting procedures, or increased willingness on the part of victims to report the crime, is an unanswerable question. However, regardless of how one interprets these statistics, they do indicate appreciable social problems.

Another widespread problem is wife abuse. Despite increased publicity and public awareness of the problem of woman battering, the 1988 U.S. Surgeon General's Report listed domestic violence as the number-one health risk among women (*Washington Post* 3 Oct. 1992).

Adult survivors of child abuse, abused women, children growing up in violent homes, and victims of rape and other crimes are all high-risk candidates for developing PTSD, and, given the prevalence of such violence, these survivors promise to be a part of many therapists' caseloads. In addition, given the persistence of war in our world, combat veterans, refugees, and other war survivors will also inevitably appear for help.

PTSD Therapy Versus Other Therapeutic Approaches

The most basic goals of PTSD therapy are to improve clients' self-confidence and their sense of being able to cope with life and with themselves. Basically, achieving these goals involves helping clients to develop and improve as many mastery skills as they can handle. Trauma renders people helpless and erodes their self-esteem, at least temporarily. Until the trauma is processed, many survivors continue to feel helpless and powerless over their lives. Your job is to restore to your clients a sense of personal power, as much as is possible.

Unfortunately, this can be as difficult to do as it is easy to say, especially in the case of family abuse survivors, prisoners of war, refugees, combat veterans, and others who have been subjected to long-term or severe trauma. As you may already know, post-traumatic stress disorder is extremely complex. Each client has a unique, perhaps virtually unbelievable, set of experiences, and an almost equally unique set of reactions to those experiences. Helping these clients will call upon your creativity and your compassion, as well as your knowledge and repertoire of therapeutic interventions. It may even cause you to reconsider some of your previous views of the world and to revise your sociopolitical perspectives. It could be the most taxing work you will ever do. Yet it is work that desperately needs to be done, and done in a manner that minimizes the retraumatization inherent in the process of reworking the trauma in a therapeutic setting.

PTSD sufferers have many of the same inner conflicts, deficits in social and vocational skills, growth issues, and self-defeating cognitions and behaviors as other clients. However, traumatized clients differ from nontraumatized clients in that, in addition to many of the familiar therapeutic concerns, they have lost their feeling of being safe in the world. Equally frightening, they have often come to feel unsafe within themselves. Concomitant to and contributing to such fears are alterations in thinking patterns, in emotional equilibrium, and in biochemistry that can result from the trauma.

Trauma also affects three important psychological abilities (Briere et al. 1992):

- The ability to modulate or temper strong feelings and the associated ability to soothe and comfort oneself

- The ability to maintain connections with others

- The ability to maintain a positive self-identity

These effects of trauma can interact to create a negative cascade in the survivor's life. For example, the inability to modulate strong affect can contribute to the survivor's difficulties in maintaining connections with others, pursuing goals, functioning at work or in school, all of which affect self-image. Conversely, lack of connection with others can create loneliness and despair, which lead to strong feelings of deprivation, rage, and self-hatred, which in turn (especially when added to the feelings born of the trauma), can make the survivor feel out of control—as if he or she were a boiling cauldron of personally aversive and socially undesirable traits. This again contributes to the survivor's loss of positive identity, difficulty interacting with others, and failure to recover from the trauma.

If a survivor has additionally been chastised, blamed, rejected, or simply ignored by important family members, friends, other loved ones, or peers, their social ties may be severely damaged as well. Consequently, trauma survivors typically have to endure not only the mental confusion, emotional pain, and involuntary physiological responses that can attend traumatization, but loneliness and abandonment as well—at the very time in life when their need for protection, care, and concern from others are at a peak.

In treating trauma survivors, you need to remember that, although on the one hand trauma is trauma, and trauma survivors, regardless of the kind or duration of the trauma they endured, have many commonalities, on the other hand there can be significant differences between the impact of childhood trauma and the impact of adult trauma. For example, childhood trauma survivors tend to look for internal solutions to their problems since in their past often their supporter was also their abuser, and hence they may fear punishment if they ask for assistance. Also, in the classic abused child paradigm, the abused child is the caretaker of the abuser. Therefore, in the client's history, it was the adult who came to the child for nurture and support, not the other way around. For the adult survivor of child abuse to ask for help is to step out of the role.

In addition, if survivors of childhood abuse come to you as young or mature adults wanting assistance with dysfunctional coping mechanisms, you will be dealing with patterns that are thoroughly ingrained, and having been practiced perhaps for decades. Consequently, your counseling goals and methods will be different from those you would use with, for example, a recent survivor of a rape or mugging, a vehicular accident, or a natural catastrophe.

Regardless of the client's history, your first task is to ascertain whether the client has been traumatized and assess for PTSD symptoms. However, if the client has not previously received adequate help, you may not see PTSD symptoms at first. Instead, you may see secondary elaborations stemming from or reinforced by the trauma or some of the client's well-practiced defenses. These disguise the underlying PTSD and can easily be mistaken for other disorders. Most commonly, long-term untreated PTSD expresses itself as a major depression, a character disorder, or in the form of psychosomatic symptoms.

You may also be exposed to clients who, until they came to you, were misdiagnosed. The average person with multiple personality disorder, for example, is in the mental health system for seven years before being properly diagnosed. Vietnam veterans, abused wives, and abused children have also been frequently misdiagnosed or had stigmatizing psychiatric labels applied to them (Sonnenberg et al. 1985; Herman 1992; Courtois 1988; Walker 1979). In fact, some of your work with trauma survivors may include correcting the effects of previous therapists and their diagnoses.

The Therapist's Role

Traumatized clients' process of regaining a sense of power and control over their lives often begins in your office. Consequently you need to structure and conduct your therapy so that you are not in the position of "superior therapist" helping an "inferior patient." PTSD therapy needs to be conducted more as a collaborative effort than as a traditional hierarchical doctor-patient relationship.

You are there to create a safe setting where the client can share about the trauma, along with other concerns. Part of creating this sense of safety is to give your client as many choices as possible within the boundaries you have established for your work. For example, from the very outset, you can make it clear that if the client begins to feel overwhelmed or extremely uncomfortable with the material being discussed, or with your questions, she or he can let you know of the anxiety or other discomfort, and you will gladly stop your line of investigation. You can then invite (not force, pressure, or insist) that the client discuss her or his reactions and why she or he needed to stop, leaving the decision up to the client.

In addition, you need to be aware of times clients feel overwhelmed and begin unconsciously to remove themselves from the session, for instance, by dissociating in some way. Signs of dissociation include blank stares, placating smiles, or other facial gestures inappropriate to the material being discussed, sudden twitching, yawning, or even falling asleep (see the "Cautions" section, below).

Although you need to give your clients as many choices and as much support as possible, this does not mean that you abdicate control of the therapy, since this would create anxiety in the client as well as defeat the therapeutic goals.

Consistency, predictability, and supportiveness are key aspects of quality PTSD therapy, as they are in any kind of therapeutic work. Ideally, you will be able to do more than be gentle and nonaccusatory; however, there will inevitably be times when all you can do is simply listen carefully, ask for more information, and show empathy for the client's predicaments and pain.

Some trauma survivors relate such horror stories that you are left speechless. When all your knowledge of psychology fails you, and when making a positive suggestion would insult the client's pain, all you may be able to do is acknowledge how you are feeling. "Your story is heartbreaking," you might say. "We therapists are supposed to have so many answers and things to say to help people, but right now I have nothing to say. Your story is so full of pain and horrible incidents that I don't know how you survived. I really admire your strength and courage. You truly are a survivor."

Cautions

You will need to constantly monitor your clients' reactions to the therapy. You also need to teach them to monitor themselves. If, in session or between sessions, a client reports any of the symptoms listed in the Warning Signs handout provided here, you need to stop whatever you are doing in therapy and attend to the symptom. In some cases, you may want to consult with a physician, a psychiatrist, or both, or urge your client to make an appointment with a medical doctor or psychiatrist. In extreme instances, you may need to rush your client to an emergency room, such as in the case of chest pains.

The symptoms listed here are among those to watch for. This list is not exhaustive—different clients will manifest problems differently. You will need to be sensitive and use your judgment. It is suggested that you photocopy this handout and give it to your traumatized clients, to help them recognize warning signs.

Also stop the therapy and focus on the symptom being experienced when clients report having so much emotional pain, anxiety, or anger that they fear they are going to die. Mild anxiety is to be expected, but extreme anxiety or despair need immediate attention.

Warning Signs

As you work to heal from your trauma, both in sessions and outside, you need to monitor your reactions. This work includes talking to your counselor, doing writing or other exercises about the traumatic events you experienced or the aftereffects, emotional effects, or subsequent related events. If you experience any of the following symptoms while doing such work (or at any other time) stop what you are doing immediately and talk to your counselor or another mental health professional.

- Hyperventilation (uncontrollable gasping for air or rapid breathing), uncontrollable shaking, or irregular heartbeat

- Feelings that you are losing touch with reality, even temporarily, for instance, having hallucinations or extreme flashbacks of the event

- Feeling disoriented, spaced out, unreal, or as if you might be losing control

- Extreme nausea, diarrhea, hemorrhaging, or other physical problems, including intense, new, or unexplainable pains or an increase in symptoms of a preexisting medical problem, for example, blood sugar problems if you are diabetic

- A desire to hurt yourself

- Self-destructive behavior such as alcohol or drug abuse, self-induced vomiting, or overspending

- Suicidal or homicidal thoughts

- Memory problems

Also call for help if you are having so much emotional pain, anxiety, or anger that you fear you are going to die. Mild anxiety is a normal reaction, but extreme anxiety or despair needs professional attention as soon as possible.

If you are unable to contact your counselor and are truly frightened, go to the emergency room of a local hospital. Meanwhile, do the following:

- Focus on something besides the trauma.

- Touch a physical object (a wall, a chair, whatever is nearby).

- Talk to someone right away.

- Avoid isolating yourself or taking alcohol, drugs, or other mood-altering substances.

- If you are angry, try expressing it in a safe way, such as talking to a trusted friend, punching a pillow, or tearing up a telephone directory.

- Do something pleasurable and relaxing: Take a hot bath, go for a long walk, listen to favorite music, pet the cat.

Even if you feel certain you do not need professional help, if you experience any of the reactions listed above, take a break from trauma work and follow one of these suggestions.

Keep in mind that having a strong reaction to thinking about the trauma or otherwise working on healing does not make you a failure. Developing symptoms as a result of being in therapy does not reflect an inability to heal or a hidden unwillingness to heal.

Instead, your reactions probably reflect the degree of traumatization you endured, which was not under your control. Your reactions have nothing to do with your strength of character.

When clients have strong reactions to therapy, it does not mean they are unwilling or unable to heal or that you have failed as a counselor. Instead their reactions probably reflect the degree of traumatization they endured, which was not under their control.

You should be aware, however, that there are those who have been so severely traumatized that they may be better off leaving the past unexamined. The memories of certain torture victims, family abuse survivors, crime survivors, prisoners of war, and concentration camp survivors may be better left buried. When clients fall into one of these categories, or if you find that the reactions listed above occur so frequently and intensely that the "healing" process is making their lives unlivable, you should concentrate your efforts on helping them find relief from their symptoms, rather than remembering and coping with the trauma itself.

Healing: Definitions and Prerequisites

For the purposes of this book, healing means that less and less of the client's energy is being drained away by the unresolved emotional and other conflicts related to the trauma, so that more and more of the client's energy can be invested in present-day activities and relationships. A variety of formulations of the healing process have been offered by well-respected professionals in the field of traumatology (Herman 1992; Courtois 1988; Smith 1985a,b; Arnold 1985). The basics of the process as presented here are these:

- The client remembers or brings forth from repression enough of the trauma that he or she can make sense of the symptoms and conflicts experienced.

- The client experiences the trauma with some of the associated emotions (not necessarily all), which may not have been experienced at the time it occurred.

- The client reproduces the trauma cognitively so as to eradicate fallacious conclusions and integrate the trauma into the client's view of themselves and the world.

Carl Jung used the metaphor of a growing tree to describe the client in therapy. The client, he said, is like a tree, naturally growing taller and fuller while its roots spread out wider and deeper into the ground. When the roots of the tree hit a large stone or other obstacle, rather than trying to shove the stone away or crack it, the roots just grow around the obstacle and keep going. The stone may have interrupted or slowed the tree's growth for a while, but no stone, no matter how large, can stop the tree from growing.

In Jung's view, the stones in the way of tree roots symbolize obstacles to personal growth. These obstacles can include an internal emotional conflict (such as loving and hating the same person) or an external stressor (such as a trauma). Jung theorized that certain emotional conflicts are never totally eliminated; they are simply outgrown. They stay a permanent part of the psyche, just as the stones surrounded by tree roots become "part of" the tree. In the same way that roots can move far past the stones in their path into new territory, clients can integrate and grow beyond their traumatic experiences.

A client's trauma may be, to one degree or another, frozen in time, outside of his or her awareness. Reintegrating the trauma can free up the powerful energy it has generated. That energy can then be used to pursue goals of the client's choosing, and the trauma can become a vital part of the client's life—just as stones can support and strengthen the tree's root structure.

However, one of the most common errors made by therapists in working with PTSD clients is that, in their desire to promote healing, they jump into the healing process almost immediately, whether or not the client is ready to do the same. In order for healing to truly begin, certain preconditions must be met. The entire healing process presented in this book is built on these foundations:

- A working therapeutic alliance between the client and the therapist
- The client feeling relatively safe in the world
- The client feeling safe within himself or herself

A "working therapeutic alliance" means that the therapist and client must trust and feel safe with each other in a relationship whose sole purpose is the safeguarding and promotion of the client's physical, emotional, and mental well-being. The second point above means that the client cannot be in a condition of current danger or victimization. For example, clients who are still in abusive relationships with violent or sexually abusive mates, parents, or other persons; clients who are subject to unpredictable assaults in a crime-ridden neighborhood; or clients who are suffering from a medical condition, but are not seeking medical attention due to survivor guilt, low self-esteem, addiction, or other aftereffects of the trauma, cannot be involved in the healing process in any meaningful manner.

The third point means that the healing process cannot take place productively—that is, without further fragmenting and frightening the client—unless the client feels relatively safe in terms of his or her own current responses to life. For example, clients who have so much leftover rage from the trauma and its aftermath that they are afraid they will commit murder the next time someone cuts them off on the highway, or whose lives are severely constricted by their avoidance of reminders of the trauma, live in fear of themselves.

Thus the major symptoms suffered by the clients need to be brought under some control—either through stress management, anger management, medication, or via some other means—before the healing process is begun. Otherwise, the therapy will inadvertently create more fear, anxiety, and stress by resurrecting the past. In learning increasingly to control their symptoms and manage their emotions, clients acquire the tools necessary to tolerating the effects generated by remembering the trauma.

Special problems arise when the client is an alcoholic, is drug-addicted or is suffering from an eating disorder. Any of these conditions serves to both block out memories and numb emotions. Since healing requires acknowledgment and processing of traumatic memories and the associated emotions, clients cannot process what they cannot remember and cannot feel feelings they have effectively numbed. Therefore, the addiction needs to be reduced or, ideally, removed, for deep healing to begin. Furthermore, these conditions present medical problems. Left unchecked, alcoholism, drug addictions, and eating disorders can reach life-threatening proportions and may require inpatient care.

Description of the Book

This book is meant to serve as an introduction to PTSD for clinicians who want to learn to work more effectively with trauma survivors. To that end, the book is divided into two parts. Part I, "Overview of PTSD," offers a broad picture of

PTSD, which you will need before beginning the therapeutic process. Chapter 1, "PTSD: Survey and Definitions," defines trauma and PTSD, stressing its uniqueness in the psychiatric classification system, presents a brief overview of some of the theories regarding the causes of PTSD, and provides a brief description of the symptoms of PTSD, associated problems, and the stages of healing.

Chapter 2, "Clinical Diagnosis of PTSD," carefully reviews each of the *DSM-IV* criteria for PTSD and gives guidelines for assessing severity. The impact of severity on treatment and prognosis are also explored.

In recent years, it has increasingly been recognized that PTSD is best understood as a bio-socio-psychological problem—that is, as a problem with significant biological and societal aspects as well as the more familiar psychological ones. Chapter 3, "The Biochemistry of PTSD," presents research regarding biochemical changes that can be caused by trauma, such as the depletion of neurotransmitters, and describes some of the potential psychological disorders that can result from these biochemical changes, including depression and substance abuse. This line of investigation began with Abraham Kardiner's observations of combat veterans. After studying these men, Kardiner (1941) called PTSD a "physioneurosis," a mental disorder with both psychological and physiological components. Since Kardiner, especially recently, considerable research has been completed on the physiology of PTSD. While some of this research is controversial, research into the biochemistry of trauma reactions is one of the major current trends in traumatology. Clinicians working in the field need to be aware of the state of art in this area and attempt to stay current.

Part II, "The Therapeutic Process," reflects in a general way the structure of the healing process. However, the healing process, like any truly creative event, seldom follows any "cookbook" prescription, set rules, or concrete pathways. Instead it is a uniquely personal flow of intrapsychic events: changes in emotional state and emotional capacity and changes in perspective. It is impossible, and highly inadvisable, to attempt to constrain the process to a set order or series of stages. Thus, the chapters in this section can be viewed as reflecting an "ideal" order.

Chapter 4, "Client Assessment," teaches you how to assess clients for PTSD and concurrent problems, including the effects of former therapists and doctors and any misdiagnoses. On the basis of the rather complete assessment recommended in this chapter, you will be guided in formulating an initial treatment plan and in modifying that plan over time. Chapter 4 also contains some discussion on using medication for controlling PTSD symptoms.

Chapter 5, "Groundwork for the Therapeutic Process," instructs you in establishing the foundation for the therapeutic process. It outlines the major elements of establishing a collaborative relationship with the client, in which she or he feels safe and valued and in which the client's self-doubt, mistrust, and hopelessness can be challenged. Also covered are the basics of educating clients about trauma, PTSD, and the cognitive and behavioral work you will be doing.

Chapter 6, "Symptom Management," provides you further tools for challenging the client's fears and negative self-evaluations and cognitions, by presenting the basics of symptom management. This chapter assists you in helping clients begin to regain a sense of control over their lives by providing guidelines that assist clients in making their present world as safe as possible, identifying and better managing situations that ignite problem emotions and memories (trigger situations), and managing their anger.

This chapter is especially helpful when clients come to you in crisis: either immediately after the trauma, when some event has triggered a memory of the trauma, or when they find themselves unable to function as they would like in some important area of life. Symptom-specific exercises and suggestions are offered.

Chapter 7, "PTSD-Related Problems," covers difficulties related to trauma and PTSD that often need to be continually addressed throughout the healing process. For example, it is important to acknowledge and deal with the way the outside world reacts to trauma survivors. Along with the trauma itself, the responses of other people to both the event and the symptoms it causes form the context in which the survivors live and seek healing. The phenomena of "secondary wounding" and "victim thinking" (or internalization of victim status), which such wounding causes, are covered.

This chapter also examines the problems of self-blame, survivor guilt, and low self-esteem, which often accompany surviving a trauma. Exercises are provided to help raise clients' awareness of these problems and their effects and to offer assistance in identifying the ways each of these problems might be ameliorated.

Chapters 8, 9, and 10 collectively cover the basic dynamics of the healing process. Chapter 8, "Uncovering the Trauma," offers guidance in helping clients remember and reconstruct the trauma mentally, as realistically and accurately as possible. Chapter 9, "Feelings Work," provides the basics of teaching clients about the nature of feelings and helping them learn to distinguish feelings from thoughts. Specific exercises and other aids assist you in helping clients work on their anger and grief, the two major emotions associated with PTSD.

If the trauma is severe, the healing process may continue for decades. However, after sufficient work is completed in remembering the trauma and coping with the associated feelings, there are areas of personal growth and reintegration into society that can be considered the latter stages of healing. Chapter 10, "Final Healing Stages," outlines and provides methods of helping clients becoming reinvolved in their community, refinding their pretrauma self, and acknowledging and working on unresolved angers, as well as identifying and accepting the limits of the therapeutic process.

Chapter 11, "Other Professional and Therapeutic Concerns," covers aspects of the therapist-client relationship and concerns specific to you as a person and a mental health professional, such as the major transference and countertransference issues that occur in work with trauma survivors, assessment of PTSD for nonclinical purposes, and the issue of false memories. Other special challenges confronting the therapist who works with trauma survivors are also discussed.

Appendix A, "A Brief History of Traumatology," gives the background of the diagnosis and treatment of what is now termed post-traumatic stress disorder. You will find it useful in educating clients about PTSD and personally in gaining a historical perspective on survivors' problems.

Appendix B, "Professional Resources and Training," discusses professional training and resources and offers a further readings list.

Client Handouts

Throughout the book are questionnaires, and exercises, set up to be photo-copied, which can serve as handouts for your clients. (The list of warning signs earlier in this introduction is one example.) They are also, however, also intended as guides for you to use in gaining needed information about your clients during your sessions. Only you can decide which handouts to use—which are applicable to a specific client and which may produce an undesired effect. It may also be that some individual questions need to be saved until a later point in therapy.

Similarly, only you can decide if a client could safely complete a handout outside of a session or if a particular questionnaire or exercise is best completed only with your assistance.

When and if you give a client a handout to take home, you need to give firm, clear instructions to the client to stop working on it whenever he or she experiences any of the symptoms listed in the Warning Signs handout above. You will also want to go over the handout in session to be sure the client understands the questions.

Stress to clients that these are not "homework assignments" that need to be completed in a satisfactory way for the therapy to continue or for you to be pleased. You could say, for example, "If—for whatever reason—you can't or don't want to work on this exercise, just stop. At our next session, simply tell me you couldn't finish it. You don't have to explain why, but if you want to share your reasons, that is fine. We will still work together whether or not you finish the exercise."

Only a Beginning

This book is not a crash course in PTSD therapy, but rather a preliminary overview of some of the many issues involved in helping traumatized persons. It will prepare you for reading some of the more in-depth books and articles listed in the "Further Reading" section of appendix B and will help in any training you decide to pursue.

You will need additional training especially if you want to work with traumatized children or individuals with multiple personality disorder (MPD). (This book does not cover the diagnosis and treatment of either MPD clients, children, or survivors of ritual cult abuse.) Trauma survivors overall are a highly vulnerable group of people, and you could make serious mistakes, despite good intentions and sincere efforts, unless you avail yourself of available workshops and reading material on PTSD in general and on the specific populations you are serving.

As you read this book, keep in mind that despite recent interest in the effects of trauma on human beings, our knowledge of the full range of human reactions to overwhelming stress is limited. Just as trauma survivors sometimes choose to deny that the trauma occurred, society sometimes chooses to deny the fact of unjustifiable human suffering. As a result, professional interest in the area of traumatology has been relatively sparse compared to research and study of other problems.

For example, despite thought-provoking research in the area of trauma physiology, the complex psychological and physiological reactions to trauma have yet to be unraveled. Experts are still searching for effective psychotherapeutic responses, and research and outcome studies regarding the use of psychiatric medications to help control some of the most troublesome symptoms of PTSD are still in the infancy stage.

To date, most of our knowledge about PTSD is based on studies of two kinds of trauma survivors: rape victims and combat veterans, especially Vietnam War and Israeli soldiers. Furthermore, outcome studies on active combat soldiers have often been oriented toward methods of helping soldiers with acute PTSD reactions to ongoing trauma so that they can return to battle, rather than toward healing on a deeper level or assisting soldiers with domestic, vocational, and other readjustment problems upon return to civilian life (Solomon et al. 1992 Avraham). Although there is a growing body of literature on abused women and children, it is still relatively small. And there are only a handful of studies on refugees, prisoners of war, and natural catastrophe, vehicular accident, and crime survivors.

Despite the limits of research in the field, however, there is ample evidence that healing is possible. According to some, the prognosis for trauma survivors has improved five to ten times in the past decades (Briere et al. 1992). The reason for this dramatic increase is a greater understanding of trauma among mental health professionals. Today more and more professionals are learning to ask about the presence of trauma in their clients' histories and to assign significance to the trauma. In the past, in many cases, healing did not occur or was stunted because the client was diagnosed as a "hopeless case" or as suffering from intractable disorder, such as implied by some *DSM-III-R* diagnoses. Simply put, when an Axis 2 diagnosis was given to people, they were essentially being told not only that they had a major problem but that they would always have it, which for some clients was easily translated into "I may as well give up." In such situations, slow therapeutic progress was the result not so much of client problems, but of the fact that the help received was insufficient or misdirected and the problem was assumed to be insurmountable.

Recovery for trauma survivors, however, is not hopeless. Therapists working with trauma survivors can take heart from the fact that individuals suffering from one of the most severe traumatic reactions, multiple personality disorder, have been found capable of healing. Thus, the promise for less traumatized persons is considerable (Cohen 1992). The therapy, however, must be intense and of sufficient duration.

You are to be commended for your interest in improving your skills to help heal people who have suffered so greatly. Working with trauma survivors is taxing, and may cause you to have nightmares, depressive moods, angry feelings and other PTSD symptoms, at least temporarily. Consequently, you will need to take excellent care of yourself. Remember to apply to yourself the advice you will want to give your clients: "You can't go through trauma alone." Try to establish a supportive network of colleagues to assist you in this difficult, but important, work.

Part I

Overview of PTSD

Chapter 1

PTSD: Survey and Definitions

Tell me, sweet lord, what is't that takes from thee
Thy stomach, pleasure and thy golden sleep?
Why dost thou bend thine eyes upon the earth,
And start so often when thou sit'st alone?
Why hast thou lost the fresh blood in thy cheeks,
And given my treasures and my rights of thee,
To thick-ey'd musing and curs'd melancholy?
In thy faint slumbers I by thee have watch'd,
And heard thee murmur tales of iron wars:
Speak terms of manage to thy bounding steed;
Cry "Courage!—to the field!" And thou hast talk'd
Of sallies and retires; of trenches, tents,
Of palisadoes, frontiers, parapets,
Of basilisks, of cannon, culverin,
Or prisoner's ransom, and of soldiers slain,
And all the current of a heady fight.
Thy spirit within thee hath been so at war,
And thus hath so bestir'd thee in thy sleep,
That beads of sweat have stood upon thy brow,
Like bubbles in a late-disturbed stream:
And in thy face strange motions have appear'd,
Such as we see when men restrain their breath
On some great sudden haste.
O, what portents are these?

—William Shakespeare, *Henry IV, Part I*
act 2, scene 3

Although Shakespeare didn't know it by name, the insomnia, depression, and other symptoms Lady Percy describes to her husband, Hotspur, in the above scene are those of *post-traumatic stress disorder* or PTSD. PTSD, one of the most common human reactions to traumatic events, is much in the news today. There is also increased professional interest in the syndrome, as evidenced by increased publications, workshops, and policy statements on the subject in both mental health and medical communities.[1] Some professionals have even specialized in trauma-related work. However, the field of traumatology is relatively new. Until recently, most mental health professionals have treated clients for the aftereffects of trauma rather than for the trauma itself.

PTSD used to be associated primarily with the struggles of Vietnam veterans, but today this term is being used to describe the afflictions of a wide variety of trauma survivors: rape and crime victims, natural catastrophe survivors, refugees, torture survivors, abused women and children, and in some cases, survivors of vehicular accidents and technological disasters. Service and medical personnel who are constantly exposed to life-or-death situations (rescue squad workers, police officers, firefighters, and medical personnel on burn wards or in trauma units), have also been described as high-risk candidates for developing PTSD (Ochberg 1988; Williams 1987a).

At first glance, combat veterans, battered women, and hurricane survivors seem very divergent populations. How can they all potentially suffer from the same syndrome? These groups do differ in many important ways. However, they, like other trauma survivors, have had at least one common experience: They have all been rendered helpless in a situation of great danger. While every individual encounters his or her trauma with a unique personal history and means of coping, and while different traumas tend to result in different sets of readjustment problems, a similar and fairly predictable set of psychological and physiological reactions potentially follows exposure to a life-threatening experience or set of experiences.

This set of reactions is what has been labeled *post-traumatic stress disorder* or, if of short duration with minimal long-term effects, *acute stress disorder*. The subject of this book, however, is post-traumatic stress disorder, or PTSD. Although PTSD has existed for centuries, under different names (see appendix A, "A Brief History of Traumatology"), and is one of the most common reactions to trauma, it was only included in the *Diagnostic and Statistical Manual of Mental Disorders* in 1980 *(DSM-III)*. (Note that full-blown PTSD, as described in *DSM-III-R* and *DSM-IV*, is not the only possible response to trauma. Psychosomatic problems, panic attacks, and other disorders are also sometimes responses. Indeed, enough is still not known about the full range of human reactions to life-threatening events.)

Insomnia, nightmares, substance abuse, anxiety, anger, depression, and the ever-present fear that the horror will return are common to those who suffer from PTSD. The nightmares and addiction problems of combat veterans have become common knowledge, and their war-related flashbacks have been glamorized in the media. Less publicized are their agonizing self-doubts, their intense fear of their falsely glamorized nightmares and flashbacks, and their sense that not neces-

---

1. In 1984, for example, the American Psychological Association conducted an in-depth survey of attitudes towards trauma survivors among a wide variety of helping professionals, ranging from policemen and physicians to social workers, psychologists, and psychiatrists (American Psychological Association 1984). The early 1990s witnessed several ground-breaking articles in journals of psychiatry and general medicine, which stressed the importance of inquiring about histories of childhood sexual and physical abuse in diagnosing and treating patients. They also noted the damaging effects of childhood abuse, regardless of its type, on the developing psyche of a child (Brown and Anderson 1991; van der Kolk, Perry, and Herman 1991; Rose 1991). Previously the majority of articles relating to childhood abuse tended to blame the "seductiveness" and "Oedipal" wishes of prepubertal children for incest and other forms of child sexual assault (Savina 1987).

war itself, but some other form of death will soon engulf either them
e they love

s well-known, but well-documented, is that battered wives and
en suffer from almost identical problems: sleeping disturbances,
addiction. Like PTSD-afflicted combat veterans and some survi-
isasters, family abuse survivors have been found to suffer from
d at least low-grade depression (Williams 1987a; Walker 1979;
tois 1988).

tal Illness

ical and mental health professionals attributed depres-
s certain other symptoms, to internal psychological
than as a response to external events. In the case
is belief is not necessarily false. (It is, however,
e into account the effect of social and economic
e stresses, on the individual.) In the case of
uma alone, regardless of any previous psy-
development of a variety of symptoms.
cute Stress Disorder are the only diagno-
s on external events rather than on in-
s are also the only ones to recognize
ing has the potential for developing
t for more than four weeks, PTSD

stress, other factors such as an
logical state, are irrelevant in
During World War II, for ex-
health and family stability
preexisting social or psy-
ariable in the develop-
he degree of stress to
2; Matsakis 1988).

Similarly, a la   victim's race, sex,
educational status,   or she would develop PTSD. Neithe   s (for example,
panic disorder, agora   mining factor
was instead the stressf   among individuals who had been th   as a burglary in which no one wa   e higher
among individuals who had   the individual or others were injure   erwise was
or appeared to be a threat to life   er Kolk 1990).

Over and over it has been fo   PTSD symptoms,
and the severity of those symptom   the intensity and duration of the stressful event than an   sonality patterns. In short,
what this means is that, although the   personality, belief system, and
values do affect reactions to and inter   ons of the traumatic event, PTSD
does not develop because of some inherent inferiority or weakness in the personality. Trauma changes personalities, not the other way around.

"These are not books, lumps of lifeless paper, but minds alive on the shelves."

—Gilbert Highet

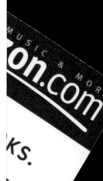

The Physiological Component

Although we use separate words for them, the mind, emotions, and body are part of one whole. When trauma occurs, it affects the whole being—not just the mind or the emotions, but the central nervous system and other aspects of human physiology. As will be further explained in chapter 3, increasing evidence indicates that many of the emotionally distressing symptoms of PTSD have a biological basis (van der Kolk 1988a,b).

For example, John, a Marine combat veteran, every Veteran's Day and Fourth of July has nightmares of the firefight that cost him his leg. He has repeatedly "ordered himself" not to have these nightmares, but to no avail. If the physiological research is correct, then his recurring nightmares are likely based in the biology of trauma and thus beyond his control (van der Kolk 1988a,b; *New York Times* 12 June 1990). In other words, the symptoms of PTSD are not "in the person's head," nor are they a play for attention. Rather these symptoms are the aftereffects of events severe enough to profoundly alter a person's thinking, emotions and physical reactions.

These events need not have gone on for years, months, or even hours. A single life-or-death incident lasting as little as a few seconds can be enough to traumatize an individual. In those few moments, an individual's emotions, identity, and sense of the world as an orderly, secure place can be severely shaken or shattered. Furthermore, an individual need not suffer permanent physical injury or losses in order to be traumatized. Although physical injuries and financial losses are often involved in trauma, even without them, trauma can cause profound ruptures in the individual's sense of self-worth and trust in the world.

Clinical Definition

DSM-IV Criteria

As discussed further in the next chapter, according to the *DSM-IV*, there are six criteria for a PTSD diagnosis. To be diagnosed as having PTSD, an individual must meet all of the following criteria:

A. Have experienced at least one trauma or life-threatening event that had the potential for bodily harm and that the individual responded to with fear, helplessness, or horror.

B. Continue to relive the trauma in the form of what are called *reexperiencing phenomena,* which include nightmares, flashbacks, and intrusive thoughts about the traumatic event.

C. Evidence a persistent avoidance of situations reminiscent of the traumatic event and a numbing of emotions (which alternates with criterion D).

D. Evidence persistent symptoms of physiological hyperarousal: startle response, irritability, difficulty falling asleep, hyperalertness, and other symptoms (alternates with criterion C).

E. Criteria B, C, and D must persist for at least one month after the traumatic event.

F. The traumatic event caused clinically significant distress or dysfunction in the individual's social, occupational, and family functioning or in other important areas of functioning.

Dynamics

As will be explained in greater detail in chapter 2, the fundamental dynamic of PTSD consists of a cycle of intrusive recall of the traumatic event (usually called the intrusive stage), accompanied by reexperiencing symptoms and physiological hyperarousal symptoms, followed by a repression of the memories (usually called the numbing stage), usually accompanied by emotional numbing and *in some cases* partial or total amnesia of the event.

Symptoms

Symptoms of PTSD include, but are not limited to the following:[2]

- Sleep disturbances: insomnia, fitful sleep, nightmares, "night sweats"
- Flashbacks: unwanted memories of the trauma and related events
- Anxiety
- Tendency to react under stress with survival mechanisms appropriate to the trauma (for example, abused children may react with placating or caretaking behaviors; incest victims with flirtatious or seductive behavior; war veterans with threats or aggressive acts)
- Emotional numbing
- Loss of interest in work or activities
- Suicidal thoughts and feelings
- Fantasies of retaliation
- Feelings of alienation and problems with intimate relationships or relationships in general
- Cynicism and distrust of authority figures and public institutions
- Hypersensitivity to injustice
- Tendency to fits of rage or to passivity (may alternate between the two)
- Hyperalertness
- Hyperventilation
- Overprotectiveness and fear of losing others
- Social isolation or emotional distance from others
- Survivor guilt
- Avoidance of activities that arouse memories of trauma
- All-or-nothing thinking
- Fear of the trauma returning

---

2. Most of this list was compiled in the Forgotten Warrior Project, conducted by Dr. John Wilson at Cleveland State University and sponsored by Disabled American Veterans (cited in Ritter 1984). I have also made contributions.

- Dissociation: trance states, denial, "out-of-body" experiences
- Organ-specific psychosomatic problems and psychosomatic problems of long-standing
- Mood swings
- Difficulty concentrating

Polarities in Family Abuse Survivors

A number of polarities have been observed in some (not all) family abuse survivors. The first of these can be labeled naivete alternating with cynicism or paranoia—a joyful "all will be well" view of life versus an extremely negative view. The naivete and optimism reflect the survivor's denial of the abuse and wish that it did not exist. The cynicism or paranoia and negative view of life reflect the survivor's recognition of the abuse and generalization of the cruelty and manipulativeness of the abuser to other persons and to life in general.

The second polarity observed is feelings of worthlessness alternating with feelings of specialness. Abusers often denigrate their victims, even to the point of relegating them to subhuman status. At other times, however, they make the victim feel special and important.

Self-punitive behavior versus self-indulgent behavior is another polarity occurring among family abuse survivors. In this polarity survivors are mimicking the abuser's pattern of first punishing then indulging the victim. In addition, the self-punitive behavior may reflect survivors' self-hatred and feeling that they "deserve" the abuse. At the same time they may reward themselves inappropriately out of feelings of deprivation or self-pity.

Intense dependency alternating with competent or excessive caretaking behavior also occurs, because, ironically, victims often function as the emotional, physical and in some instances the financial or sexual caretakers of their abusers. Abusers foster the victim's dependencies through forced isolation and appeals to the victim's sympathies.

Masked Presentations

The terms *secondary elaborations, epiphenomena,* and *masked presentations* all refer to the psychological syndromes and problems that evolved to cope with trauma. These problems do not present as PTSD, but they suggest possible PTSD and should be carefully explored by the clinician for underlying causes. The longer the individual has suffered from untreated PTSD, and the longer and more severe the trauma, the more likely the clinician will first observe a secondary elaboration or epiphenomenon of the traumatic event rather than clear PTSD syndrome. This is especially the case when clients are in the numbing stages of PTSD and may have difficulties remembering the trauma that range from partial recall to complete amnesia.

Secondary elaborations include:

- Alcohol or drug abuse
- Eating disorders: bulimia nervosa, anorexia nervosa, compulsive eating
- Compulsive gambling or compulsive spending

- Psychosomatic problems

- Homicidal, suicidal, or self-mutilating behavior

- Amnesia

- Phobias

- Panic disorders

- Delinquent or criminal behavior

- Depression or depressive symptoms

- Dissociation symptoms

- Fainting spells

- Psychotic episodes

- Previous diagnosis of a depressive disorder (a major depression, single episode; major depression, recurrent; dysthymia or depressive neurosis; depressive disorder not otherwise specified)

- Previous diagnosis of a dissociative disorder (hysterical neurosis; multiple personality disorder; depersonalization disorder; psychogenic fugue; or dissociative disorder not otherwise specified)

- Borderline personality

- Sleepwalk disorder

The Process of Healing

Paul Hansen (1992), a therapist who works with adult survivors of childhood sexual abuse and who is a survivor of childhood sexual abuse himself, has identified three stages of recovery for individuals who have undergone trauma: the victim stage, the survivor stage, and the thriver stage. Of course, as with all "stage theories" of any psychological process, the stages are not clear cut, and a given individual may not follow the stages linearly or literally. For example, a trauma survivor may have a traumatic memory breakthrough from repression and then once again lose memory of the event.

Also, in cases where a person has been severely traumatized over many years, there is a tendency for the least traumatic memories to emerge first and the most traumatic memories to emerge later in the healing process. As each new level of memories begins to emerge, the survivor may be plunged (temporarily) back into some "victim" thinking, feeling, and behaving.

Furthermore, an individual may not be in the same stage in all areas of life. For example, she or he may be in the thriver stage regarding certain relationships but in the victim stage in others.

According to the *American Heritage Dictionary*, a victim is "someone who is harmed or killed by another" or "someone who is harmed or made to suffer from an act, circumstance, agency, or condition." A victim is also "anyone who suffers as a result of ruthless design or incidentally or accidentally" (*Webster's Third New International Dictionary*). The suffering and losses can be physical, psychological, or both.

People raised in poverty, and those subjected to racial, sexual, religious, or other forms of discrimination, are often viewed as victims of social and historical forces beyond their control. Similarly, people who acquire life-threatening or chronic illnesses or permanent disabilities can also be considered victims. For the purposes of this book, however, *victim* is defined as someone who has suffered from at least one "particularly negative ... intensely disruptive" event (Janoff Bulman and Frieze 1983).

Victimization, which means the process of becoming a victim, can be considered to occur on three levels (McCarthy 1986):

1. The traumatic event itself.

2. Secondary wounding experiences. These are experiences in which the institutions, caregivers, and others to whom the trauma survivor turns for emotional, legal, financial, medical, or other assistance respond by:

   • disbelieving or discounting the victim's experiences

   • blaming the victim for the traumatic event

   • stigmatizing or negatively judging the victim for the trauma or for any long-term symptoms he or she may suffer

   • denying the victim promised or expected services

3. The acceptance of the victim label. On this level of victimization, the victim internalizes society's perception of victims as incompetent, inferior, careless, or immoral or as having some other (usually negative) quality that caused the trauma to occur.

The Victim Stage

Individuals who experience trauma *are* victims in that they have been victimized in at least one, if not more, of the ways listed above. As level 3 indicates, however, the individual can, to one extent or another, remain a mental or emotional victim of the trauma long after the trauma has ceased.

The victim stage itself consists of three stages: prediscovery of the trauma, early awareness, and discovery (Hansen 1992). During the prediscovery stage, writes Hansen, trauma victims suffer PTSD symptoms with little understanding of their origin or relationship to the trauma. Consequently, victims experience their symptoms as inner chaos, and there is usually chaos in their relationships as well. Often they also have poor recall, if not total amnesia, of parts or all of the traumatic event.

When the victims suffer from low self-esteem due to lack of awareness of the trauma and its impact on their lives, or when they are emotionally, physically, and/or financially vulnerable due to the trauma, they are at high risk for revictimization by others. To seek relief, victims may engage in escapist activities, for example, substance abuse, moving from one geographical location to another, changing jobs frequently, running from relationship to relationship, and so forth.

During the early awareness stage, victims have a vague sense that they experienced a traumatic event, which leads to increased anxiety and some depression, irritability, and dissatisfaction with themselves and others. When the trauma begins to come into awareness, there is initial disbelief and shock, vacillation between denying the trauma and allowing it to come into awareness (even in fragments), and an increase in PTSD symptoms such as flashbacks and nightmares.

The Survivor Stage

In one sense, the essence of being a victim is being out of control—either of the situation at hand or of one's inner life. Given that, then the essence of being a survivor, and subsequently a thriver, is increased control over one's environment and one's inner self (as much as possible, of course). In the survivor stage, Hansen (1992) says, the survivor makes a commitment to therapy or some other healing effort. Here the trauma is confronted, in whole or in part, and the intense feelings associated with it begin to emerge from repression and find constructive expression. As the survivor moves the trauma and its associated affect from repression into awareness and begins to examine the trauma and its emotional, mental, and other aftereffects, the traumatic memories and formerly repressed feelings which used to control her or his inner life, relationships, and external behavior lose much of their former power.

The Thriver Stage

In the thriver stage, personal goals, not the trauma, become life's central organizing principle. The survivor begins to pursue "new education, job, and life goals, with resulting changes in family life." There are fewer and fewer emotional upheavals in relationships, and the thriver experiences greater inner peace and serenity (Hansen 1992).

Although some symptoms of PTSD may persist, they are fewer in number and less intense. Also, the survivor has acquired some skills by which to manage the symptoms. Consequently he or she experiences considerably less anxiety and panic in response to the symptoms.

Contributing Factors

Those who would argue against the validity of the PTSD diagnosis often point to predisposing factors, such as family history, genetics, and personality variables, to explain why some individuals succumb to the disorder. Yet study after study shows that when the stressor is sufficiently great, almost any individual will develop PTSD. The degree of impact of the trauma, however, is not uniform.

Some individuals suffer longer-term impairment and more severe symptoms than others, but this individual variability only highlights the fact that PTSD is complex and its manifestation subject to numerous individual personality and social factors. For example, Judith Lyons (1991b) found that those who recover from trauma more readily are those with the following advantages:

- Good health that is not significantly impaired by the trauma

- No physical disfigurement as a result of the trauma

- Adequate financial support or services

- The ability to resume functioning in some, if not all, pretrauma roles

- A supportive network of significant others

A reasonable approach to the question of who gets PTSD includes consideration of antecedent variables, as well as the trauma itself, with a special emphasis on how their interaction might have created extra stress on the individual. For example, people with histories of emotional or other deprivation, previous trauma, or other significant emotional problems are probably more vulnerable to trauma and may be more likely to develop PTSD. Individuals who must face their trauma alone, without a comforting or nurturing friend or relative, have also been shown to suffer more than individuals who have at least one source of consistent human concern and affection.

Antecedent Variables

Taking into account relevant childhood or pretrauma characteristics helps provide a fuller picture of the meaning and impact of the trauma on the client. However, the consideration of pretrauma factors should not be distorted to blame trauma survivors for their own pain or to support the predisposition theory, which attributes the development of PTSD to the client's "predisposing" personality and other antecedent variables. As mentioned earlier, this theory has been disproven by numerous research studies on Vietnam veterans and veterans from earlier wars. These studies showed, for example, that PTSD developed among even the most mentally healthy and dedicated of soldiers (Sonnenberg, Blank, and Talbott 1985).

Corroborative evidence exists in the case of the twenty-six children kidnapped and buried alive in their school bus. All twenty-six survived and escaped, but all of them also suffered symptoms of PTSD. The most severe symptoms tended to occur in children from families with preexisting pathology, those who lived in communities with relatively poor bonding, and those who had individual vulnerabilities which caused them to react with greater intensity to the kidnapping. However, four years later, all of the children still evidenced PTSD symptoms. Even those children with no known preexisting physical or psychological problems, who came from intact, functioning families, and who lived in supportive communities were symptomatic. Furthermore, and this is significant, the PTSD symptoms of all the children were amazingly similar despite the difference in their backgrounds and ages, which ranged from five to fourteen (Terr 1983).

Although a negative experience may have a devastating impact on one person and only a mildly distressing effect on another, sufficiently high stress levels will cause almost anyone to develop acute or long-term PTSD. Consider the following examples:

- About 30 percent of those who are burned, at least one quarter of Vietnam combat vets, and most of those involved in the partial collapse of the Kansas City Hyatt House experienced symptoms of PTSD (Silverman 1986).

- A study of a tanker-freighter collision in the Delaware River found that "preexisting personal or family background did not predict post-disaster psychopathology." The same conclusion has been reached in other studies of maritime and vehicular disasters (Silverman 1986).

- Numerous epidemiological studies of natural disasters, technological disasters, and criminal victimization have consistently found PTSD and other symptoms in those who survived such experiences, regardless of demographic characteristics or preexisting psychiatric problems (Keane 1990).

Taking the position that only individuals who are predisposed to PTSD by inherent weakness or deficiency will develop the syndrome is one of the most destructive acts a mental health professional can commit. This blaming response not only humiliates the client, it is based in ignorance. To date, the "precise interaction between trauma, constitutional factors, level of personality development, cultural factors and the ultimate expression in the form of altered affect, behavior, pain, perception and somatic functioning remains an unexplored territory" (van der Kolk 1984).

Client Deficits

As with the consideration of pretrauma conditions, client deficits should in no way be construed to blame the victim for her or his own pain. However, it must be acknowledged that clients come for help not only because they are haunted by the trauma on some level, but also because they are having difficulties within themselves, with interpersonal relationships, with their health, with the law, or with some other present area of life. Some difficulties are clearly and directly trauma-related; others are not. Some problems may have been created by the trauma, while at the same time the trauma exacerbated certain minor difficulties and made them into major life obstacles. For example, a person who was an occasional binge drinker might cross the line from social drinker to alcohol abuser due to his or her devastating experience. Or trauma could cause an individual who had been making a minimal living to join the ranks of the homeless or an individual who had been functioning marginally in both job and social contexts to become dysfunctional on the job and alienated from his former friends and family. Trauma can also bring to the surface latent problems with depression, paranoia, manic-depressive illness, and other psychiatric disorders, as well as any of a host of medical problems including diabetes, hypertension, tumors, and heart problems.

Many times trauma survivors experience emotional and cognitive changes that are appropriate to the situation of the trauma. These changes often hold survival value and may even save lives during the traumatic episode. Afterwards, however, these survival mechanisms are no longer useful. They can, at worst, be harmful; at best they may prevent the survivor from leading a fulfilling life.

For example, a woman who learned as a child to bury her emotions to protect herself from an abusive parent, might find in the present that being out of touch with her feelings deprives her of the comfort of friendship or the experience of falling in love. Similarly, a former prisoner of war who, to protect himself from physical abuse, learned to ask permission from authority figures for every small act, might find that in a white-collar work setting his constant requests may not be functional. Instead of his behavior being seen as appropriate, it might be seen as annoying and as a sign of undue dependency, which would make promotion unlikely and could lead to his losing his job.

Nowhere is the issue of client deficits more apparent than in survivors of incest and other forms of child abuse. Family abuse survivors who practiced dissociation or learned to "tune out" while being beaten, raped, or abused, may continue to practice dissociation in the present and hence be vulnerable to revictimization by others since the dissociation covers up warning signs of possible danger. Revictimization among family abuse survivors is "appallingly common" (Kluft 1992a). Furthermore, revictimization may not be limited to physical or sexual abuse, but may include economic exploitation. Those family abuse survivors who have "blind spots" cannot pick up the usual warning signs that another individual may be malevolent or exploitative.

While it is important to have clients identify and take pride in their strengths and assets, it is also important to take an honest unflinching view of their problem areas. The purpose of identifying and working on problem areas is not to further degrade the client or lower her or his already wounded self-esteem, but to help with problem areas so that she or he is not hurt or traumatized again (Kluft 1992a).

Chapter 2

Clinical Diagnosis of PTSD

As discussed briefly in chapter 1, *DSM-IV* establishes six criteria for the diagnosis of PTSD. The sections that follow explain each of the criteria in detail.

Criterion A: A Traumatic Event

> The person has been exposed to a traumatic event in which both of the following have been present:
>
> 1. the person has experienced, witnessed, or been confronted with an event or events that involve actual or threatened death or serious injury, or a threat to the physical integrity of oneself or others.
>
> 2. the person's response involved intense fear, helplessness, or horror. Note: in children, it may be expressed instead by disorganized or agitated behavior (*DSM-IV*)

In life, there are many crises, large and small, ranging from the loss of a wallet to the death of a loved one. Yet these events, although stressful and often called traumatic, and not considered trauma. True *trauma*, in the clinical sense, refers to situations in which one is rendered powerless and great danger is involved. Trauma in this sense refers to events involving death and injury or the possibility of death and injury. Trauma also encompasses events of such intensity or magnitude of horror that they would overtax any human being's ability to cope.

For example, Mr. and Mrs. Jones lost two children and four nieces and nephews in a car accident. Even though Mr. and Mrs. Jones were not in the car at the time of the accident, and the car carrying their family members was not at fault, they felt responsible for the accident and were plagued by "if-onlys": "If only we had been with them . . . " "If only the car had had a tune up . . . " "If only we had at least kept some of the young ones home instead of letting them all go."

Following the accident, Mrs. Jones gained sixty-five pounds and Mr. Jones developed diabetes. They visited the accident site nearly every day, withdrew from their regular church and social activities, and suffered from insomnia and other sleep difficulties. Though their lives had not been threatened and they had not witnessed the car accident, they developed PTSD due to the magnitude of their loss.

In general, the word *trauma* is reserved for:

- Natural catastrophes—hurricanes, floods, fires, earthquakes, and so on

- Man-made catastrophes—war, concentration camp experiences, physical assault, sexual assault, and other forms of victimization involving a threat to life and limb

Victims of vehicular accidents and crimes other than those listed can also develop PTSD, as can individuals injured on the job if they sustain severe injuries. Depending on the situation, witnessing death or injury or its aftermath can also lead to PTSD.

People are in a traumatic situation when they know or believe that they may be injured or killed or that others about them may be. For example, if a mugger says he will shoot someone, that person has every reason to believe he or she is in danger. Such a situation would definitely be classified as a trauma. However, if the mugger says nothing, but the person senses from the look on his face or certain gestures that he is capable of murder—or for any other reason the person believes he or she might die or be seriously injured during the mugging—he or she is also being traumatized.

PTSD can also develop in persons who witness trauma on a daily basis or are subject to nearly constant and unabated stress as part of their job. This statement holds true even for individuals who are carefully screened for mental health problems prior to admission to their field. For example, PTSD has been found among rescue workers, firefighters, health care teams, and police officers, as well as nurses and doctors who served in Vietnam and other wars.

Trauma Means Wounding

The question of what constitutes trauma in the context of PTSD requires careful consideration. In medicine, trauma has two meanings. The first is that some part or particular organ of the body has been suddenly damaged by a force so great that the body's natural protections (skin, skull, and so on) were unable to prevent injury. The second meaning refers to injuries in which the body's natural healing abilities are inadequate to mend the wound without medical assistance.

On the psychological and mental levels, trauma refers to the wounding of the emotions, the spirit, the will to live, beliefs about the self and the world, one's dignity, and one's sense of security. The assault on one's psyche is so great that normal ways of thinking and feeling and the usual ways the individual has handled stress in the past are now inadequate.

Being traumatized is not like being offended or rejected in a work or love relationship. Such events can injure a person's emotions, pride, and sense of fairness, but they are not of the order of magnitude of trauma. During trauma, a person touches his or her own death or the deaths of others and at the same time, is or feels helpless to prevent the death or injury.

Yet even those experiences by themselves do not constitute true trauma. As human beings, we must all confront the fact of our mortality. We and our loved ones will die some day, no matter who we are or what we do. Usually this awareness becomes most powerful in our middle or later years, when we see parents and their contemporaries dying or when we ourselves acquire an illness. Even the loss of a child, though an unexpected life event in societies with relatively low child mortality rates, does not generally lead to PTSD unless additional factors are involved (Rynearson 1988). So far only the loss of a child by homicide is considered a traumatic stressor (although parents and family members who lose a child due to terminal illness have been found to be at high risk for developing emotional problems).

Similarly, although abortion, adultery, divorce, chronic illness of a parent, and similar events have been defined as trauma by some clinicians—because some individuals who have undergone these experiences have developed some symptoms of PTSD (as well as other symptoms) (Catherall 1992)—in most cases the PTSD symptoms that developed are insufficient in number, intensity, or duration to constitute even a diagnosis of partial PTSD. Abortions, loss of a love relationship, and betrayal can be highly distressing; however, such events cannot be considered traumas in the *DSM-IV* sense of the word. Nor do such events, on their own, lead to full-blown PTSD.

Depersonalization and Entrapment

Two elements that serve to clarify the definition of trauma in relation to PTSD are those of depersonalization and entrapment. *Depersonalization* refers to the stripping away of one's individuality and humanity. The sense of being depersonalized or dehumanized is especially strong when the injuries sustained or the wounding and death witnessed seem senseless or preventable.

At the moment of attack, whether the assailant is a mugger, rapist, enemy soldier, or a hurricane, the individual does not feel like a valuable person with the right to safety, happiness, and health. At that moment, one is more like a thing, a vulnerable object subject to the will of a power or force greater than oneself (Haley 1984). When the assailant is a natural force, such as a tornado, the catastrophe can be explained away as an accident of fate (provided human error was not involved). However, when the assailant is another person, trust in other human beings and in society in general can be severely shaken or shattered entirely. Loss of sense of self, of safety and trust, and of a logical predictability to life are all elements of PTSD.

Another related loss is that of feeling that one has some control over one's life. Traumas vary from a single traumatic event, such as a tornado, train accident, rape, or mugging, to repeated traumatization over time, such as happens to hostages, torture victims, some combat soldiers, battered wives, and abused children. Regardless of the duration and severity, however, all traumas carry with them the element of *entrapment*, or the reality that all escape routes are extremely dangerous or costly—morally, economically, or in some other sense.

Victims of vehicular accidents and natural catastrophes are trapped in concrete, physical ways. They can wish or struggle all they want, but there is little to no escape from an oncoming car or a tornado. In other traumas, there may be an escape route, but that route may seem or actually be just as treacherous as the trauma itself, if not more so.

For example, soldiers in World War I engaged in trench warfare did not have the choice of simply leaving their trenches for a safe place. Nor did combatants during the Vietnam conflict have the option of hopping a plane or boat to leave the country. In most wars, save for some of the elite, the majority of soldiers are trapped in the combat situation. The only ways out are to physically mutilate themselves or commit suicide, go AWOL, or declare themselves mentally ill, after which they risk having a stigmatizing psychiatric label placed on their record, a label which could severely limit their vocational options for the rest of their lives.

It is sometimes argued that rape and crime victims have a choice—to submit without resistance or to fight back. These are not real choices. If one submits, one will be victimized. And if one fights back, one risks both failing to overcome the attacker and incurring the criminal's retaliatory wrath either at the time or later.

In other cases there are emotional and sometimes moral aspects of the trauma that are entrapping, in that none of the choices are desirable. In fact, in severe trauma any choices that exist are often morally reprehensible and emotionally devastating. Having the "choice" of a series of unacceptable options is really no choice. This is one of the factors which makes trauma so destructive.

As an example, consider a battered woman who must choose between her abuser's sexually abusing her (by forcing her into some form of sexual activity she finds degrading), his economically exploiting her (by taking her paycheck), or his physically abusing one or more of her children. She knows through experience that defying him in any way almost always leads to vicious retaliatory action, either against her or her children. Yet she is not naive enough to believe her compliance will guarantee the absence of abuse. Still, the probability of a beating or some other form of misuse is lower if she complies; therefore, the "safest" alternative, although highly unacceptable to her, is surrender to the abuser's wishes (Walker 1979). If she leaves her abuser, she may not find legal and police protection and she may or may not find assistance in starting a new life. The abuser may stalk or hunt her down, kidnap the children, or otherwise harass her. Some women consequently decide it is safer and easier to live with the abuser (and thus be able to observe his behavior and have some forewarning of abuse and some possibility of placating or diverting him) than to leave and have absolutely no control over him.

In such a situation the abused woman is trapped between her integrity and her safety, between her moral code and the safety of her children. In a parallel manner, some incest survivors accommodate their abuser's sexual demands because the abuser has threatened to sexually abuse a younger sibling if they do not comply. In fact, many incest survivors finally expose the abuser when he or she breaks a promise made not to harm a younger sibling or relative (Courtois 1988). Similarly, many abused women finally leave their abusers once all their self-sacrificial efforts to protect their children from harm fail (Walker 1979).

Natural catastrophes can also lead to entrapping emotional and moral dilemmas. For example, during the 1991 hurricane in Bangladesh, a father had to choose which of his children he would attempt to save. His wife and other relatives had already drowned, and he was not physically capable of carrying all three of his children in his arms while he swam to safety. "Better to save one than none," he thought. Yet after the hurricane subsided, he was so tormented by the image of the two children he had left behind and his surviving child was so riddled with guilt that at times both wished they had died along with the others. Combat medics, doctors and nurses, and medical personnel in other settings who frequently must make choices between who will live and who will die struggle with the same dilemma and emotional pain as the Bangladeshi father.

Soldiers, especially those in guerilla warfare, are frequently faced with dilemmas of having to kill women, children, or elderly people who might be spies or who might have been boobytrapped or otherwise armed to destroy them. "Kill or be killed" is their rule of survival, yet for some soldiers, killing women and children is morally objectionable. On the other hand, allowing themselves or their units to be injured or killed is also unacceptable. Such soldiers face a morally and emotionally unresolvable conflict similar to that facing other trauma survivors.

The elements of physical, moral, and emotional entrapment inherent to trauma reach their ultimate expression in situations where people become virtual (if not literal) captives. As psychologist Judith Herman (1992) points out, these situations include prisoner of war camps, hostage situations, concentration camps, formal and informal prisons (for instance, some brothels and some homes). "Political captivity is generally recognized," writes Herman, "whereas the domestic captivity of women and children is often unseen" and is usually less recognized. The elements of captivity may or may not include physical confinement, such as with bars or chains, but usually involve the perpetrator attempting to take total control of the victim.

Dominating the victim includes eroding if not breaking the victim's former attachments; isolating the victim from others; attempting to psychologically dominate or "brainwash" the victim into the perpetrator's mode of thinking; and making the victim emotionally, as well as financially, dependent on the perpetrator so that the perpetrator becomes the center of the victim's life. Other elements of captivity include denigrating the victim's family of origin and other significant former attachments; forcing the victim to violate his or her moral principles, which can involve hurting others as well as other immoral or illegal activities or activities the victim finds repulsive for personal reasons; and forcing the victim into secrecy about these and other activities, especially the abuse. Captivity can also involve the power-holder's dominating and prescribing the details of the victim's life, such as the victim's eating, sleeping, urinating, and defecating habits; sexual and recreational activities; and clothing, hairstyle, and body weight and form (Herman 1992; Shay 1992).

At the same time, the power holder tries to subdue the victim's rebellion against captivity by giving the victim certain rewards and attentions and trying to create in the victim a mindset that the abuser is wiser and more knowledgeable than the victim and therefore knows what is right and true. All challenges to the power holder's version of reality are forbidden or strictly punished (Herman 1992; Shay 1992; Walker 1979).

Under conditions of such extreme control, victims are often coerced into betraying their own values. For example, prisoners of war, torture victims, and concentration camp victims have historically been faced with morally and emotionally horrendous choices: POWs and torture victims have often been forced to choose between being tortured and killed themselves and torturing or killing a member of their family, a friend, or comrade. During World War II, gypsy musicians, on pain of their own death were forced to sing while their fellow gypsies were being killed and buried in mass graves (*Washington Post* 2 Nov. 1991).

In a parallel manner, on threat of being brutalized themselves or of having a favorite pet or relative hurt or injured, some abused children are coerced into watching, initiating, and/or participating in the physical or sexual abuse of their siblings or other children (Herman 1992; Courtois 1988). The choice of either abusing or being severely hurt oneself (or watching as a loved one is hurt) hardly constitutes a choice. (For an excellent discussion of the element of captivity in prolonged trauma, see chapter 4 "Captivity," in Herman 1992.)

Criterion B: Reexperiencing the Trauma

> The traumatic event is persistently reexperienced in at least one of the following ways:
>
> 1. recurrent and intrusive distressing recollections of the event, including images, thoughts, or perceptions. Note: in young children, repetitive play may occur in which themes or aspects of the trauma are expressed
>
> 2. recurrent distressing dreams of the event. Note: in children, there may be frightening dreams without recognizable content
>
> 3. acting or feeling as if the traumatic event were recurring (includes a sense of reliving the experience, illusions, hallucinations, and dissociative flashback episodes, including those that occur upon awakening or when intoxicated) Note: in young children, trauma-specific reenactment may occur
>
> 4. intense psychological distress at exposure to internal cues that symbolize or resemble an aspect of the traumatic event
>
> 5. physiologic reactivity upon exposure to internal or external cues that symbolize or resemble an aspect of the traumatic event (DSM-IV)

The fundamental dynamic underlying PTSD is a cycle of reexperiencing the trauma, followed by attempts to bury memories of the trauma and the feelings associated with the trauma. This cycle of intrusive recall, followed by avoidance and numbing, has a strong biological component, which you will read about in the following chapter.

During the recall stage of the PTSD cycle, memories and the emotions associated with them emerge, in conscious or unconscious awareness, over and over again in a variety of forms. The client may have intrusive thoughts or images, dreams and nightmares, even flashbacks about the event. Or the client may suddenly find him or herself thinking or feeling as if back in the original trauma situation. All of these phenomena are part of the process of reexperiencing the trauma.

According to Freud, reexperiencing the trauma, including repeating it in present-day life, are ways of dissipating the intense psychic energy generated by the trauma and of trying to gain mastery over it. It is as if the client were watching a movie that ended sadly. The movie is replayed in hope that perhaps this time the ending will be a happy one. It isn't, of course, but the movie is nonetheless replayed as if with enough repetitions the desired ending will come to pass. Some trauma survivors become so absorbed with the unresolved trauma of their past that they have less psychic energy to devote to work, friends, and family, and most importantly to themselves, in the present.

Sleep Disorders

Sleeping difficulties may be forms of reexperiencing the trauma. Dreams or nightmares about the traumatic event are common. During these dreams the client may shake, shout, and thrash about. The client may or may not remember the dream upon awakening; however, the feelings of terror and fear experienced in the dream may persist for quite some time.

Some dreams or nightmares are almost exact replays of the traumatic event or are very similar. Other dreams, however, simply contain the feelings experienced during the trauma: helplessness, fear, anger, and grief.

Insomnia can also be a symptom. As a result of dreams, falling asleep and staying asleep may be major problems for the client. Or it may be that at night, without the distraction of the activities of the day, thoughts of the traumatic event begin to surface. The client might start thinking about the event itself or about other events involving losses and threats to safety. He or she might experience vague anxiety, nameless fears, or a generalized irritability.

Alternatively, sleep problems may indicate that the client is suffering from a biochemical depression in addition to PTSD. Alcohol and drug use (often associated with PTSD) can affect sleep patterns. Insomnia is also associated with increased arousal, or *hyperarousal*—another symptom of PTSD (see Criterion D).

Flashbacks

A *flashback* is a sudden, vivid recollection of the traumatic event accompanied by a strong emotion. During a flashback the client does not black out or lose consciousness, but temporarily does leave the present and reexperiences the original traumatic situation. The client may see the trauma, smell it, and hear its sounds. He or she may or may not lose awareness of present reality and may or may not act as if actually in the original traumatic situation. Or the client may alternate between the current reality and experiencing the past. A flashback can last anywhere from a few seconds to several hours.

A client need not be a combat veteran to have flashbacks. Flashbacks have been documented among survivors of Nazi concentration camps, World War II aviation personnel, crime victims, victims of occupational and technological disasters, and rape and incest survivors (Carmen 1989; Bard and Sangrey 1986; Herman 1989; T. Williams 1987a). Flashbacks tend to occur among persons who have had to endure situations where there was an "intense, chronic or pervasive loss of security" and lack of safety (Blank 1985).

Clients are often reluctant to acknowledge or tell anyone that they are having a flashback for fear of sounding "crazy." Flashbacks are not indications that the client is on the verge of a psychotic break or some other loss of emotional or mental control, but rather that some traumatic material is coming into consciousness. (The hope is that the more the traumatic material is made conscious, through verbal discussions or "creative therapies" such as writing, dance, or art therapy, the less need there will be for it to emerge in flashbacks, nightmares, or other dreams.)

A flashback is to be differentiated from a psychogenic fugue, during which an individual travels away from home or work and finds him or herself in a new location, unable to remember his or her previous identity and history. For example, Oliver K., a combat veteran, had a flashback of burning heads calling to him after the shooting death of a neighbor. He had been in therapy for over a year for symptoms of PTSD and had suffered from frequent nightmares regarding his combat experience, however he had never before had a flashback. Furthermore, even after a year of therapy, he could only recall his first and last weeks of combat duty. "Everything else is a fog of blood and dust," he stated. Nor could he recall the names of his buddies or anyone in his combat unit; he often also had difficulty remembering the names of other veterans in the therapy group he was attending. The flashback frightened him because he could not relate it to any experience in his memory. However, discussing the flashback in therapy reminded him that his unit frequently fought at night, with the backdrop of burning buildings or flares providing the only light. The "burning heads" were not actually heads that were on fire, but visions of the heads of men he had killed in areas where fires had been set.

Individuals with PTSD may also suffer from fugue states. However, the PTSD must be severe in order for such an event to occur. Such fugue states are not the same as flashbacks. For example, the flashback experienced by Oliver is not the same as the psychogenic fugue state experienced by Brenda, a family abuse survivor, who woke up in a hotel in a different state without knowing how or when she arrived there. She would have not remembered her name except for her driver's license and other papers.

Physiological Reactivity

Physiological reactivity as a form of reexperiencing the trauma can include symptoms such as sweating, rapid heart beat, nausea, dizziness, dry mouth, hot flashes, chills, frequent urination, trouble swallowing, and diarrhea or other abdominal problems. The source of these problems is frequently in the fight-or-flight or freeze reaction described in greater detail under "Criterion D: Hyperarousal Symptoms."

Other Forms of Reexperience

Another form of reexperiencing the trauma, that is considered by some to be a kind of unconscious flashback (Blank 1985) occurs when the client suddenly has painful or angry feelings that do not seem clearly related to any particular memory of the traumatic event. For example, the client may experience irritability, panic attacks, rage reactions, or intense psychic pain, without any conscious thought of the traumatic event.

"I can understand why I sulk or explode about hearing about another cop being killed in the line of duty. But many times I get moody or angry for no reason at all," explains a police officer. What this man may not fully appreciate is that often there is a reason for the emotional upset, even though that reason may not be obvious. The reason may lie in the intensity of his repressed feelings about the deaths or injuries of other police officers or in the very real possibility that someday he will be injured or killed on the job.

Like this policeman, other PTSD clients are often puzzled by these periods of irritability, panic, rage, or emotional pain. The unexplained shift in mood makes many clients feel out of control of themselves, as they did during the original traumatic event. Educating clients about the possibility that their mood shifts may be a form of unconscious flashback, during which their psyche attempts to dispel the tremendous energy aroused by the danger, anger, grief, and other feelings associated with the trauma, often helps to restore client self-esteem.

Criterion C: Numbing and Avoidance

> Persistent avoidance of stimuli associated with the trauma or numbing of general responsiveness (not present before the trauma), as indicated by at least three of the following:

1. efforts to avoid thoughts, feelings, or conversations associated with the trauma

2. efforts to avoid activities, places, or people that arouse recollections of the trauma

3. inability to recall an important aspect of the trauma

4. markedly diminished interest or participation in significant activities

5. feeling of detachment or estrangement from others

6. restricted range of affect (e.g., unable to have loving feelings)

7. sense of a foreshortened future (e.g., does not expect to have a career, marriage, or children, or a normal life span) *(DSM-IV)*

Reexperiencing the trauma can be cyclical, or it can be sporadic. The client may be symptom-free for many weeks or months but then begin to suffer as anniversaries of events associated with the trauma approach. A personal loss or other current-life stress or change—even positive changes such as the birth of a baby or a wedding—can call up memories or flashbacks. In addition, sometimes *triggers* in the environment—people, places, and things that remind the client of the trauma—can set off a memory.

Whenever or however the client reexperiences the trauma, it is usually pure agony. As a result, both emotionally and physically the client alternates between being hyper (see Criterion D) and being numb or shut down.

Emotional Shutdown or Psychic Numbing

What happens when a client enters a state of *psychic numbing*, often called shutdown, is similar to what occurs when the human body is injured. The body is able to emit a natural anesthetic which permits people some time to take care of their wounds and to do whatever is necessary to protect themselves from further injury. For example, due to this natural anesthetic, severely wounded soldiers have walked miles to safety. Similarly, abused women and battered children sometimes report experiencing minimal pain from their injuries during or immediately after being attacked.

In a similar way the psyche in self-protection can numb itself against onslaughts of unbearable emotional pain. During whatever traumatic event was endured, it was probably essential for the survivor to put aside his or her feelings since at the time those emotions could have been life-threatening. For example, if a rape victim began to connect with her feelings while being assaulted, she would be less able to assess the dangerousness of her assailant or figure out how to escape or otherwise minimize the threat of injury. Similarly, in the midst of a hurricane or tornado, the victim would most likely be preoccupied with how to stay safe, not with his or her emotional reactions.

This deadening, or shutting off of emotions is called psychic or emotional numbing. It is a central feature of PTSD and has been found among survivors of all forms of assault, survivors of natural catastrophes, survivors of the bombing of Hiroshima and the Nazi holocaust, and other war-related situations. Many researchers believe that, like the body's natural anesthetic, emotional numbing may be partially biological (van der Kolk 1990a).

Avoidance and Triggers

During the times the trauma is reexperienced, the client may have some of the feelings associated with the trauma that were not felt, or only partially felt, due to the psychic numbing which attends trauma. These feelings of fear, anger, sadness, and guilt may shake the client to the core. In response to the power of these feelings the client may shut down, just as he or she did during the traumatic event. Shutting down serves as a means of reducing the intensity of the affect generated by the trauma.

In addition, having flashbacks, being in a state of hyperalertness, and the opposite, being in a state of psychic numbing, are not only personally painful conditions, but conditions that can be easily misunderstood and misinterpreted by the client's family members, friends, and associates. In order to avoid possible social judgments and social rejection, PTSD-afflicted clients may begin to avoid situations that they have found bring forth (or that they fear will bring forth) either symptoms of numbing or hyperalertness. This avoidance may lead to various degrees of mental, social, and physical retreat from society.

For example, just as rape survivors may stay inside their homes at night, hurricane survivors may stay inside when only a minor thunderstorm is predicted. Flood survivors may avoid water-related activities, and car- or airplane-accident survivors may drastically limit their travel. Medics, nurses, and doctors who have worked in high-stress environments may seek work in nonmedical fields. People who have suffered massive injuries on the job may change their line of work.

Similarly, crime victims may avoid the site of the crime or places that remind them of the crime; if the crime occurred in a restaurant, they may have great difficulty dining out for some time. War veterans may avoid the sound of popcorn popping because it reminds them of airplanes or helicopters. Or they might avoid plastic trash bags or fires because they are reminded of body bags or burning villages.

Every trauma survivor has his or her own set of triggers that can touch off memories of the trauma. Avoiding trigger situations makes utter sense—clients are trying to prevent a resurgence of their PTSD symptoms. However, the avoidance can generate yet another set of problems, particularly in relationships. For this reason, as with flashbacks clients need to be educated as to the purpose of their numbing states. Otherwise, they may begin to feel "out of control" of themselves and subsequently either berate themselves, lash out at others, or isolate from others. (Exercises to help clients understand and manage trigger situations and avoidance behaviors are presented in chapter 6.)

Other Criterion C Symptoms

Memory impairment is a common feature of PTSD sufferers. Unlike amnesia caused by head injuries, the kind of memory difficulties tapped in this criterion are psychological in origin. Because the traumatic event was so traumatic, the individual needs to repress all or parts of his or her memories to maintain sanity and the ability to function. Ordinary forgetfulness can not explain this degree of forgetfulness. For example, some survivors have simply "forgotten" certain months, or even years, of their lives, depending on the extent of the abuse. Or they may remember some traumatic episodes but not all, or parts of the episodes but not the entire series of events.

PTSD sufferers frequently report loss of interest in one or more activities of former significance to them, for example, family and social activities, once-favored hobbies, and what are usually pleasurable activities, such as eating, sex, and recreational activities. If they were involved in a political, social, or religious activity of some importance to them, interest in this activity may also have waned.

Regression to previous states of development sometimes characterizes survivors of extreme trauma. For example, adult survivors sometimes display relatively infantile behavior. Such regression also can characterize traumatized children, who may regress to previous states of psycho-social development. For example, children who have recently been toilet trained may lose the ability to control themselves following a traumatic incident. Or children may lose recently acquired advances in reading and speaking abilities, or in certain motor skills, following trauma.

Trauma survivors, especially survivors of long-term or severe trauma, often suffer from a sense of doom about the future. Because they were powerless during the trauma, they may feel they are powerless to achieve their life goals, such as marriage and family. If, in addition, they suffer from clinical depression or from debilitating PTSD symptoms which make it difficult for them to achieve their personal or vocational goals, these realities contribute to their sense that there is no hope of their achieving life dreams, whatever those dreams might be.

Criterion D: Hyperarousal Symptoms

> Persistent symptoms of increased arousal (not present before the trauma), as indicated by at least two of the following:
>
> 1. difficulty falling or staying asleep
>
> 2. irritability or outbursts of anger
>
> 3. difficulty concentrating
>
> 4. hypervigilance
>
> 5. exaggerated startle response *(DSM-IV)*

This fourth PTSD criteria concerns symptoms of increased physical alertness or, in psychological terms, *hyperalertness* or *hyperarousal.*

Fight-or-Flight and Freeze Reactions

Trauma involves life-threatening situations, which naturally give rise to feelings of terror and anxiety. If the individual is not threatened personally, he or she may feel horror and grief at seeing others being injured or dying. There may also be anger at the circumstances causing the devastation. All of these trauma-generated emotions—fear, anxiety, and anger—are emotions that have strong physiological components and can actually change the body's chemistry.

In a dangerous situation, the adrenal glands may begin to pump either adrenaline or noradrenaline into the body. Adrenaline causes a state of hyperalertness in which the heart rate, blood pressure, muscle tension, and blood sugar levels increase. The pupils dilate and the blood flow to the arms and legs decreases, while the flow to the head and trunk increase so that the individual can think and move better and more quickly. This is called the *fight-or-flight reaction.*

Alternatively, if the adrenals pump noradrenaline into the system, the individual may have a *freeze reaction,* during which moving or acting is difficult, if not impossible. Some PTSD sufferers have described their freeze reactions as moving or thinking in slow motion. Others find themselves temporarily unable to move at all. However, even if a person freezes, he or she will most likely be experiencing some of the other symptoms of hyperarousal.

The persistent hyperarousal symptoms experienced by those with PTSD are caused by an adrenaline surge analogous to the one they likely experienced during the trauma. Symptoms of hyperarousal or autonomic hyperactivity include insomnia, irritability or outbursts of anger, difficulty concentrating, hypervigilance and exaggerated startle response, diarrhea or other abdominal distress, hot flashes or chills, frequent urination and trouble swallowing.

Criterion E: Duration

> Duration of the disturbance (symptoms in B, C, and D) is more than one month. (*DSM-IV*)

After undergoing any experience that is dangerous, frightening, or distressing, it is normal to experience shock, fear, confusion, helplessness, anxiety, and depression. These immediate reactions are covered in the diagnosis of Acute Stress Disorder, described under "Factors Affecting Severity." PTSD, however, is something more. PTSD includes these reactions, but on a deeper, more complex, and more enduring level, as indicated by the *DSM-IV* criteria.

According to *DSM-IV*, these symptoms must persist for at least 30 days in order to be considered PTSD. This is, of course, just a rule of thumb. There isn't much difference between 29 days and 31 or 32 days. However, if the symptoms persist much longer than five or six weeks, the individual can be assumed to have PTSD and should be treated accordingly.

Criterion F: Impaired Functioning

> The disturbance causes clinically significant distress or impairment in social, occupational or other important areas of functioning. (*DSM-IV*)

In order to qualify as having PTSD, an individual must not only have experienced a traumatic event and reacted with the symptoms described in Criteria B, C, and D for over a month, but the symptoms and other reactions to the trauma must have significantly diminished the individual's capacity to work, love, and play. For example, if an individual is having frequent flashbacks while driving and on the job, that person will need to stop driving and may need to stop working. His or her ability to maintain employment, and even social and family relationships, can also be severely impaired. Similarly, if an object that symbolizes or reminds the individual of the trauma is commonly present in a variety of settings, and that individual tends to react physiologically to such a degree that he or she is almost incapacitated, that individual will be severely restricted socially and occupationally.

For example, if an individual who has developed PTSD as a result of being in a fire has symptomatic reactions to fire extinguishers that are unmanageable or all consuming, he or she will have great difficulty being employed in an office, attending movies and theaters, or visiting homes where fire extinguishers are present. Such individuals suffer from severely crippling effects of the trauma and would definitely meet Criterion F. On the other hand, a fire survivor who also displays symptoms in the presence of fire extinguishers, but whose reactions are of short duration or minimal intensity, so that she or he is soon able to complete the task at hand or continue with a social interaction, would probably not meet this criterion (depending, of course, on the presence or absence of other factors).

Acute vs. Chronic PTSD

> PTSD is considered acute if the symptoms exist for less than three months; chronic, if the duration of symptoms is three months or more. (*DSM-IV*)

Delayed Onset

> **Delayed onset:** the onset of symptoms was at least six months after the trauma. (*DSM-IV*)

In delayed-onset PTSD, the symptoms occur anytime later than six months after the traumatic event. This can be 1 year, 20 years, or even 40 years after the traumatic event. For example, previously asymptomatic 60-year-old people can develop PTSD in response to having been sexually or physically abused as children.

Factors Affecting Severity

The Three Levels of Traumatic Response

In general, there are three levels of PTSD (Herman 1992). The first is a crisis-level response, which can occur immediately or within four weeks of the traumatic event. This crisis level response, called acute stress disorder in *DSM-IV*, includes PTSD symptoms, but the symptoms disappear or abate before the month specified in Criterion E for PTSD. Although acute stress disorder is similar to PTSD in many of its symptoms, this book concerns the treatment and diagnosis of PTSD, not acute stress disorder.

A supportive family or community environment or crisis intervention work by a trained professional or layperson can be critical in preventing the crisis reaction from becoming a more long-term problem.

The second level of PTSD conforms to the *DSM-IV* definition. Here the symptoms match the *DSM-IV* criteria in a straightforward fashion, and the individual's psychological profile is relatively free of other disorders.

The third level of PTSD, long-term untreated PTSD, is usually suffered by people who were not so fortunate to have had either community or family assistance immediately following their traumatic experience or adequate professional help at a later time. Here PTSD symptoms coexist with other disorders, which in some cases may appear to be the dominant problem. However, as will be explained in more depth in chapter 4, "Client Assessment," some of the concurrent disorders may be the result of the untreated PTSD. This statement is not meant to imply that all concurrent disorders in complicated, long-term PTSD cases are PTSD-related; many individuals merit dual diagnoses.

Nevertheless, clinical experience, as well as recent research (Courtois 1988; Herman 1992), indicates that many individuals do not receive help for the trauma underlying their PTSD because the symptoms that developed in the absence of positive intervention have come to dominate the PTSD symptoms. Thus the client presents to the mental health professional a diagnostic picture other than that of PTSD. As a result, the client is given a diagnosis that does not take into account the traumatic experiences and resulting PTSD. And treatment is geared toward the more obvious symptoms, rather than the less obvious or perhaps almost hidden PTSD symptoms and trauma. Consequently, the client frequently "never gets better," which reinforces his or her sense of helplessness which originated in the trauma. Clients in this category frequently need particular help in overcoming the low self-esteem and hopelessness about recovery that the misdiagnosis has exacerbated.

Single-Trauma vs. Multiple-Trauma Survivors

The extent of PTSD is also influenced by whether the client has been exposed to one or to more than one traumatic incident. For instance, although rape is traumatic, incest, which typically involves multiple rapes or molestations over an extended period, is more traumatic. Similarly, seeing people die in a car accident, although traumatic, is generally not as traumatic as being in combat or being a policeman in a deteriorating neighborhood and seeing death and violence day in and day out.

Several prominent researchers and therapists who have worked with trauma survivors have noted differences between individuals subject to a single isolated traumatic event—a rape, earthquake, or car accident—and those subject to repeated threats to their life and psyche such as incest, battering, and prisoner of war or concentration camp experiences. Lenore Terr (1991), who has extensively studied PTSD in traumatized children, has suggested that individuals who have endured a one-time or "Type 1" trauma suffer from different effects that those who undergo repeated or "Type 2" traumas. For example, people who have experienced Type 2 traumas are more likely to exhibit dissociation and other forms of self-hypnosis as well as extreme mood swings.

In some cases, an earlier trauma will remain repressed until a subsequent trauma unearths it. For example, after the Persian Gulf war a number of returning veterans were traumatized not so by their combat experiences as by the memories of childhood trauma that the war brought to the forefront of their minds.

If a client was physically or sexually abused as a child or had previously been the victim of a crime or other trauma, but somehow avoided dealing with the earlier trauma, the current trauma may put the client on overload. The client then suddenly needs help with not just one but two traumas. For example, Richard lived in an area struck by Hurricane Hugo. He was not directly injured by the hurricane, nor were his property losses significant. However, he did see the body of a woman who had died in the storm, which caused him to begin dreaming about his early childhood. When Richard was four years old, his father beat Richard's mother to death. Richard had witnessed both her death and earlier beatings, and had been abused himself. But he had successfully blotted out those memories until the sight of the woman's mangled body brought them back.

Herman's (1992) observations regarding the entrapment of individuals subject to long-term trauma are similar to those of Terr. For example, Judith Herman found that long-term trauma survivors evidence a greater tendency to dissociate or enter trance states and have somatic problems such as abdominal pain and nausea, tension headaches, pelvic pain, and other such symptoms. They also show more profound ambivalences and distrust of themselves and others.

Herman has also found that long-term trauma survivors are more vulnerable to repeated victimization in that they are more likely to be exploited by others. For instance, if someone has used dissociation and denial to cope with abuse, then he or she may have significant trouble recognizing dangerous people and situations outside of the original abuse situation. If that person is abused again, and once again practices dissociation in order to cope, she or he is not developing a warning system for protection against danger. In essence, instead of learning and becoming "smarter and smarter" about potentially abusive situations and people, the chronically abused, dissociative individual becomes "dumber and dumber" (Kluft 1992a).

The multiply traumatized person is also more vulnerable to subsequent harm because he or she is more symptomatic than most people. The more symptomatic a person is, the greater the need for reassurance and affirmation, which makes that person easy prey to manipulative or exploitative personalities.

On yet another level, long-term trauma survivors are more vulnerable to subsequent harm because they tend to be more harmful to themselves than single-trauma survivors. Substance abuse problems, eating disorders, self-mutilation, suicide attempts, and suicide itself are more common among long-term trauma survivors than single-trauma survivors (Courtois 1988; Herman 1992; Walker 1979).

Therapists vary in their ability to understand victims of extreme trauma. Although it may be easy to be empathic toward, for example, Jews who endured horrors under the Nazi regime, it may be harder to be empathic toward soldiers who, under the stress of war, engage in atrocities and senseless acts of killing. Likewise, it is easy to feel empathy toward survivors for psychic wounds and terror they have suffered, but more difficult to be understanding of their socially unacceptable thoughts and behaviors, their seemingly irrational fears and compulsions, and their passivity or aggression.

As Herman explains, part of therapists' difficulty in understanding victims of extreme trauma is that "the diagnostic categories of existing psychiatric canon are simply not designed for survivors of extreme situations and do not fit them well. The persistent anxiety, phobias, and panic of survivors are not the same as ordinary anxiety disorders . . . " Neither are their somatic complaints or depressions the same as ordinary ones.

Duration and Severity of Trauma

The more severe and longer in duration the trauma, the higher the risk for the development of subsequent PTSD in the survivor. This general statement has been shown in research on war veterans, as well as other populations, and has been confirmed repeatedly in numerous studies (Sonnenberg, Blank, and Talbott 1985; Courtois 1988; Herman 1992; van der Kolk 1988a,b, 1990a; Wolfe 1990). For example, statistically the greater the exposure to combat, the more likely a veteran will develop PTSD. Similarly, veterans who were exposed to or participated in abusive violence or atrocities during their tour of duty have higher rates of post-war PTSD than veterans who were not (Sonnenberg, Blank, and Talbott 1985).

However, the effects of other factors also play a role in determining the impact of the trauma. These factors include presence or absence of emotional support or other positive experiences associated with the trauma and the presence or absence of blame or stigmatization. For example, veterans who credit their military experience with helping them to mature and develop a sense of discipline and purpose, or who feel grateful to the military for vocational training and other forms of education, tend to experience less severe stress reactions than those who feel that their war experiences impaired both their mental and physical health.

Just as the experience of all combat soldiers is not alike, all abusive families are not the same. Some abusers are more vicious than others, verbally and/or physically. Abusive families also vary greatly in their degree of dysfunction and in the amount of emotional and financial support they provide the abused child. Child abuse and incest are rarely isolated problems, usually they coexist with other family problems: substance abuse, marital discord, prior trauma in the abuser or the nonabusing parent. Thus some families in which child abuse occurs are more dysfunctional and nonresponsive to the child's needs than others. The presence of a supportive loving grandparent, aunt or uncle, sibling, or an outside nurturing adult, can help to mitigate some of the damaging effects of child abuse.

For example, Rodney was sexually abused by his mother and three brothers and was also "lent out" to his brother's friends for a fee. The abuse began when he was three and ended when he left home at age seventeen. Yet Rodney had a great aunt who continuously demonstrated her love for him throughout his childhood although she could not intervene to save him from the abuse. Among other gifts, she paid for his college tuition, which enabled him to leave home without facing destitution.

Rodney was abused several times a week by several family members for more than a decade. In contrast, Shawn suffered relatively less abuse, in that he was "only" beaten by his father (with whips, rods, and so on) at most once a week for less than seven years. However, there was no nurturing adult in Shawn's life, so at age fifteen, he ran away from home and survived by doing odd jobs and living in a friend's basement. Even though Rodney's abuse was longer and more severe than Shawn's, Shawn suffers from more intense PTSD symptoms than Rodney. Some of the difference between the two men's PTSD can be attributed to almost the total absence of any affection or emotional support in Shawn's life, as opposed to Rodney's, during the time of the abuse.

The existence and preservation of an attachment system is also important following, as well as during the trauma, as is explained in a later section.

Ongoing Traumatization or Its Threat

Some trauma survivors have not only endured a traumatic experience or set of experiences in the past, but continue to live in threat of danger or are being actively abused or victimized in the present. For example, crime victims may continue to live in high-crime neighborhoods or have vocations that expose them to danger. Or a client may be a family abuse survivor who is still being physically or sexually abused either by a family member or another perpetrator even though he or she is in treatment. It goes without saying that it is almost impossible for someone who is still in danger or is being currently victimized to heal from PTSD.

In many cases, however, clients do not tell their therapist of the current trauma, either because the trauma is in repression or because they fear the therapist will be rejecting or judgmental. Incest survivors in particular are often extremely ashamed to reveal that they are still being abused. They sometimes feel that they would be betraying their family by telling the therapist about the abuse. Also, frequently they have been trained not to tell by the abuser or other family members.

In a parallel manner, physical abuse victims may feel ashamed to tell their therapist of ongoing abuse. In addition, they, like incest survivors, may have significant amnesia about the abuse, or, as another form of defense, they may minimize its severity and impact on their lives. Similarly, some refugees who are torture or refugee camp survivors may fear or be threatened with deportation, further torture, or even extermination. They may also fear that the therapist will "inform" on them.

Ongoing abuse (as well as PTSD) may also be difficult to detect because paradoxically, some of the most traumatized individuals who present for therapy, for example, battered wives and abused children, may present as high-functioning, creative, normal people. Because of the caretaker aspect of the battered woman and abused child roles, often these categories of survivors are adept managers of families, productive workers on the job, and contributors to society. Their PTSD may not be recognized because of their external abilities, because they are amnesic regarding the abuse, or because they may come to therapy in the numbing or constrictive phase of their PTSD, which sometimes closely resembles normal functioning (Courtois 1988; Herman 1992).

Spiritual or Moral Concerns

As suggested in the discussion of depersonalization and entrapment, part of the severity of the trauma involves the degree to which the survivor has had to transgress his or her moral or spiritual values or betray important emotional bonds in order to survive. The abused child who is forced to injure a sibling in order to please the perpetrator suffers a greater degree of traumatization than the abused child who receives the same kind and degree of abuse but is not forced to imitate the aggressor.

Similarly, the abused wife who is forced into activities she feels are immoral will suffer more intense PTSD symptoms and greater self-loathing than the abused wife whose misery consists "only" of beatings and economic deprivation. Prisoners of war, concentration camp survivors, and other kinds of prisoners who are made to deceive, hurt, torture, or kill family members or other prisoners will suffer longer-term depression and other PTSD symptoms than those in almost identical situations who somehow escaped the humiliation of such absolute surrender to the individuals who held life and death power over them.

It is one thing to allow one's body or material possessions to be exploited by another and quite another to have one's inner life invaded and raped as well. The autobiographies of survivors of extreme stress, for example, slaves, prisoners of war, and concentration camp survivors, often speak of their captors' being able to rob them of everything except their inner dignity. However, when the situation forces people to surrender their moral identities to the perpetrator, extreme self-hate, guilt and loss of self follow. The self-abasement of such survivors, however, may be hidden by the numbness or an aggressive "macho" or "macha" facade, which they adopt in order not to experience the full magnitude of their loss (Herman 1992).

Not only do such survivors hold themselves in contempt, often others do as well. Many persons, including some mental health professionals, assume that under similar circumstances they would have behaved more courageously. Consequently, trauma survivors who have engaged in corrupt acts are often the objects of extremely negative moral judgments. Even less egregious acts are subject to such judgments. Although many people have some understanding and empathy for individuals in concentration and prison camps who succumbed to the mind-control procedures of their captors, there is also widespread condemnation of victims who "gave in" to the enemy. As cases in point, Herman (1992) points out that even the Jews in Nazi concentration camps were blamed for their "passivity" and prisoners of war have frequently been considered "traitors" for having given in to the enemy's will.

If there is a lack of understanding of concentration camp survivors and prisoners of war, there is even less understanding of the analogous conditions that occur in many domestic violence situations. Even when the pressures on an abused wife are comprehended, such as when she is threatened with great harm or the death of another if she does not comply with the abuser's wishes, there is always the lingering suspicion on the part of many that the woman must have been emotionally disturbed to have chosen the perpetrator as a mate in the first place.

The same holds true for abused men. Although statistically fewer men are abused than women, the dynamics of abuse are quite similar. Public misunderstanding of the dynamics of abuse exists regardless of the sex of the victim or perpetrator.

Few understand, for example, that the perpetrator starts off in an intimate relationship not by displaying abusive or otherwise negative qualities, but by displaying charming and positive qualities. Only after gaining some power over their victim, for example, by establishing some economic control, does the abuser make evident a more negative side. Meanwhile, the abuser might have been steadily using the victim's vulnerabilities and affections to erode the victim's autonomy and sense of self to establish the abuser as the sole authority in the victim's life.

By the time the mental health professional meets such a survivor, the survivor may be numb to her or his acts of moral compromise, which further serves to earn the survivor the negative judgment of the mental health professional as well as the suspicion of characterological pathology or other mental illness. This can make the mental health professional even less sympathetic toward the survivor. However, the moral corruption of such survivors needs to be seen as an indication of the degree of traumatization, rather than as a sign of pretrauma mental illness.

In this area of spiritual and moral values, one must also be especially cognizant of the role of personal and societal values in passing judgment on such survivors. For example, atrocities occur in all wars. In recent history they were largely swept under the rug regarding World War II and the Korean War, yet they received great attention during and after the Vietnam conflict.

The same actions were evaluated quite differently depending on the political climate and the social popularity of the war. Vietnam veterans were frequently called "babykillers," yet the killing of women and children civilians during other wars was seldom mentioned. Consequently, as would be expected, a higher percentage of Vietnam veterans suffered guilt and moral pain over their killing than men who fought in other wars.

However, even in "popular wars" such as World War II, the "normal" killing required in combat constituted a moral transgression for some (but not all) soldiers. Some of these men experienced a deep conflict between their patriotic loyalty, which led them to join the military, and their moral abhorrence of killing. The conflict was only exacerbated when the killing extended beyond acceptable limits to include nonmilitary targets such as children.

Man-made vs. Natural Catastrophe

Survivors of man-made catastrophes are often believed to suffer from longer-term and more intense PTSD than survivors of natural catastrophes. This thinking reflects the common view that, in general, survivors of natural phenomena such as earthquakes and floods suffer less psychological devastation than survivors of traumas such as war, crime, and domestic violence.

There are two reasons for such thinking. The first is that natural catastrophes tend to be shorter in duration than man-made ones. A tornado can last less than fifteen seconds, for example, whereas a war can last months or years. The second reason is based on the assumption that natural catastrophes do not involve human error, betrayal, or violence. Because natural catastrophes can be explained away as acts of God or bad luck, natural catastrophe survivors are thought to be less likely to lose their trust in other human beings and in society than are survivors of man-made catastrophes.

For example, crime victims are violated not by the impersonal forces of nature, but by one or more of their fellow human beings. In the case of family violence, the trauma is not perpetrated by a stranger, but rather by one's own flesh and blood. Hence victims of these and other man-made disasters must deal with the issue of trust in the healing process.

In contrast, survivors of natural catastrophes are presumed not to have to grapple with the issue of trust. However, such reasoning does not take into account two significant aspects of natural disasters: the man-made elements involved in most natural disasters and the impact of the recovery environment on the natural disaster survivor. Both the recovery environment and the recovery process usually are, in today's world, heavily influenced by both individual human beings and governmental and other institutions. To make matters worse, both domestic violence and stranger crime tend to increase following a natural catastrophe.

Although we cannot control weather or geologic events such as earthquakes, modern technology has made tremendous strides toward preventing or lessening much of the death and destruction that used to result from natural catastrophes, as well as assisting survivors in the recovery process (Lindy 1985). However, warning systems, emergency services, and disaster-relief agencies still have limitations. In some cases, these limitations can be experienced as betrayal by survivors of the catastrophe. Natural catastrophe survivors face long lines, delays, and considerable red tape before they receive promised compensations for their losses. And in many cases, when the promised compensation appears, it is not adequate to cover the losses suffered.

In addition, warning systems and other parts of an infrastructure sometimes simply fail. For example, in April 1991, the failure of a tornado-warning siren in Andover, Kansas contributed to over a dozen deaths (*Washington Post* 30 April

1991). Similarly, the freeway collapse that caused numerous deaths during the 1989 Loma Prieta earthquake in Northern California can be seen as a technological failure, though its direct cause was the earthquake. In sum, from the survivor's point of view, there are few purely natural disasters. Consequently, natural disaster survivors may have more in common with survivors of man-made catastrophes than is often thought.

However, survivors of natural disasters do in fact differ from other survivors, especially abuse survivors, in that they tend to be less stigmatized. Natural catastrophe survivors in general are spared the "blame-the-victim" attitudes that frequently afflict survivors of man-made catastrophes. As mentioned earlier, in many cases victims of rape, incest, and other types of abuse are blamed for either provoking the abuse or for accepting it, as if it had been their choice. Furthermore, survivors of man-made catastrophes are much more likely to be seen by others as lacking in strength, caution, intelligence, or moral integrity.

Immediacy and Quality of Assistance

It cannot be overstressed that PTSD is a bio-socio-cognitive phenomenon as well as a psychological one. Consequently, restorative experiences play a major role in the recovery process. When traumatized individuals receive adequate psychological, economic, and other assistance as soon as possible following the incident, the effects are less severe and of shorter duration than if assistance is delayed, unavailable, or laced with shame, degradation, and rejection. This statement has been verified in research studies completed on war veterans in this country, Israel, and elsewhere; on rape and incest survivors; and on survivors of other forms of assault (Silver 1991; Courtois 1988; Sonnenberg, Blank, and Talbott 1985).

In addition, the responses of significant others, important social groups and institutions, and the community at large to which trauma survivors turn for assistance or protection can be critical in determining the effect of trauma. As Lyons (1991b) points out, following trauma, survivors either move toward people or against them. When a social support system turns against trauma survivors, the negative effects of the trauma are compounded.

Meaning and Attachment Systems

Bessel van der Kolk (1984) writes that the effects of trauma are significantly mitigated if the survivor's meaning system is not significantly damaged. When survivors can make sense of the trauma, they can better understand their reactions to it. Consequently, they do not become as confused and disparaging of themselves as do survivors who feel their pain has no meaning or makes no sense. For example, a trauma such as physical or sexual abuse is stripped of logic and sensibility when victims are told (by their abuser or others) that they provoked the abuse because they like it, that they deserve it, that the abuse is a figment of their imagination, or that the abuse isn't really so bad. Any one of these messages contradicts victims' sense of self-worth and their inner knowledge that they didn't provoke the abuse, that they don't like and don't deserve it and that the abuse is real and painful. Survivors' meaning systems can also be challenged or destroyed by blame-the-victim messages and other secondary wounding experiences.

The second mitigating factor emphasized by van der Kolk (1990b) is an attachment system. As long as the survivor has at least one person to turn to who can provide some assurance and emotional stability, recovery from the trauma is expedited. In some circumstances, however, a survivor's attachment system is destroyed. For example, combat soldiers may have continually lost their attachment systems to casualties in battle. Refugees, concentration camp survivors, torture victims, and survivors of vehicular accidents and natural catastrophes also frequently lose their attachment systems.

People who lose their families or other loved ones suffer a double loss. In losing friends or family, they lose not only a major attachment system, but part of their meaning system as well. To the extent that their role as family member or friend held an important meaning in their life, they lost that meaning when their relatives or friends died. They can never again be daughter, wife, mother, husband, son or father if their family was destroyed.

What Severity Means in Terms of Treatment and Prognosis

The severity of the trauma has numerous implications for treatment and prognosis. The severity must be considered on two levels, the physical and the psychological, although the two are intimately related. In instances of what Krystal (1978) calls catastrophic trauma—torture and mass violence—the physical trauma may be extensive. In these situations, as well as in prisoner of war or family abuse situations where repeated physical injuries were inflicted on the survivor, the nature of the physical assaults, including the extent of any starvation or malnutrition, sleep deprivation, and exposure to extreme temperatures, needs to be assessed.

Clients whose trauma had a strong physical component may need to be referred to a physician for medical attention and to a psychiatrist for assessment for possible clinical depression. Clinical depression often results not only from prolonged untreated trauma but from physiological stress, such as hunger and exposure. Other possible aftereffects of starvation and malnutrition are self-absorption, social isolation, propensities towards both aggressiveness and helplessness, stealing, and, in extreme situations, self-mutilation. Since these aftereffects are also symptoms of various psychiatric disorders, it can be easy to confuse the effects of trauma with a psychiatric disorder.

Individuals with histories of battering or sexual abuse may present with an eating disorder, which also may need medical attention as well as a psychiatric referral. Similarly, any individual with a prolonged history of substance abuse is at risk for medical problems, clinical depression, or other problems secondary to the substance abuse.

At this point, our knowledge of trauma is too limited and each traumatic event and individual survivor too unique to make any general statements about prognosis, treatment length, or treatment modality by trauma type or severity. In general, however, the more severe the trauma, the more intense the recovery period. For clients with acute reactions to a recent crisis, supportive counseling, education about the nature of PTSD, and crisis intervention counseling, along with eliciting family and community supports for the survivor, may be all that is needed to assist the client.

The length of the recovery period is also influenced by the severity. For example, one-time rape survivors who get good help soon after the rape can recover in six months to a year. In contrast, incest survivors, depending on their age and the duration and severity of their molestation, may require anywhere from two to three years or longer to heal.

For clients with classic PTSD, the healing process as outlined in this book is a good beginning. However, the therapist will need to acquire skills and knowledge in the specific trauma area suffered by the client. For example, if treating childhood abuse survivors, the therapist will need to be knowledgeable about the dynamics of dysfunctional, abusive families and the specific problems in the area of relationships (sexuality, self-care, and so on) that often attend survivors in this category.

Terr's (1991) Type 1 survivors may be helped on an outpatient basis. In contrast, Terr's Type 2 survivors and Herman's (1992) complicated PTSD survivors (survivors of long-term or repeated trauma), may require a period of inpatient care, followed by outpatient care. Similarly, combat veterans with severe stress reactions may require more than outpatient help, even if they are fortunate enough to recognize the signs of PTSD soon after their combat experience.

In treating individuals with PTSD compounded by years of lack of treatment and the development of a host of dysfunctional defense and coping mechanisms, the therapist will need all of the above skills and will also need to take special care not to in any way replicate aspects of the trauma in the therapeutic situation. Survivors of catastrophic trauma are also especially sensitive to triggers which remind them of the original trauma. (But survivors of what Krystal calls partial trauma can also be highly reactive to such triggers.)

Keep in mind that most of the above discussion is based on knowledge of only three kinds of trauma: rape, combat, and natural disaster. Our knowledge of appropriate treatment for other kinds of trauma is much sparser and often presents a bewildering array of possibilities to the clinician. In treating refugees, torture survivors, and other survivors of catastrophic stress, the success of treatment depends a great deal on the cultural background of the victim and the psychotherapeutic approach (Mollica 1988; Kinzie 1989).

Chapter 3

The Biochemistry of Trauma

The pain of being a trauma survivor is not limited to coping with the traumatic incident or series of incidents. Indeed, for many survivors, understanding what occurred and their reactions to it is only the first step towards recovery. Another major challenge is understanding and coping with those current life situations that, consciously or unconsciously, remind them of the trauma. Almost automatically, survivors may find themselves either overreacting or underreacting to these situations. Either way, their responses are usually socially inappropriate and personally problematic. Indeed, many survivors come to therapy because they realize their responses are inappropriate and pose serious obstacles to their personal happiness, interpersonal relationships, and vocational goals. They want to change some of their reaction patterns.

The self-esteem of some survivors is damaged not only because they have been unjustly stigmatized by society, friends, or family, but because they greatly fear and grossly misunderstand their own trauma-related responses to present-day events. When these people do not understand the causes of their reactions, they may feel not only like failures but like social misfits or as if they are emotionally aberrant.

"So-and-so died. I loved them, but I didn't feel a thing," I have heard dozens of combat vets say in therapy. And their next statement inevitably is "What's wrong with me, Doc? Why can't I feel? Why can't I cry? Why can't I be sad at funerals and happy at parties like other people? Am I a weirdo? What's happened to me? Is this how I'm going to be forever?"

Adult survivors of child abuse often make similar statements. For example, Joshua, who had been beaten, kept in a cage, starved, force-fed alcohol and drugs beginning at age five, and made to kill his pets by his extremely possessive father, came to therapy with one wish. The first words out of his mouth were "I want to love. I want to be able to love a woman, my neighbors, my friends, without flying into rages at them and driving them away from me. I want to love without becoming frightened and paranoid, to fit in somewhere, to be able to go to parties and family events without being on guard for danger and without having to drink or drug to feel comfortable and relaxed."

Trauma survivors in therapy, like Joshua, often want to change the way they react to certain situations, but feel powerless to do so. The powerlessness experienced with regard to their own emotional responses and behavior only reinforces the powerlessness experienced during the original traumatic event.

However, some of this powerlessness may be out of the survivor's control, in that, to one degree or another, overreacting or underreacting to situations reminiscent of the trauma may be biochemically determined. Consequently, when clients say "I couldn't help it," they may not be making excuses; they may be stating the truth. They truly may not be able to control experiencing heightened anxiety, feelings of rage, tuning out, or other reactions appropriate to traumatic situations but not to normal life events.

In recent years, it has become increasingly recognized that post-traumatic stress disorder is best understood as a bio-socio-psychological problem, that is, as a problem with significant biological and societal aspects as well as the more familiar psychological ones. PTSD is also a cognitive problem in that certain mindsets that may have been functional during the trauma, are not always functional in nontraumatic settings—for example, anger as a problem-solving technique for war veterans or passivity and lying for abused children.

This chapter explores the physiological aspects of PTSD, with an eye toward their implications for the survivor's self-esteem and relationships. The ways in which aspects of PTSD can perpetuate themselves and thus create vicious cycles are also presented in an effort to help explain the chronicity of PTSD and other living problems in some clients. The societal and cognitive aspects of PTSD are explored in later chapters.

It cannot be overemphasized, however, that the biochemical shifts that can occur as a result of trauma do not happen to every trauma survivor. Many of the biological changes discussed here may not apply at all to one-time trauma survivors, or they may apply only under very limited conditions. There are no hard and fast rules. For example, children who witness the violent deaths of family members or friends can suffer from biological changes just as readily as soldiers who spent time in prisoner-of-war camps. In general, incest survivors, refugees, battered wives, abused children, prisoners of war, combat soldiers with extended tours of duty, and others who have endured long-term, repeated, or severe trauma are those most likely to be affected.

Bear in mind that the ideas presented in this chapter are all tentative and that they are simplified explanations of complex processes that have yet to be fully understood. Research in the area of the physiology of trauma is relatively new and is still sparse. Until recently, the majority of the research on the biology of mental illness investigated the genetic aspects of certain mental disorders and excluded the impact of actual life events on mental health. The reality is that human physiology is a product not only of genetic inheritance but of environmental factors as well. The complexity of these interactions has yet to be defined.

The bulk of this chapter is based on the work of Dr. Bessel van der Kolk of Harvard University. His work is groundbreaking; however, even he regards it as only a beginning effort.

The Physiology of Trauma

When Abraham Kardiner first described, in 1941, the full syndrome of what is now called post-traumatic stress disorder (PTSD) he called it a "physioneurosis," a mental disorder with both psychological and physiological components. He noted that sufferers from PTSD continued to live in the emotional environment of the traumatic event, with enduring vigilance for and sensitivity to environmental threat. Following an even earlier tradition of Charcot and Janet, he noted that the bodies of traumatized individuals continue to be on the alert for a return of the trauma and tend to react to even minor stresses with physiological emergency responses. . . .

Over the years, a small literature has accumulated describing the human response to child abuse, incest, rape, wars, and concentration camp experiences. Only recently has it become clear that the response to trauma is relatively consistent across various traumatic stimuli: the central nervous system has a limited and rather consistent response to overwhelming life experiences. (van der Kolk 1987)

According to van der Kolk and others who have studied traumatized persons and animals, the severity of the initial trauma (intensity, duration, and frequency) and the severity of the initial emotional and physiological reactions to the trauma are important predictors of the long-term impact of the trauma on the survivor. In addition, the trauma survivor may also suffer from the effects of certain biological shifts that occurred during the trauma. In many cases, these biological shifts continue to influence the survivor's physical and emotional functioning and serve to perpetuate the trauma or the trauma mentality. Kardiner, for example, hypothesized that the following features of PTSD had physiological bases: persistent startle response and irritability, rage reactions, "fixation on the trauma," "constriction of the general level of personality functioning," and an "atypical dream life" (van der Kolk 1988a).

These biochemical shifts also have been found to create difficulties in four other areas of a survivor's current life: in thinking clearly, in regulating the intensity of emotions, in relating to other people, and in sustaining hope for the future. Trauma-induced biological changes can also lead to or contribute to the development of clinical depression and substance abuse problems.

Emotionally, the traumatic stressor gives rise to four affects which are, during the trauma, unbearable: fear, grief, rage, and heightened anxiety at confronting one's powerlessness and the possibility of death. These emotions can be so painful and intense that the survivor needs to repress them, either totally or in part.

Physiologically, trauma can give rise to a host of bodily changes. These changes can include increases in heart rate, blood sugar, muscle tension, and perspiration; dilation of the pupils; and hyperventilation (rapid shallow breathing from the upper lung versus more normal gentle breathing from the lower lung) (Wilson 1987).

The possible effects of hyperventilation include irregular heart rate; dizziness; shortness of breath; choking sensations; lump in the throat; heartburn; chest pain; blurred vision; numbness or tingling of mouth, hands, or feet; muscle pains or spasms; nausea; shaking; fatigue; and confusion or inability to concentrate (Wilson 1987).

The adrenaline increases, in turn, can lead to a fight-or-flight or a freeze reaction, as well as to biochemical shifts in certain neurotransmitters. Since these neurotransmitters are involved in regulating emotions, changes in their functioning have serious consequences for the survivor's ability to handle subsequent intense emotional experiences and life stresses.

Adrenaline Reactions

The adrenal glands are highly reactive to life-threatening situations. These two diamond-shaped organs, located on top of the kidneys, secrete large doses of either adrenaline or noradrenaline in response to the threat of danger. Adrenaline provides a supercharge of energy, which enables people to move with more speed and power than usual. In contrast, noradrenaline makes people freeze or go numb. This reaction is similar to the way some animals play dead when threatened.

During adrenaline surges, the heart rate increases, the pupils dilate, digestion slows down, and blood coagulates quicker, to prevent too much blood being lost. The lungs become more efficient, providing the increased oxygen necessary to fight back or run away as powerfully as possible. The increased oxygen can also vastly improve the acuteness of the senses and the mind's alertness. Sounds, smells, and other sensory data are perceived more vividly, and the brain uses this sensory data to assess the situation, thus maximizing the chances for survival.

Due to the increased oxygen, the brain can work more quickly and efficiently to make the best decisions possible. Consider the following examples: On her way to the babysitter's house with her small daughter, Mary realized she had forgotten to bring diapers, so when she passed a convenience store, she decided to run in and buy some. Thinking it would only take a second, she left her baby in the car. But when she came out of the store minutes later, her car was rolling backwards down the hill, toward a busy intersection. Although Mary was fifty pounds overweight, had not exercised in years, and the glasses she needed to distance vision were in the car, the adrenaline surge she experienced enabled her to clearly see the traffic at the bottom of the hill and she was able to run fast enough to stop the car before it rolled into traffic. Not only that, but by herself she pushed the car back up the hill into the parking lot.

Remembering the incident she said, "I didn't think; I just reacted. I felt like a wild animal being chased by tigers. Knowing that my baby was in that car made me run faster than I've ever run in all my life. I guess it was stupid of me to shove the car all the way back up the hill. I could have really hurt myself, but I had all this energy. I was so charged up I just didn't think."

If, on the other hand, Mary's adrenals had pumped her with noradrenaline, instead of having a fight-or-flight reaction, she could simply have frozen, as Sarah did. Sarah was sitting by her living room window watching her husband show their baby daughter the roses twining on the fence, when suddenly a dog jumped over the fence and attacked the child. Although Sarah was a pediatric nurse who had seen many injuries and illnesses, at the sight of her own child being harmed, she became immobilized, unable even to call for help. Fortunately, her husband had an adrenaline reaction that enabled him to save the child. Afterwards, however, Sarah's self-recriminations for her temporary paralysis were enormous.

Similarly, soldiers in battle, victims of rape and battering, survivors of natural catastrophes, and victims of mugging sometimes report having frozen or been unable to act. Combat medics, rescue workers, firefighters, and others on whom people depend for quick, decisive action, frequently suffer massive guilt because during a particular episode they "went limp," "couldn't think," or "couldn't do anything." The truth is, however, that these individuals, like Sarah, probably couldn't help it. They were not experiencing a failure of courage or a lack of dedication, but were most likely having an involuntary noradrenaline freeze reaction.

At first glance, an adrenaline surge may seem preferable to a noradrenaline response. However, adrenaline surges can be highly problematic, because they cannot be turned off at will. Just as Mary used her excess adrenaline to push the car up the hill, soldiers in battle are easily tempted to discharge their excess adrenaline through abusive violence, needless killings, or other acts of destruction. And the same dynamic might apply to some police officers and others involved in security work. Although the adrenaline surge does not excuse excessive violence, even in battle, the hyperalert adrenaline surges triggered by pursuit or combat do play an undeniable role in incidents of excessive violence.

Depletion of Neurotransmitters

Under conditions of severe stress there is an initial massive secretion of certain neurotransmitters. However, if the stress is prolonged, there a depletion of these neurotransmitters occurs "presumably because utilization exceeds synthesis" (van der Kolk 1988b).

Some of the major neurotransmitters that tend to be depleted as a result of continuous or intense stress are norepinephrine (noradrenaline), dopamine, serotonin, endogenous opioids, and catecholamines. These neurotransmitters are significant because they serve as emotional buffers and help individuals regulate the intensity of their feelings. Thus when these neurotransmitters are depleted, the trauma survivor is subject not only to clinical depression, but to difficulties in modulating emotions, leading to the much-publicized mood swings, explosive outbursts, startle response, and hyperreactivity to subsequent stress. Another possible effect is the development of "learned helplessness" syndrome: diminished motivation, clinical depression, and a decline in optimal functioning. Depletion of some neurotransmitters can result in overdependence on other people, feelings of "I can't make it without you," or in the opposite, an unrealistically independent or counterdependent stance of "I don't need anyone; I can make it on my own" (van der Kolk 1983, 1986; van der Kolk et al. 1984).

In research, primates subject to the trauma of maternal separation and other animals subjected to inescapable shock (IS) develop similar depletions in the above-mentioned neurotransmitters. Not unexpectedly, animals subject to maternal separation have also evidenced a subsequent pattern of aggressive outbursts alternating with despair and listlessness.

Human beings subject to parental neglect exhibit similar reactions. For example, incarcerated teenage boys convicted of murder who had histories of many years of nearly continual gross parental neglect were found to respond with listlessness and boredom when told that they would not be subject to the death penalty. At times, however, the pain of their childhood would break through "the false bravado" and the boys would "call out for a counselor, call him Dad or call her Mom. 'Please take me home with you' they'll ask" (*Washington Post* 8 Nov. 1992).

Furthermore, animals subject to IS have evidenced difficulties in learning how to escape new aversive situations, decreased motivation for learning new contingencies, chronic subjective stress, statistically increased tumors and decreased immunity to physical illness, and the learned helplessness syndrome.

In addition, artificially lowering the serotonin, endogenous opioid, catecholamine, and other neurotransmitter levels in nontraumatized animals has produced physiological "emergency responses" in these animals, as well as psychological distress, as measured by changes in their ability to play, mate, and otherwise positively interact with other animals (van der Kolk 1988a; Roth 1988).

Learned Helplessness

In a famous series of experiments conducted by Martin Seligman (1975), animals were subjected to electric shocks from which they couldn't escape. No matter what they did, or didn't do, they couldn't stop the pain. At first the animals fought, tried to get away, and uttered cries of pain or anger. Then they sank into listlessness and despair. Later on, in a second set of experiments, the same animals were given shocks again—only this time, by pressing a certain lever or completing some other simple task, they could stop the electric current. But they made no effort to do so. The animals had learned to be helpless. Due to their previous experiences, even when a means of escape from the pain was provided, these animals were too defeated, or too changed neurologically, to take the simple action that would end their suffering.

The result of these experiments was Seligman's learned helplessness theory. This theory has been applied not only to traumatized animals, but to human beings trapped in inescapable negative circumstances—individuals who have been traumatized. According to Seligman, "When an organism has experienced trauma it cannot control, its motivation to respond in the face of later trauma wanes. Moreover, even if it does respond and the response succeeds in producing relief, it has trouble learning, perceiving, and believing that the response worked. Finally, its emotional balance is disturbed; depression and anxiety, measured in various ways, predominate" (Seligman 1975). Since Seligman's original studies, much more work on learned helplessness has been completed. This new research shows the neurotransmitter depletions and numbing and hyperalert stages of PTSD (van der Kolk 1988b; Rossi 1986).

A variety of trauma survivors, notably abused women and children, prisoners of war, concentration- and refugee-camp survivors, and torture survivors, have been shown to be especially vulnerable to developing learned helplessness syndrome. For example, one major reason abused persons have difficulty leaving their abusers and striking out on their own is because of learned helplessness. Similarly, prisoners of war and some combat veterans also struggle long after they have been released from prison camps or military duty with the passivity, anxiety, and depression that comes with having learned to be powerless. Clients subjected to ongoing physical or sexual abuse or other forms of repeated trauma are at special risk for having acquired the learned helplessness syndrome to one degree or another. However, learned helplessness is not irreversible. These clients can, with effort and support, unlearn what the trauma ingrained. One step at a time, they can learn to take more and more control over their lives, and each small success will encourage them to take the next risk and the next step. Exercises in chapter 7 on victim thinking and on empowerment are specifically designed to help clients unlearn learned helplessness and take stock of their progress.

However, if as a result of the biological aspects of PTSD a client has developed a clinical depression or a major substance abuse problem, then he or she must first get special assistance with these problems. The client will be severely impeded in achieving her or his goals if either of these problems is left untreated.

The Biological Basis of the PTSD Cycle

The results of animal research confirm clinical observations of PTSD sufferers and helps to establish a physiological basis for some of the basic characteristics of PTSD: the tendency to react to relatively minor stimuli as if the trauma were recurring; the visual and motor reliving of the trauma through nightmares, flashbacks, intrusive thoughts, and behavioral reenactments; and the emotional numbing with various forms of attendant passivity, listlessness, and despair.

Because physiological arousal is paired with traumatic memories (and subsequently with stimuli associated with the original trauma), being physiologically aroused over any stimulus, whether related to the trauma or not, can precipitate remembering or reliving of the trauma. For example, states of physiological arousal can result in flashbacks, anxiety, or rage reactions; a numbing response may occur; or the hyperalert and numbing states may alternate.

The reverse is also true: Any stimulus that reminds the trauma survivor of the trauma, whether a person, place, thing or emotion, can precipitate a state of physiological arousal and emotional overload, especially when the emotion-buffering neurotransmitters are lacking. The simple lack of sufficient serotonin, catecholamines, and so on, with the consequent inability to regulate emotions, can make a major crisis out of a relatively small matter.

Since both hyperalertness and numbing can be painful, clients may begin to avoid situations that remind them of the original traumatic event. Such avoidance behavior may limit their opportunities and options. On the other hand, staying away from or minimizing contact with situations that trigger PTSD symptoms makes perfect sense emotionally. In either case, there may be trigger situations clients cannot or do not wish to avoid because they are potentially life-enriching or because doing so jeopardizes their personal and professional relationships and goals.

Implications for Intrapersonal and Interpersonal Relationships

Because hyperarousal and reliving the trauma are connected, the survivor learns to avoid situations of intense emotion or stress. When such situations cannot be avoided, the individual may need to shut down, emotionally and/or physiologically. The physiological relationship between hyperarousal and traumatic memories and feelings helps to explain why PTSD is more than an list of symptoms. Rather, PTSD is a pattern of phasic alteration between intrusive recall of the traumatic event and associated emotions—which lead to extreme anxiety and other forms of hyperarousal—followed by the numbing response.

The cyclical nature of PTSD can create problems in dealing with other people and with the client's own self-concept and self-esteem. It is not just the specific emotions themselves, but the way the client views or evaluates his or her emotions that can create confusion and emotional pain. That is, it is not just the feelings but the conscious or unconscious cognitions about those feelings that can create psychological pain.

Clients, for example, may view themselves as crazy, weak, or out of control because one day they feel hyper or manic and the next day, dead inside or unable to cope. This cycle may be particularly difficult for men who adhere to the stereotypic view that being emotional and having emotional fluctuations are solely female traits and that "real men" are in control of their feelings at all times and under all circumstances.

Healing often begins when clients become educated about the nature of trauma and its possible emotional and physiological consequences, and when they begin to accept, rather than deny or fight, the ways their traumatic experiences have affected them. If they can view their emotional fluctuations, their aggressive impulses, their need to isolate and numb themselves, in terms of physiology and psychology of PTSD, they may be less likely to label themselves the "crazy," "weak" or "defective." On the other hand, it is important that knowledge of the possible effects of trauma should not be interpreted as meaning there is no hope for healing. Nor should this information be used as an excuse to avoid responsibility for one's life, to abuse others, or to continue to abuse oneself.

The cyclical nature of PTSD also creates problems in clients' relationships with employers and coworkers, family members and friends, and so on, especially relationships where emotional communication and intimacy are involved, as is discussed in some detail below.

Difficulty Modulating Emotion and Poor Affect Tolerance

PTSD-afflicted survivors may respond to emotional stimulation with an intensity appropriate to the original traumatic situation, or they may not react at all. Because of the trauma, heightened emotions are paired with physiological hyperarousal and the possibility of reliving the trauma, both of which can lead to heightened anxiety. This anxiety can in turn easily create cognitive and emotional disorganization, which only creates further anxiety. Both the depletion of the neurotransmitters responsible for helping individuals to modulate their emotions and any negative views clients have about emotional intensity and expressiveness can play a critical role in this process.

As a result of their heightened anxiety and resulting emotional and cognitive disorganization, PTSD clients can literally be unable to make a realistic appraisal of their situation. The clients' awareness that they "can't think" (that they can not assess the situation or respond to it appropriately) only creates more anxiety, more self-disparagement, and more avoidance. In short, having anxiety creates its own anxiety.

Under such circumstances, clients may respond to the situation with action, with somatic symptoms, or by shutting down and avoidance, rather than with thought. Their spouses, friends, employers, and coworkers may interpret survivors' behavior as a sign that they are "crazy" or "don't care" and may consequently feel angry and abandoned.

This tendency of PTSD sufferers to respond in an "all-or-nothing" fashion is part of the fight-flight-freeze reaction, which is one of the physiological reactions to trauma. Interpersonally, the fight-flight-freeze reaction translates itself into all-or-nothing responses to other people (either numbing or rage); avoidance of others (psychologically, as a defense, and physically, as a way to reduce the anxiety and the bodily discomforts associated with being overstimulated); and fixation on the trauma and a consequent fear of new situations and people.

Regression: Inability to Differentiate Emotions

PTSD can contribute to psychological regression. As the human being matures, emotions become more specific and differentiated. When there is regression, as a result of trauma, for example, there can be loss of differentiation and emotions may express themselves physically, in terms of psychosomatic illnesses.

Individuals who have regressed emotionally are in danger of becoming over-whelmed by their responses and may have to block their feelings completely. Ideally, emotions could be used as a signal (that communication, change, or some action is needed), but when there is panic at the emotion, a deadly anxiety arises and the emotions are blocked entirely, or almost entirely (van der Kolk 1984a,b).

Difficulty Modulating Dependency and Intimacy

Spouses of PTSD-afflicted survivors complain of their partners' rage reactions, but they also complain of their "submissive" personalities and inability to be assertive or take care of problems. They resent making financial and other deci-sions by themselves and in other ways taking the major responsibility for the welfare of the family.

As discussed above, this "surrender" pattern, or learned helplessness, is uni-versal throughout the animal kingdom. The paralysis of initiative can be fol-lowed by various degrees of immobilization, which can also lead to automatic obedience or a numbing process by which all affective responses are blocked.

As van der Kolk (1988a) writes, the biological shifts that can result from trau-ma play a major role in creating depression, poor affect tolerance, and inability to modulate intimacy and dependency in survivors. These biological shifts often cause survivors to feel not in control of their lives because many times they are not in control of their emotions. They decry their "overreactions" to some situ-ations and their "underreaction" to others. Survivors' awareness of the inappro-priateness of their responses, may in turn cause them to either cling to a caretaker and become overly dependent or to isolate, shun relationships, and adopt a counterdependent stance. These two opposing reactions form what van der Kolk (1988a) calls the dependence-independence spectrum.

When survivors isolate, they inadvertently "perpetuate the central role" that trauma plays in their lives and diminish the richness of their lives by excluding the benefits of human ties (van der Kolk 1988a). Other possible relationship problems stemming from trauma-induced biological changes are a proclivity to rage following relatively minor incidents, self-blame for any physical or emo-tional abuse endured in the relationship, and a tendency to view oneself as being victimized in many social interactions.

Depression as a Secondary Elaboration

Depression is by far the most common psychiatric problem in our country. Many mental-health professionals estimate that one third of adult women and one tenth of adult men can expect to suffer from at least one bout of depression in their lifetime (Beck 1973; Rovner 1991). Unfortunately, very few of these indi-viduals recognize the symptoms. Even if they do, they often fail to get help. Like PTSD, depression is a highly treatable condition. There is no necessity for, or purpose in, these clients' continuing to suffer needlessly.

It will be your role as therapist to assess clients for depression using the of-ficial *DSM-IV* criteria and to make an appropriate referral to a psychiatrist if warranted. If your client does suffer from depression, you will need to encour-age him or her to seek psychiatric help and to continually remind the client that depression is a curable condition. You will also need to teach your client about what depression is and is not, just as you need to teach her or him about PTSD. Like PTSD, depression is a problem shrouded in stigma and shame. You can mediate the client's self-loathing or other negative feelings about having depression with information and a strong didactic approach. For example, in addition to "lecturing" on depression, you can point out when the client's feelings or thoughts reflect the illness of depression rather than reality. You can counter statements of hopelessness with comments, such as "That's depression talking. Depression says there is no hope. The truth is, there is always some hope and you have several choices in this situation. Also, if depression has weakened you—which it does—then you can ask for help. Here I am, start with me. How can I help you with this?"

To do this, however, you must be familiar with depression as a clinical entity and be able to distinguish it from normal "blues," from grieving, and from other emotional states with depressive components.

The following description of depression provides a brief overview, along with some information about its relationship with trauma and PTSD. However, it will be necessary for you to undertake further study of the various depressive disorders listed in *DSM-IV* on your own.

Definitions and Causes of Depression

Everyone has the blues from time to time, and when it happens, people often say they are depressed. There is a difference, however, between those feelings and biochemical or clinical depression.

For example, depression is part of the grieving process. However, the depression that is part of the five stages of grief (denial, anger, bargaining, depression, and acceptance) does not constitute true clinical depression. Normal grief is a response to a real external loss—that of a loved one, a pet, or a home, car, or other valued object—that is consciously recognized. In contrast, in clinical depression the grieving may be unconscious or only partly conscious. Furthermore, in clinical depression, as opposed to normal grieving, there is usually grief over psychological or spiritual loss, such as a loss of innocence, a loss of a belief once held dear, or the loss of self-respect.

In normal grieving, the depression tends to lessen over time, although it may take years. In clinical depression, however, the sadness tends to grow over time. Other components of clinical depression include mixed feelings towards oneself and others or active self-hatred and physiological problems such as sleep disturbances and fatigue.

In clinical depression, the negative feelings are so overwhelming that they impair the ability to function. One can't make it to work, or it is a struggle to do so. One stops going out and one avoids socializing. The smallest task seems like a monumental chore and one can't concentrate enough to finish a newspaper article, much less a book. One has trouble meeting the most basic obligations to one's family or oneself.

Clinical depression can also impair reality testing. For example, one becomes hypersensitive to the reactions of others and consequently may have a distorted view of others' feelings. Or one may also feel utterly hopeless about situations in which there is, in fact, considerable hope.

Clinical depression is not only widespread, but numerous studies suggest it is on the rise in all age groups and especially among young adults. Experts attribute the rise in depression, in part, to increasingly difficult economic conditions. Increased depersonalization and the breakdown of traditional support structures during the past two decades also contribute to the rise in depression.

Depression rates are especially high among groups who are oppressed in some manner, for example, the poor, minority groups, women, and the handicapped. Depression is also prevalent among victims of abuse, violence, or other traumas.

Trauma survivors are at risk for developing a clinical depression. Or they may already have a clinical depression of which they—or you—are unaware. Some studies indicate that at least 50 percent of individuals with PTSD also suffer from depression. This depression is frequently, but not necessarily, a result of the trauma. But whether the depression predates the trauma or developed afterward, the effect is the same.

There are many different explanations for what causes clinical depression. No one of these theories is 100-percent accurate in all cases, but they all have some validity in some instances. Clinical depression is caused by many factors, some of which are beyond individual control. Several of these causes can be directly related to trauma.

As you read the following sections, keep in mind that causes for depression may vary over time—a given depressive episode may have an entirely different cause than the ones preceding or following it, and the theory that explains one person's depression will not apply to another's.

Biological Theory

One way of looking at depression is as the result of disturbances in the neurotransmitter system, usually caused by the depressed person having been subject to severe stress for a prolonged period of time—as discussed above. Due to the stress or trauma, the person's biochemistry becomes so strained that it cannot perform its functions as it did before the traumatic event. Breakdown of the neurotransmitter system can lead to low self-esteem, hopelessness, and other forms of negative thinking, and to difficulties with concentration, sleep, and decision making. It can also lead to irritability, anxiety, loss of the ability to experience pleasure, and hypersensitivity to the reactions of others—all of which are classic symptoms of depression.

Depression is also associated with physical illnesses, especially those of a chronic or severe nature such as cancer and heart disease. In addition, depression can result from severe injuries and permanent disabilities or from the multiple medications that might be needed due to these problems. Physical illness, disability, and medication tax the neurotransmitter system immensely. They also put a strain on other bodily functions. Physical injury or illness also often creates other problems—financial, social, sexual, emotional. These stresses further disturb biochemical balances and negatively affect the central nervous system.

A client who was already ill or disabled when the traumatic event occurred, was suffering from malnutrition or sleep deprivation, or was seriously injured during the trauma is at special risk for developing depression. The risk is especially high if a part of the person's body essential to her or his work or interests was affected. For example, a dancer who lost the use of her legs in an accident would lose not only her work but her means of creativity as well—a double blow that would almost certainly lead to depression.

Loss and Grief Theory

The dancer's depression over her loss in part fits Freud's view of depression. He believed that depression was the result of grief over the loss of a love object. However, the kind of grief he was referring to was not normal grief, but grief that was mixed in with anger and hostility towards the loved one. Freud also felt that the loved one need not be dead. Death of the relationship with the loved one was sufficient to cause depression.

The concept of the loved one can be extended to include a cherished ideal, such as patriotism, certain spiritual values, or self-respect. Consequently, losing a long-held value or ideal or one's dignity can also lead to depression. If a client's dignity or self-respect was assaulted not only by the trauma but subsequently by others' negative reactions to the client's feelings, he or she may be at a special risk for depression. Similarly, if the client's assumptions about the goodness and justice of the universe or other values were shattered by the trauma, her or his subsequent grieving may also develop into depression.

For example, in all of this century's wars, some soldiers have become disillusioned with the government or the military after observing hypocrisies, incompetence, and errors that resulted in needless deaths among their comrades. Many of these soldiers lost faith in military authority; some experienced a lessening of their patriotism as well. The resulting feeling among these men was not only anger but grief. They had lost the very ideals that caused them to join the military in the first place.

Behavioral Theory

The behavioral view of depression states that depression is the natural result of inadequate reinforcement, rewards, or recognition. Depression can easily develop among people who are inadequately rewarded or appreciated by others. Depression also results when people are unable to adequately appreciate, reward, or lovingly care for themselves.

Some popular self-help books espouse or imply the idea that if one can only accept oneself, one doesn't need love and acceptance from others. Nevertheless, people do need the recognition, love and approval of at least a few other people as well as self-love and self-appreciation.

Trauma survivors are sometimes deprived of both: They lack reinforcement from others as well as self-reinforcement. Vietnam veterans and police and other service workers are prime examples of depression caused by lack of reinforcement. In general, until recently, the Vietnam veteran was far from appreciated by our society. Instead of a welcome-home parade like that which greeted the Persian Gulf veterans, the Vietnam veteran was castigated and rejected for his sacrifices. Similarly, some rescue workers work long hours for relatively low pay and receive little recognition for their many heroic efforts on behalf of others. Such situations are the breeding grounds for depression.

If your clients, as trauma survivors, were denigrated or not properly acknowledged for their efforts to survive or to help others survive, or if they withstood long-term traumatic conditions for which they received few rewards, they may be at risk for depression.

Learned Helplessness Theory

Part of learned helplessness is a belief that one cannot exert control over the important events in one's life. This feeling of helpless resignation or fatalism can lead to a clinical depression. Due to direct experience with powerlessness, and because of the biochemical changes that can occur during trauma, trauma survivors are especially susceptible to learned helplessness and consequently to depression.

Cognitive Theory

The cognitive view of depression is similar to the learned helplessness theory. However, cognitive theory states that depression is a problem of thoughts and beliefs, rather than feelings. Once someone begins to think or believe he or she is helpless or ineffectual, then such thinking controls her or his behavior. Negative thinking can result in negative events, which further reinforce the negative thinking and view of life.

Cognitive theory further states that depressed people misinterpret life events and thus distort their view of the world, themselves, and the future in a hopeless direction. Such distortions and misinterpretations are often directly related to trauma, which in some cases teaches survivors that they are ineffectual, incompetent, or powerless (Burns 1980).

"Anger Turned Inward" Theory

People who do not know how to express their anger, are afraid to express their anger, or feel they do not have the right to express it, often turn that anger on themselves—resulting in depression. Turning their anger inward is frequently a cause of depression in trauma survivors for whom expressing anger could have caused their death (crime victims, refugees, and other captives) or could have led to physical abuse or other forms of punishment (abused women, children, and elderly persons). Even when the abuse or captivity is over, the "habit" of suppressing anger can be difficult to unlearn.

Anger is also often turned inward when there is no clearly identifiable target for the anger—when there is no one person or identifiable group to express anger toward, as, for example, when a large bureaucracy or institution is non-responsive to a survivor. Likewise, toward whom do Holocaust survivors, survivors of torture and totalitarian regimes, and mistreated Vietnam, Korean War and World War II veterans direct their rage? In these cases, as one survivor put it, "Everybody was responsible, but nobody was responsible."

Similarly, at whom or what can natural catastrophe survivors vent their anger? Yelling at nature is less than satisfying. Blaming God or other supernatural forces poses a similar problem, complicated by the fact that those who direct their anger at a spiritual being often turn to that same being for protection, direction, and love. For those people it may be easier or safer to turn their anger inward than to risk a loss of faith by blaming God.

Unrelated Causes

Depression can also be caused by events unrelated to trauma. These include an acute brain syndrome, some other organic mental disorder, or a psychiatric problem such as schizophrenia or paranoia. In some cases, depression is hereditary. If a client has a family history of clinical depression or manic-depressive illness, it does not automatically mean that she or he will develop that problem. However, the strain of the trauma can bring forth these and other latent genetic-based psychiatric disorders. Therefore, if one or more of the family members has suffered from depression, watch carefully for symptoms of depression in your client.

Depression over Depression

Some depressed people tend to get "depressed about being depressed." They interpret their symptoms of depression as signs of personal inadequacy and failure, and feel great shame and guilt over being depressed. Their feelings are reinforced by three factors: societal attitudes that blame people for their own pain, societal ignorance about depression, and cultural norms that view any person in emotional pain as weak or deficient. These are the same attitudes that oppress people with PTSD, but these attitudes do not reflect reality. Rather, they reflect people's ignorance about mental health matters and their fears about themselves, which underscores the need for educating clients about depression.

Substance Abuse and Compulsion as Secondary Elaborations

Addictions and compulsions are complex phenomena. They have many possible causes, ranging from genetic and biochemical factors to social pressures to dysfunctional family backgrounds. However, in the case of trauma survivors, in many instances addictions and compulsions serve as forms of self-medication for the symptoms of PTSD.

Sometimes it is difficult for those who do not suffer from PTSD to comprehend the pain and frustration involved in being hyperalert and unable to sleep or the agony of being constantly on guard against others and against one's own mind. At any time, memories and nightmares can pop into one's brain, destroying, at least temporarily, any semblance of mental and emotional self-control.

Equally painful is the numbing stage of PTSD. To feel bored, shut down, more like a stone than human being, can be almost intolerable. Then to further feel as if there is nothing one can do to feel normal again is cause for even more despair.

It is for such reasons that some survivors reach out to mood-alerting substances, such as alcohol, drugs, and food, or to mood-altering activities, such as compulsive gambling, shopping, or sexual behavior. Although this statement is not intended to justify illegal or self-destructive activities, the fact is that these substances and activities can and do provide comfort and relief. Often they are the only "friend" a survivor feels she or he can turn to, especially late in the night when one is most vulnerable to fear and loneliness.

However, the friend eventually becomes an enemy. Usage can quickly develop into dependency, and as the dependency grows, it can eventually consume the survivor's life and wreak havoc in his or her body, mind, relationships, finances, and, worst of all, his or her self-esteem.

Many survivors disparage themselves for being "addicts" or involved in compulsive activities, but the majority fail to see the connection between their substance abuse or compulsion and the original traumatic event. One goal of therapy is to help clients make this connection. It often helps to point out to clients that high percentages of trauma survivors suffer from substance abuse problems and other addictions and compulsions. The populations studied thus far include war veterans, natural catastrophe survivors, fire and technological disaster survivors, and abused persons, including men, women, and children. Although much more research needs to be completed in this area, studies thus far have found rates such as the following:

- Approximately 50 to 60 percent of women and 20 percent of men in chemical dependency recovery programs report having been victims of childhood sexual abuse. Approximately 69 percent of women and 80 percent of men in such programs report being victims of childhood physical abuse (Kunzman 1990b; Bigham and Resick 1990).

- Anywhere from 40 to 60 percent of women in recovery for bulimia, anorexia, and compulsive overeating report victimization experiences (Slogan and Leichner 1986; Kunzman 1990a,b; Bigham and Resick 1990; Zweben 1987).

- The trauma of war has been implicated in the relatively high rates of substance abuse among combat veterans, with anywhere from 50 to 65 percent of PTSD-afflicted Vietnam combat veterans reporting alcohol and/or drug abuse. High rates of alcohol abuse have also been noted among World War II and Korean War combat veterans (Jelinek and Williams 1984; Keane et al. 1983; Matsakis 1988; Lacoursiere, Godfrey, and Ruby 1980).

- Severe trauma has also been documented among compulsive gamblers seeking help, among runaway and delinquent children and adolescents, and among both male and female prostitutes and actresses and models in pornographic films and magazines (Taber, McCormick, and Ramirez 1987; Courtois 1988; Finkelhor 1979; Brown and Finkelhor 1986).

- Researchers have also noted increases in alcohol consumption among survivors of fires, floods, and other natural disasters.

Ironically, drugs, food, and compulsive behaviors can serve as both stimulants for the numbing phase and sedatives for the hyperalert stage of PTSD. For example, a drink, a pill, a snack, a sexual encounter, or a shopping spree can induce some feeling during the numbing phase. Or that same drink, drug, or binge can produce a calming effect on the hyperalert symptoms. (However, these same substances also may lower inhibitions against expressing frustration and rage in a verbally or physically abusive manner.)

Drugs and food can also help fight insomnia, bad dreams, and intrusive thoughts. Alcohol helps induce sleep, for example, as well as suppressing the stage of sleep during which most dreams and nightmares occur. Food and drugs can quell the anxiety, anger, and other strong feelings of the hyperalert stage.

Addictions and compulsions can also be used by PTSD sufferers to handle the avoidance symptoms of PTSD, which include the tendency to isolate from others. "I couldn't handle the people at work (at parties, at home) if I didn't drink (do drugs, binge)," some trauma survivors say. Their addiction or compulsion gives them the courage and confidence they need to feel comfortable with others. Without it they might choose to be virtual hermits, limiting their contact to their immediate families and needed professionals.

Addictions, Compulsions, and Depression

PTSD can also lead to substance abuse via depression. If the PTSD has contributed to the development of a biochemical depression, substance abuse or compulsive activity can medicate not only the PTSD but also the depression.

Recent research has shown a substantial correlation between alcoholism and depression and between eating disorders and depression. In some studies, for example, over 80 percent of alcoholic men have been shown to suffer from biochemical depression (Anixter 1990). Experts are, however, not clear about which comes first—the alcohol abuse or the depression. On the one hand, alcohol can serve to make tolerable some of the symptoms of depression. On the other hand, prolonged alcohol use, with its debilitating effects on the body and on the individual's ability to function, can actually create a biochemical depression.

Also some of the initial symptoms from alcohol observed in detox treatment programs are similar to depressive symptoms. Thus the only way to tell if an alcohol-addicted person also suffers from depression is for him or her to be assessed for depression two or three weeks after the withdrawal stage. For the nondepressed individual, the symptoms of depression may largely disappear after two or three weeks of sobriety. However, for the dually affected individual, the depressive symptoms persist for at least two weeks following withdrawal and sobriety.

In the area of eating disorders, several studies have shown that over half of bulimic and anorectic women suffer from depression or come from families with histories of depression. As with alcoholism and depression, sometimes it is not clear which came first—the eating disorder or the depression. The eating disorder may have begun as a means of coping with the sad, lonely, angry, hopeless, and otherwise negative feelings associated with depression. However, prolonged dieting can create biochemical depression by stressing the neurotransmitters and by depriving the body of adequate nutrients. Such dieting is common among all who suffer from eating disorders, whether anorexia, bulimia, or compulsive overeating.

For people with eating disorders, the only way to determine whether they suffer from clinical depression is to wait until they have achieved some mastery over the disorder itself. Ideally, the overeating, self-starvation, or binging and purging will have stopped, or at least be at a manageable level, before it is determined whether the person also suffers from depression.

Further evidence of the relationship between depression and addiction lies in recent research that shows anti-depressants to be exceptionally successful in controlling binge drinking and binge eating (Wadden, Stunkard, and Smoller 1986; Liberman, Wurtman, and Chew 1986; Wurtman and Wurtman 1989; Lee, Richards, and Mitchell 1985).

Case Example

At first glance, the following portion of an interview between a counselor and a male incest survivor does not appear related to the biochemistry of trauma. However, the client's presenting concerns—fear of losing control of his anger and substance abuse—are extremely common readjustment problems for many survivors. The difficulty many trauma survivors have in modulating their emotions is, as this chapter shows, at least to some degree the result of biochemical shifts that occur as a result of trauma, especially prolonged or repeated trauma. As you read the following excerpt, keep in mind that the client has already undergone many months of therapy and has made significant gains in self-understanding.

Client:	My wife is angry at me and my children are terribly disappointed, but I refuse to go to Thanksgiving dinner if Jack is going to be there.
Counselor:	Why? What happens when you see Jack?
Client:	Jack is the stupidest, most disgusting man in the world. He's my wife's first cousin, but he looks just like the uncle who abused me.
Counselor:	Tell me more.

Client:	Jack just says the most vicious, stupid things.
Counselor:	Give me an example.
Client:	At the last family party, Jack had too much to drink and started singing "East is east and west is west, but all around the world, incest is best." Everybody laughed and thought it was so funny. Then he went on and on with incest jokes. Jack knows I'm an incest survivor. He knows how much therapy I've been through and how much I hurt. I thought he understood. But that night it became clear that he was just like everyone else. He thinks that because incest involves sex, it's a big joke.
Counselor:	How sad you had to endure such an experience. Jack's remarks were outrageous and he, like those who laughed with him, are terribly misinformed, aren't they? They simply have no idea how much suffering is involved in being an incest survivor, do they? How did you feel when everybody started laughing?
Client:	I couldn't stand it.
Counselor:	Of course you couldn't stand it. It reminds me of the times you told me about when your uncle laughed at you while he was abusing you. You were alone then, with no one to protect or help you. It sounds like you were alone at that gathering with Jack too ... Didn't anybody ask him to stop? Not even your wife?

(*Client shakes his head.*)

Counselor:	How awful. How absolutely awful.
Client:	(*Weeping*) I felt like punching him and yelling at him, but I didn't want to embarrass my wife.
Counselor:	So what did you do?
Client:	I just smiled in my usual sickening people-pleasing way and told my wife we had to go home right away. She felt I was overreacting and wanted to stay. Then I went into a rage, almost slapped her, and shoved her into the car. We argued all the way home, and she threatened to leave me if I ever shoved her again. This has happened before, you see. That night I drank a fifth of vodka. After a whole year of being sober, I blew it. Then I got so mad at myself for drinking, I drank some more. Then I started thinking about how sweet death would be. I wouldn't have to deal with any of this anymore.
Counselor:	No wonder you don't want to go to Thanksgiving dinner this year.
Client:	The last time Jack made his comments, my children weren't there. But if he makes comments like that in front of my children, I'm afraid I'll do more than shove my wife ... I just lose it.
Counselor:	What do you mean by "lose it"?
Client:	I'm afraid I'll hit him and that I won't stop there. Once I get into him, I could hurt him badly, even kill him without meaning to.
Counselor:	Have you ever lost control like that?
Client:	More than once.
Counselor:	Do you want to share about those times, or would you rather not?
Client:	I'd rather not. Do I have to tell you everything?
Counselor:	No. Of course not. However, your fear of losing control is something you might want to talk about sometime because it bothers you so

much and affects so many areas of your life. But, if you don't wish to talk about the specific incidents where you lost control right now, or ever, that's fine.

Client: Listen, I told you I don't want to talk about it. Stop pressuring me.

Counselor: I feel you are tremendously upset right now. Am I reading you right?

Client: Yes, because you're pressuring me to talk.

Counselor: Maybe you didn't hear me before, so let me repeat to you clearly: You don't have to talk about anything you don't want to talk about in here. Do you believe me?

Client: No, because you might be mad at me if I don't answer your questions.

Counselor: And if I'm mad at you, what will happen next?

Client: You'll throw me out. You won't help me anymore. (Sobbing) You'll beat me, put sticks in my privates like my uncle, make me talk about sex things like he did, make me . . . (*Client continues to sob.*)

Counselor: What you endured is beyond belief. How awful that a little boy had to endure all that. How trapped you were. If you didn't please your uncle, he would have hurt you physically, and emotionally too, by abandoning you. He pressured you in so many ways and held such power over you. No wonder you don't like to be pressured today.

Client: I'm sorry, Doc. I know you're on my side. But see how I am? One minute I'm a rational man, then I'm an angry man. I can't even hear what my own counselor is telling me. If it wasn't you, and we were somewhere else and something like this happened, I'd probably be all over that person. It would only be their good luck or if somehow someone intervened that I didn't really hurt, or even kill, them. I get that urge to hurt people all the time.

Counselor: And you fight it all the time, and most of the time you win. Wow! What a battle. What a struggle. How hard it must be for you to simply live. Do you appreciate that?

Client: I guess I don't. Honestly, Doc, I don't want to hurt anyone. I'm tired of hurting people because of my problem, but I'm being pressured to go to this dinner. My eight-year-old is already in tears because I mentioned not going. But if I go, I might do something I'll regret later. What should I do?

Counselor: You're in quite a bind here. But I think the question we should be asking is not what should you do, but what can you do? Can you handle Jack or someone else making insensitive remarks?

Client: No. I can't handle it, which makes me think I should stay home. But I hate myself for being like this. I want to be normal. I want to have a normal life. I want to be able to go to a Thanksgiving dinner with my family just like everyone else.

Counselor: You would, if you felt safe. And there may well come a day when you can listen to comments like Jack's and be able to manage your reaction. But what you're saying today, and correct me if I'm wrong, is that for now you don't feel safe. You don't trust that you can control your anger, and you want to stay home. If you're afraid you will lose control, then maybe you should consider staying home. If that is your decision, I will support you.

Client: But what about my family? They'll be so disappointed.

Counselor: True, but they'll be more disappointed if you attack Jack or if you stifle your anger by drinking and return to being alcoholic. Unfortunately, the truth is that having PTSD does impose certain limits on your life. But you're here to work on those limits, to stretch them as far as they can go so that you are free to do the things you want to do.

Client: Yes. But what do I do now?

Counselor: Are there options other than going or not going at all, for example, going only for an hour or two or making an arrangement with your wife that you will leave at once if someone says something insensitive? Or, could you consider standing up to Jack? Or would that single you out and make you feel worse? Do you want to brainstorm some options and then see if you think any of them would actually work for you?

At this point, if the client wishes, the therapist could explore the pros and cons of various options. But equally important, to help reduce the client's self-blame about his reaction to Jack and Jack's remarks, either in this session or the next, the client needs to be told about (or provided educational materials that explain) some of the reasons for his intensely aggressive responses to certain situations. This would include information on the biochemistry of PTSD and help with triggers and trigger situations (discussed in chapter 6).

In some cases, medication might also be considered. Many of the negative effects of PTSD, the sleep disorders, the mood swings, the aggressive outbursts, and other troubling symptoms can be ameliorated by a variety of psychotropic medications, such as MAO inhibitors, tricyclic anti-depressants, lithium, beta-blockers, and others (Roth 1988). This option is discussed further in chapter 4.

Part II

The Therapeutic Process

Chapter 4

Client Assessment

Ideally, clients should be assessed for PTSD early in the therapeutic process, usually after five or six sessions. It is useful not only to you, as the clinician, but to your clients so that they have some definition of their major problem area or areas. (If your agency or practice has different requirements, for example, if a diagnosis is required by the end of the first interview, you will have to adhere to the policy as best you can, revising or refining your diagnosis as you obtain additional information about the client.) Diagnosis of the problem area gives the clinician at least an initial focus. At the same time, diagnosis also provides relief and direction for the client. "I only have PTSD. I'm not totally crazy," or "I have PTSD and depression with an eating disorder. That's not good, but at least I'm not a basket case," is the sentiment of some clients. At least (and perhaps at last) their malady has a name, and having a name makes it an identifiable problem rather than a mystery, which greatly reduces its power. This can automatically give clients hope by making their inner turmoil seem more manageable. In sum, the diagnostic process itself, if completed sensitively and accurately, can be a positive therapeutic intervention. At the very minimum, clients will realize that they are not alone in having their problem.

The purpose of diagnosis is *not* to label clients for the sake of labeling, but to provide proper care:

> Diagnosis in psychiatry is a very imperfect science with a very limited range of usefulness. Like a powerful drug, it is best used sparingly and only when it clearly benefits the patient. Diagnosis does not lead to cure, and where improperly applied can actually interfere with the person's getting better. Initial diagnoses are frequently incorrect or incomplete, and even when accurate, provide us with little more than a first approximation, a rough guide, to treatment decisions. A diagnosis should not be thought of as answer to a problem, but rather as a hypothesis to be tested and reviewed where indicated. It should assume increasingly less importance in therapy as the work proceeds. In our profession, we treat fellow human beings, not symptoms. (Newman 1987)

This is a point it is well to bear in mind at all times, especially with traumatized clients.

You need to assess whether or not your client has PTSD according to the *DSM-IV* guidelines. If your client does have PTSD, you need not only to ask about the traumas experienced and the existence of the various PTSD symptoms, but also to obtain as much detail as you can about the frequency, intensity, and history of these symptoms. You also need to put together as full as possible a picture of the other difficulties, including coexisting problems such as substance abuse, depression, and medical problems. If the client engages in self-mutilation or has had significantly positive or significantly negative experiences with former therapists or doctors, these aspects of the client must also be included in the clinical picture (as well as discussed with the client at some point). The client's potential for suicide or homicide must also be assessed.

Although it is desirable to conduct a thorough assessment for PTSD in the first few sessions, this may or may not be possible, or even advisable. If the clients come to you in crisis, either due to the trauma or some other life event, your primary role may be to help them understand and contain their feelings, to help them deal with their fears and anxieties, or to direct them to outside medical, legal, social, or other sources of assistance, as needed. If there is time, you may be able to ask a few pertinent questions regarding PTSD. Or the clients themselves, in their self-description, may provide you with evidence of PTSD. This information may or may not be sufficient for you to make a conclusive diagnosis.

Assessing for Trauma and PTSD

Inquiry about trauma needs to be a routine part of your intake procedure with *all* clients—not just those you suspect may be trauma survivors. As basic as this may sound, numerous research studies show that typically therapists fail to inquire about trauma in completing a client history.

In fact, perhaps the most common error in diagnosing trauma survivors is failure to detect that they *are* trauma survivors. Their trauma may have been so severe, or have taken place long ago, that they present to you with a host of symptoms that reflect secondary elaborations rather than PTSD. Even if you ask certain clients about trauma in their history, the trauma may be so repressed that they do not remember it.

Severe repression or amnesia is most often found in individuals who were severely traumatized, who were traumatized at the preverbal level or before the age of five, or who were threatened with harm if they disclosed the traumatic incident. For example, as psychologist Christine Courtois (1988) points out, incest survivors were usually instructed not to tell about the incest, under any circumstances. Consequently, sharing the incest secret with a therapist may feel like a betrayal of the family. In addition, many incest victims survived and continue to survive by keeping tight control of themselves, including control of "the secret." Survivors may fear that divulging their secret may open the floodgates to unbearably painful feelings and memories, to suicidal or homicidal thoughts, and to fears of insanity, being killed or punished by family members, being blamed for the abuse, or never being able to stop crying. Consequently, even if the survivor has conscious memories of the incest, she or he may need to keep them secret in order to retain internal strength and cohesion (Courtois 1988).

Amnesia regarding the trauma, fear of harm, or fear of loss of personal control if the traumatic incident is shared have also been found among battered adults (Walker 1979), prisoners of war, and other survivors of war. Refugee and torture survivors, for example, have been found to have difficulty sharing their secret, whether it is rape, torture, or some other horror. Like incest survivors, these persons were instructed that if they told, they or their loved ones would be punished or even killed (Kinzie 1989; Lee and Lu 1989).

You will also have difficulties detecting PTSD or a history of trauma if you encounter a client during the numbing-avoidance phase of the PTSD cycle. In such cases you may not recognize PTSD until the intrusive recall stage emerges. Some clients stay in numbing for years, if not decades. These are the clients who often function quite normally and do not display any aberrant behavior or thought patterns. Yet they seek therapy because of a vague sense of emotional pain and difficulties with intimacy and human relationships. Even if the client has had years of therapy, he or she may not be in touch with or have adequately processed the core trauma.

In sum, it is highly unlikely that you will uncover the core trauma during your initial assessment, especially if the client is new to therapy. Consequently, in working with PTSD clients at any phase of treatment, it is vital that you make no assumptions. Keep an open mind. It is not unheard of for individuals in their forties or fifties, or even their sixties, to recall childhood traumas and develop PTSD as an overlay to whatever other concerns brought them to you for help. Indeed, it may be precisely because they have made such significant progress in other areas or because their life is somehow free of other stresses or pressures that they now have the psychic energy or readiness to have a childhood (or other) trauma come to the surface.

The client, for example, needs to have sufficient ego strength and other supports (inner or outer) to cope with the new information in a constructive manner. Consequently, in some cases, the client will need to have undergone treatment with you for some time period before she or he gains the psychological capacities to have the traumatic memories surface. In cases where memories are repressed, treatment may need to come before diagnosis (Courtois 1988).

The Assessment Process

In assessing for PTSD, structured questions that are based on the *DSM-IV* work well. The Self-Assessment Questionnaire that appears on the following pages lists questions you should ask clients. Be sure to familiarize yourself with them thoroughly.

The more organized you are, the more secure clients will feel. Clients will also feel more secure if you, at each juncture in the therapy, share with them what you are doing and why. In PTSD therapy, there should be as few secrets as possible. At as many points as you can, without its being cumbersome, advise clients as to what you are attempting to do and why. Such sharing helps restore to clients the sense of control they lost in the trauma and builds faith in you as a therapist.

When assessing for PTSD, you can say, "It's time for us to assess whether or not you suffer from post-traumatic stress disorder, or PTSD. The purpose of assessing you is not to put a negative label on you or to put you in a box. You are a unique individual, who is far more than any problem you may have. However, in order to help you, we need to find out if you suffer from PTSD and, if so, from what degree of PTSD. We also need to determine which PTSD symptoms are causing you the most problems so that we know how to proceed."

You can then give the client a copy of the handout presented here, saying "This questionnaire is based on the official definition of PTSD found in this

Self-Assessment Questionnaire

This questionnaire will help you determine whether or not you suffer from post-traumatic stress disorder or PTSD. The questions in it are based on the official definition of PTSD in the *Diagnostic and Statistical Manual of Mental Disorders (DSM-IV)*, the handbook used by all mental health professionals. As you answer these questions, *be sure to write down your responses* so that you can go over them with your counselor.

The first set of questions asks you to identify all the traumatic experiences you have had that you can remember. You can be as brief or as detailed as you want in answering the questions. Keep in mind that answering just yes or no is enough. In some cases your reply might be "Maybe" or "I'm not sure."

If, and only if, you want to and feel you can emotionally handle it, you may write specific and detailed descriptions. You may also stop writing these descriptions at any point. You should definitely stop if you begin to experience any of the warning signs your counselor has told you about.

Answering these questions may bring up memories you would rather forget. It may also give rise to pain, anger, sadness, or remorse. However, your purpose for being in counseling is to better understand what happened and how what happened has affected your life. This understanding will enable you to increase your control over your present and future life experiences.

Questions for Criterion A

According to *DSM-IV*, you must have experienced a traumatic event or series of events in order to qualify as having PTSD. And, either initially or later on, you must have responded to those events with intense fear, helplessness, or horror. In your life, you may have experienced several frightening, sad, or unhappy events, and many major losses. However, only certain events can be categorized as traumatic. By answering the following questions, you can determine whether or not you have been traumatized.

If you don't understand what some of the words mean, are unclear whether some of your life experiences "count" as answers, or if you are afraid to answer any of the questions honestly or completely, stop working on these questions until you see your counselor.

1. Have you ever been in a natural catastrophe, such as an earthquake, fire, flood, hurricane, tornado, volcano, landslide, or a dangerous dust-storm or windstorm? Have you experienced a community or work-related disaster, such as an explosion or chemical spill?

2. Have you ever lived in a refugee or concentration camp or been tortured?

3. Were you ever sexually or physically assaulted, either by a stranger, a group of strangers, a family member, or anyone else?

    Sexual assault includes fondling and molestation; oral, anal, or vaginal sex; and any other forced sexual activity. Physical assault includes any form of physical contact intended to intimidate or cause pain. Being hit, slapped, thrown down stairs, beaten with fists or objects, or being threatened with a weapon are all considered forms of assault.

4. As a child, were you physically maltreated with excessive beatings or spankings? Were a parent's or caretaker's disciplinary measures sadistic?

    For example, were you ever forced to eat worms or insects, to stand nude in the cold or in front of others, or to injure a pet, sibling, or another person? Were you ever confined in a cage, a closet, or tied up? Were you deprived of adequate nutrition and medical care?

5. Have you ever witnessed the death, torture, rape, or beating of another person as part of war or crime? Have you ever seen someone die or be badly injured in a car, airplane, or other such accident?

6. Has anyone in your family or a close friend been murdered?

7. As a child, did you ever witness the beating, rape, murder, torture, or suicide of a parent, caretaker, or friend?

8. Have you ever been in a war, either as a combatant, a medic, a prisoner of war, or a member of a support team or grave registration unit? Were you ever, in any way, exposed to combat, enemy or friendly fire, or atrocities?

9. Have you ever been kidnapped, abducted, raped, burglarized, robbed, or mugged?

10. Were you ever injured in a burglary, robbery, mugging, or other criminal episode or in a car, boat, bicycle, airplane, or other vehicular accident?

11. Have you ever been involved in a situation in which you felt that you or a member of your family would be harmed or killed? Even if your life or the lives of your family members were not directly threatened, did you distinctly fear that you or they were in serious danger?

    It does not matter if, in retrospect, you realize your fears were unfounded. Neither does it matter if, later on, you decided you were overreacting or foolish for your fears. The critical issue is whether at the time of the trauma you perceived the situation as life-threatening to yourself or others.

12. Were you ever a member of a medical team, a firefighting team, a police force, a rescue squad, or a rescue operation that involved at least one of the following conditions:

    • danger to your safety and life

    • witnessing death and injury

    • making life-and-death decisions

    • high-stress working conditions (long hours, unsafe conditions)

If the answer to any one of these questions is yes, then you have experienced trauma. However, in order to meet the *DSM-IV* criteria, in addition to not having witnessed or been directly involved in a traumatic event or series of events, you must have responded to the situation with intense fear, feelings of helplessness, or horror. If these events occurred when you were a child, you might have begun to behave in a disorganized or agitated manner. If you were involved in a trauma and also responded with the feelings listed above, then you have met the first criterion for PTSD. This doesn't mean you necessarily have PTSD. However, it does place you at high risk for suffering from or developing PTSD or some symptoms of PTSD.

In order to have PTSD, you also must meet four other criteria: You must reexperience the trauma, show evidence of numbing or other avoidance behavior, and exhibit signs of hyperarousal. In addition, your response to these events must have been so distressing, or your PTSD symptoms so frequent or severe, that your ability to function at home, at work, with friends, or in other areas of life has been damaged.

Questions for Criterion B

According to the official definition of PTSD in *DSM-IV* you must be able to answer yes to at least one of the following questions. Write about the ways you reexperience the trauma, again, trying to be as specific as possible. Include information on frequency, duration, and so on. Also, as closely as possible, note the date you first began to reexperience the trauma.

1. Do you, on a persistent or recurring basis, find yourself having intrusive or involuntary thoughts of the traumatic event? Do you find yourself thinking about the trauma when you don't mean to or when you are trying hard not to think about it? Do visions or pictures of the trauma pop into your mind?

2. Do you have dreams or nightmares about the event?

3. Do you have dreams or nightmares that are not replays of the actual event but that take place in the location where the event occurred, contain some of the actions involved in the event, or include some of the feelings you felt during the event?

   For instance, if you were raped in a parking lot, you may dream about the parking lot without any vision of the rape. Or you may dream about being attacked in some other way or about drowning, suffocating, falling into a well, or watching your house catch on fire. These are not rape dreams, but they capture the feelings of helplessness, fear, anger, and anxiety you most likely experienced during the rape. PTSD-related dreams also include those about a life-threatening event happening to a member of your family or someone you love.

4. Do you find yourself suddenly acting or feeling as if you were back in the original trauma situation? For example, do you have flashbacks, visions, or hear sounds of the event? Do you have waves of strong feelings about the trauma or otherwise feel as if you have just lived through the trauma again, even without having a flashback or a vision?

5. Do you become extremely upset (angry, teary, confused, frightened, anxious, or panicky) around people, places, or events that resemble an aspect of the original trauma?

6. Do you become distressed around the anniversary date of the trauma?

7. Do you have physical reactions when exposed to events that are similar to or symbolize the traumatic event?

   Such physical reactions include hyperventilation, sweating, vomiting, dizziness, muscle or stomach cramping, shaking, or physical pain not related to any medical condition. For example, someone raped in a green car might feel faint when she sees a green car. A medical staff person who served in a combat zone might start sweating when he sees pictures of wounded soldiers or articles on treating war casualties. If the traumatic event occurred in May, you might start having stomach cramps around that time of the year.

How many of the above questions were you able to write about? If you had an affirmative response to at least one of these questions, then you have met the reexperiencing criterion for PTSD.

However, even if you answered no to all of these questions, continue on with the rest of the questions. Quite possibly, you do not suffer from full-blown PTSD but from some PTSD symptoms, and even they require healing.

Questions for Criterion C

The following questions concern psychic numbing and avoidance behavior. Answer yes to the following questions only if the symptoms described presented themselves *after* the traumatic event (and make a note of the date they began). If you practiced any of the numbing or avoidance behaviors listed below prior to the traumatic event, that behavior is not a symptom of PTSD. Describe your yes answers in detail.

1. Since the traumatic event, have you ever had periods of time when you felt emotionally numb or dead inside? Have you ever had periods of time when you have had great difficulty feeling tender, loving feelings or any feelings at all except perhaps anger, resentment, or hatred?

2. Have you tried not to talk about the event or avoided thoughts or feelings associated with it?

3. Since the traumatic event, have you felt alienated and apart from others?

4. Have you had a sense of doom or foreboding since the event? Do you feel that you will die young or never experience the rewards of living? For example, do you feel you will never have a family, a career, the love of others, financial security, and so on?

5. Have you lost interest in activities that used to involve you or give you pleasure? These might include sports, hobbies, and other recreational activities; participation in a group; activities involving socializing with others; and eating, dancing, sex, and other activities.

6. Are you unable to remember certain aspects of the trauma? For example, do you have difficulty remembering when it began or how long it lasted? Are there certain details or entire episodes you can't recall? Are there hours, days, weeks, months, or years you can't remember at all? Do you have difficulty remembering the names, faces, or fates of any of the other people involved in the trauma?

To how many of these questions did you answer yes? If you have answered yes to at least three of them you have met criterion C for PTSD. Remember, only those avoidance or numbing symptoms that appeared *after* the traumatic event count. If you had one of these symptoms prior to the traumatic event, you cannot include it as a yes response.

Even if you answered yes to less than three of the above questions, continue with the following questions. It may well be that even if you don't suffer from full-blown PTSD, you have troublesome symptoms that need attention.

Questions for Criterion D

According to *DSM-IV*, PTSD sufferers must have at least two of the following symptoms of increased arousal:

- Difficulty falling or staying asleep
- Irritability or outbursts of anger
- Difficulty concentrating
- Hypervigilance or overprotectiveness towards oneself and others
- Exaggerated startle response (jumping or otherwise overreacting to noises or the sudden appearance of a person)

Answer yes to the following questions only if you experience the symptoms relatively frequently and you came to experience these symptoms persistently *after*, not before, the traumatic event. Record and describe any yes answers in writing along with the approximate date you first experienced the symptom.

1. Do you have difficulty falling or staying asleep? Is your sleep fitful or disturbed in any other way?

   Insomnia may be a particular problem for you if you were traumatized or abused while in bed, reclining, or asleep. Due to your experience, an association has been made in your mind between being asleep or lying down and being in danger. Therefore, you may feel you have to be on alert at bedtime. Insomnia tends to be a special problem for war veterans, incest survivors, crime victims, and anyone else who has been physically or sexually attacked while sleeping.

2. Do you suffer from periods of irritability that are not directly associated with any present stress or problem in your life? Do you feel tense much of the time? Does your high tension level ever lead to outbursts of anger, such as smashing dishes, punching holes in the wall, throwing objects around the house, yelling at other drivers, or shouting at family members, friends, or coworkers? Do you frequently have to restrain yourself from lashing out at others?

3. Do you have difficulty concentrating? Can you concentrate enough to read an entire magazine article or book, or can you read only a few paragraphs or pages at a time? Are you easily distracted when trying to complete a job or listen to someone talk?

4. Are you overprotective or in psychological terms, *hypervigilant*? Are you extremely concerned with your safety and the safety of your loved ones?

   For example, when you enter a room, do you stand by the door or some other exit for a while in order to scan the room for potential danger? Do you examine people to see if they might be carrying a weapon or be dangerous in some other way? Do you identify places where it would be safe to hide in case of trouble? Whether with others or alone in your home, do you situate yourself so that you can keep frequent surveillance over your environment or make a quick escape in case of danger? Do you carry or sleep with a weapon?

Do you try to restrict the comings and goings of people you care about, for fear they will be injured? Do you have an "anxiety attack" if a family member is late coming home? Do you insist that family members and friends call you when they arrive at their destination or if they plan to be even five or ten minutes late?

Do crowds make you anxious? Do you avoid shopping malls, parades, movie theaters, concerts, circuses, or large parties? Do you avoid situations where it is difficult to control your level of safety? Do you drive in an excessively cautious manner, even by the most conservative standards? Do you double- or triple-check seatbelts before setting out?

5. Are you easily startled? Do you jump at loud or sudden noises or at noises that resemble some aspect of the trauma?

For example, if you are a combat veteran, do you dive to the floor if you hear an airplane overhead? Do you jump if someone touches you from behind or wakes you from your sleep? If you were a victim of a crime committed by an intruder in your home, do you jump when someone unexpectedly comes into the room?

To how many questions did you answer yes? If you have answered yes to at least two of the above questions, and the symptom did not exist before the trauma, then you have met the hyperarousal criteria for full-blown PTSD. Whether or not you have met the hyperarousal requirement, continue on to the next sections to determine the severity of your PTSD symptoms.

Question for Criterion E

Have the symptoms you identified above persisted for more than a month? If so, you meet Criterion E.

Questions for Criterion F

All PTSD cases are not the same. PTSD symptoms take different forms in different people, depending on their personality, their spiritual or religious beliefs, their culture, and the meaning they ascribe to trauma. You can have PTSD symptoms without having them take over your entire life. The crucial question in assessing the severity of your symptoms—and whether you meet criterion F for having PTSD—is, "How much do they affect your ability to work, love, and play?"

Criterion F states that to be diagnosed as having PTSD, your symptoms must cause "clinically significant distress or impairment in social, occupational, or other important areas of functioning." If you have met Criteria B, C, and D for PTSD, it is likely that your symptoms cause you considerable difficulties at times. However, if in general, you feel satisfied with life and are able to hold down a job and have fulfilling relationships with other people, you will probably not be considered to have PTSD as defined by the *DSM-IV*. Even if your symptoms sometimes become worse in situations or times of stress, so long as you "bounce-back" and there are no long-term aftereffects, then you will most likely not be diagnosed as having PTSD.

Symptoms that could cause social and vocational problems include:

- Difficulty concentrating

- Anxiety and panic attacks

- Memory loss (short-term or long-term)

- Flashbacks and intrusive thoughts

- Insomnia and other sleep problems

- Overwhelming feelings of anger or sorrow

- "Freezing"—being unable to move, speak, or interact

- Withdrawal

- Depression

Your answers to the following questions will give you and your counselor an idea of the degree to which your symptoms affect your present life functioning. It is very important that you record the details of any "yes" answers. For example, if your symptoms cause you to withdraw from people, describe the situations in which you withdraw and how frequently those situations occur.

1. Do your PTSD symptoms affect your ability to work and, if so, to what degree? For example, are you unable to complete tasks on time? Does an inability to communicate with or relate to coworkers or others make it difficult or impossible to perform effectively? Do your symptoms indanger yourself or others because of the nature of your work? Does work itself worsen your symptoms to such a degree that you must leave the job?

2. Do your PTSD symptoms make it difficult ot impossible to maintain friendships or relationships with family members or intimate others? For example, have your symptoms significantly contributed to a divorce or
estrangement from those you had been close to? Have your symptoms
or your fears about how others might react to your symptoms caused you
sever old ties or avoid new relationships?

3. Have your symptoms affected you to such a degree that, in addition to
preventing you from holding a job and having fulfilling relationships, you
are unable to take care of your basic living needs, such as health care,
personal hygiene, proper diet, paying bills, using the telephone?

4. As a result of anger, anxiety, depression, or other symptoms, do you stay
at home whenever possible and avoid contact with other people? Do you
have thoughts of suicide or homicide so that you feel you are a danger
to yourself or others?

If you have met Criteria A, B, C, D, and E, and you feel these symptoms
have had a significant adverse effect on your life, you will likely be diagnosed
as suffering from PTSD. If you have met some but not all of the criteria, it is
likely that you are suffering the aftereffects of trauma and have PTSD symptoms
that would benefit from treatment. In either case, the ultimate decision about
whether you can be diagnosed as having PTSD will probably be made by your
counselor, perhaps in conjuction with other mental health workers.

book." You can then show them the *DSM-IV*, open to the pages describing PTSD and explain what the *DSM-IV* is (a handbook that lists and codes various psychological problems).

At this point, you could simply offer some very preliminary information about PTSD. Alternatively, you could use the diagnostic interview as a more extensive educational session. For example, you can provide your client with a brief history of PTSD (see appendix A) and explain its nature and the reasons for the various symptoms. Some therapists prepare an audiotape or a written handout on PTSD. For some types of trauma survivors, such as Vietnam veterans and battering and sexual abuse survivors, videotapes are available commercially or through government agencies. During this session, you could also address any fears or questions the client might have about being diagnosed with or about having PTSD.

You can have the clients begin the assessment process themselves, if they desire, by giving them the questionnaire as a homework assignment, with the following exceptions: Because the questionnaire itself can trigger some powerful feelings and memories, using the self-assessment questionnaire as homework is *not* advisable for nonfunctional or semifunctional clients, for clients with psychiatric problems or histories of psychoses, for clients whom you feel are capable of psychotic episodes, or for clients who are so regressed, anxious, or depressed that strong emotional response to the questionnaire might overwhelm them. You also need to review the cautions listed in the introduction. If a client begins to exhibit any of the symptoms listed there, you need to postpone the assessment.

Even when clients are relatively functional and emotionally stable, you need to exercise extreme cautions before allowing them to take the questionnaire home. Clients might complete the questionnaire only partially, or they might misunderstand some of the wording. Therefore, before the questionnaire is given as a homework assignment, you will need to review it with clients and you will need to have them begin to work on it under your supervision or the supervision of another trained mental health worker. This may include their beginning to answer the questions on paper in a quiet area near your office. After a half hour, they should return so that you can ask them how it felt to work on the questionnaire.

Clients may tell you, "I thought it would be easy, but I'm getting more upset than I thought," or "There's no way I can do this at home, or alone." On the basis of client feedback and your own observations of the client's reaction to answering the questions, you can then determine if it is safe to allow the client to complete the questionnaire as a homework assignment.

Be certain, however, that you have reviewed cautions listed in the introduction with the client and that he or she fully understands that it is imperative to stop working on the questionnaire as soon as any of the listed symptoms are experienced.

It cannot be overemphasized that the maxim "Better safe than sorry," applies here. Better to underestimate a client's ability to write about traumatic material without support and supervision than to risk the client's becoming retraumatized by the assignment.

If you do not give the questionnaire as homework, you can give clients a copy during your diagnostic session, so that they can read the questions while you go through the list. This helps reinforce the definition of PTSD and also assures the clients that you are being honest with them. If, for some reason, you prefer not to give the questionnaire to your client, you will still want to ask those questions in your diagnostic interview.

In your homework directions, or in the diagnostic interview itself, preface your inquiries about traumatic events by stating that although you are asking about trauma in the client's past, you are not going to press for detailed descriptions. This might be a good time to set the stage for your future work with the client by stating that in healing from trauma, details of the trauma are extremely helpful and that you would be more than willing to listen to a detailed description of the traumatic event. However, for purposes of background information, all you need to know for now is the type of trauma endured, if any, and its time, place, and duration, if the client can remember.

State that you will accept "I don't know" or "I'm not sure" or "I don't want to talk about it" as acceptable replies to your questions. You can also indicate to clients that if any of the questions make them uncomfortable, or if they start to become angry, tired, anxious, or sad, you would like to know about such reactions. Furthermore, if they tell you they feel extremely uncomfortable, especially if they feel the questions might make them feel as if they might explode, hurt themselves, or hurt someone else, you are willing to stop immediately. Review with your clients the cautions section of the questionnaire, asking them if they have any questions about the terms used or what they are to do if they experience any of the difficulties outlined in that section.

Although you can ask clients for feedback on their reactions, keep in mind that they may not be aware of how they are feeling or able to articulate their feelings, especially if they are in numbing. Therefore, it is incumbent on you to watch clients for signs of anxiety, sadness, and dissociation. If any of these non-verbal cues becomes significant, you need to stop the assessment and ask the client how he or she is feeling. When clients stare blankly or nod, when they have forced smiles on their faces, or when their eyes dart anxiously around the room, ask if they are with you or if you have lost them. "I can't help but notice that you are . . . " "Are you able to concentrate now, or is something else on your mind?" and "If you aren't feeling comfortable or you need to talk about something else, we can continue this line of questioning at another time," are all approaches you could use.

Do not even assume that your clients necessarily know what the word *trauma* means. Define it for them. Even if a client is well-educated or psychologically sophisticated, list the various kinds of experiences that qualify as trauma and ask for at least a yes or no answer.

Be prepared for clients who say, "Sure, that happened, but I don't understand why you call it trauma. It didn't bother me then and it doesn't bother me now." Your response should *not* be, "You're in denial. Someday soon you will see how truly traumatized you are and that the trauma is the root of your problems today." In the first place, the client may be right. What occurred, although technically a trauma, may not have, for one reason or another, generated long-term scars. Secondly, if you are right and the client is in denial, the client is unlikely to accept your insight and your remark will only create antagonism.

In addition, some clients have experienced such a variety of traumas that they consider their more minor ones to be ordinary experiences. A war veteran may consider his combat experiences so traumatic that being sexually abused as a youngster pales in comparison. Similarly, an incest survivor may consider the incest so devastating that she doesn't consider having been raped by a stranger worth discussing. Labeling such an attitude as denial would only be destructive to your relationship with the client and otherwise.

On the other hand, there will be clients, such as torture victims, prisoners of war, refugees, and survivors of concentration camp or mass violence experiences, who probably wish intensely for the respite of denial. Such clients can be automatically classified as trauma survivors. It is not necessary, and it might be highly destructive, to ask for details of their traumatic experiences during the diagnostic interviews or during the initial stages of therapy. If you know already that a client has been a prisoner of war or a torture victim, you can simply say, "I understand that you suffered torture and many cruelties as a prisoner. These experiences are considered trauma, without exception. If you wish to tell me about your experiences now, you can. Or you can tell me about them later. Or you never, ever have to talk about them with me. I am ready and willing to listen, but the decision is entirely up to you."

Regardless of any curiosity you might have, the focus of assessment of such individuals should be more on their symptoms than on their story. Your trauma survivor clients, as much as your other clients, need to be given the choice to share or not to share as much of their history as they desire. With all your clients, you must always bear in mind that you are not the author but a facilitator of their healing. While you can play a critical role in lending support and offering positive direction for the healing process, it is usually best if the client, not you, determines the pace, including the pace at which the trauma is revealed during diagnostic sessions. One of the most common errors made by therapists is to push the client to reveal traumatic material.

You also need to explain to clients that the severity of PTSD varies from one person to the next and may vary in severity in the same person depending on reminders of the trauma and other stresses. It may be helpful to use a medical example, like the following, which compares PTSD to a cold.

> All people who have colds are not alike. Some people's colds are so bad they have to stay home from work, whereas others' colds are just a nuisance.
>
> In the same way, all people with PTSD do not have the same degree of PTSD. The crucial questions we are concerned with are to what extent your PTSD interferes with three important life activities: your abilities to love, work, and play.
>
> If you have PTSD symptoms, but they don't really interfere with your ability to love, work, or play, you don't have so much to be concerned about—just as having a simple runny nose doesn't prevent you from going about your life relatively unimpeded.
>
> But if the runny nose becomes a bad cough or an ear infection, then you need to get medical attention and plenty of rest to get over your illness. Similarly, if your PTSD is severe, you will need to attend to it so that it doesn't get worse.
>
> For many people, PTSD symptoms get worse around anniversary times or when there are other stresses in their lives, such as a death in the family, economic pressures, or problems in important relationships. This is like having a relatively minor cold that turns into bronchitis when the weather gets cold and damp.

A Note on Criterion F

If a client is applying for PTSD disability, the ultimate judge of whether her or his symptoms classify as PTSD and whether they are socially or vocationally disabling will be decided by a specialized committee or board, such as that of the Social Security Administration. This determination will depend much on the particulars of client's situation and the discretion of the evaluating mental health professionals. In matters of financial and legal claims for disability, if the client's condition does not fall at either extreme (functional most of the time with sporadic symptoms versus dysfunctional in almost every area of life) what qualifies as being "clinically significant distress or impairment" may be cause for debate.

Considering Family History

In addition to determining whether clients themselves have suffered a traumatic event, you need to inquire about any family history of trauma. Were any parents, grandparents, siblings, or other close relatives of the client ever traumatized? Research evidence substantiates two phenomena: the transgenerational transmission of PTSD symptoms and secondary traumatization. The transgenerational transmission of PTSD symptoms occurs when one family member's symptoms give rise to similar symptoms in other family members. One process involved here is imitation learning. A two-year-old, for example, might learn to hide under the bed when an airplane flies over because her combat veteran father does. The child could even learn that airplane sounds are to be feared, acquire startle reactions to these sounds, and continue to react as her father does toward airplane sounds even into adolescence or adulthood.

In contrast, secondary traumatization occurs when young children internalize a parent's or other relative's trauma to such a degree that they actually become traumatized by the events that traumatized the family member. For example, if the same child were exposed to detailed descriptions of her father's war experiences or in other ways acquired a vivid picture of the airplane-related combat events that cause the father to startle, she would be considered to be suffering from secondary traumatization. In this situation, the child's startle response would stem not so much from imitating her father, but rather from a deep sense of the emotional meaning of the airplane sounds.

Another example of these phenomena is the transmission of anger. An adult trauma survivor who vents anger destructively in the home is teaching his or her children to do likewise. In addition, the child is probably not exposed to ways of dealing with anger other than verbally or physically abusing others or destroying property, and he may consequently manifest outbursts of rage similar to those of the adult trauma survivor. This is an example of transgenerational transmission of symptoms. However, if this same child were subject to secondary traumatization, he could manifest the similar outbursts of rage. Yet in this case, the rage would arise from the presence of a trigger or from some event related to the adult's trauma, not solely from lack of training in handling anger constructively. If your client grew up with a trauma survivor, you need to be alert to the possible impact of that relative's trauma on your client.

In sum, assessing for PTSD can be very complex and, given the special problems with recalling trauma, assessment may follow rather than precede treatment in many cases—the reverse of the usual method and trend in doing therapy. Nevertheless, an attempt should be made to assess for PTSD as early as possible. Even if a client is in complete denial or numbing, the fact that he or she has learned about various kinds of traumas and been introduced to the types of symptoms associated with PTSD helps to open the door to the client's confiding in you when and if traumatic memories begin to emerge.

Assessing for Concurrent Problems

Dual Diagnosis—Coexisting Mental Disorders

Formerly the diagnosis of PTSD tended to be ignored in favor of more traditional diagnostic categories. Today, however, there is increased recognition that PTSD can coexist with other mental disorders.

In some cases, PTSD is not the primary diagnosis. The individual may have had a preexisting mental disorder that was exacerbated by the trauma and the resulting PTSD. In such cases, the trauma issues can be treated, but any preexisting problems will remain. Conversely, untreated PTSD can develop into personality disorder, depression, or some other mental health problem. In these cases, the PTSD symptoms may be hard or even impossible to detect until significant strides have first been made in treating the other disorder.

Another complicating factor in diagnosing PTSD is that its symptoms overlap with the symptoms of a variety of other disorders, for example, personality disorders such as borderline personality disorder, antisocial personality disorder, and multiple personality disorder (MPD). Some clinicians view MPD as a form of chronic PTSD; others see MPD as a special form of borderline personality; still others contend that borderline personalities are actually multiple personalities but consider both of them forms of PTSD (Courtois 1988).

Arthur Blank (1989), a psychiatrist who served in Vietnam and who heads the Readjustment Counseling Program for veterans of the Persian Gulf, Panama, Grenada, and Vietnam has outlined five ways in which PTSD can interrelate with the diagnosis of personality or character disorder:

- The personality disorder preceded and coexists with PTSD.

- The personality disorder preceded the trauma and therefore predisposed the individual to PTSD due to inadequate coping skills.

- The individual had a latent tendency toward personality disorder that was crystallized by the trauma.

- The PTSD masques as a personality disorder. This is more likely if the PTSD is chronic.

- The personality disorder was not present prior to the PTSD. Due to lack of or inadequate treatment, the PTSD caused the personality disorder.

The same relationships between PTSD and other diagnoses are possible. *Substance abuse, clinical depression, paranoia, paranoid states,* and other diagnoses may each be substituted for *personality disorder* in the preceding statements. This will give you an idea of the range of impacts PTSD can have on your clients' other diagnoses.

The hallmarks of individuals with a primary diagnosis of PTSD are the intrusive recall-numbing cycle accompanied by excessive guilt, irrational self-blame, and an avoidance of situations reminiscent of the trauma. Some PTSD sufferers also avoid all discussion of their experiences or similar traumas; others are "fixated" on the trauma, as evidenced by frequent discussion and other forms of preoccupation with the trauma, to the exclusion of meaningful involvement with their present lives. Another hallmark is a fear of loss of control. Such individuals are typically aware that their behavior is dysfunctional, offensive to others, or self-destructive. They take responsibility for their behavior, and feel guilty and ashamed of it, even though they feel powerless to change. In addition, they have, to one degree or another, internalized our culture's blame-the-victim attitudes and suffer from some degree of depression as a result.

At the same time, they suffer from powerful feelings associated with the trauma, for example, deep grief and survivor guilt (often experienced as intense anger), recurring feelings of rage and desire for revenge, feelings of helplessness, and self-destructive impulses. They do their best to hide these emotions from others and to keep them from emerging. Yet it is impossible to contain such emotions under all circumstances. Every now and then, these "relatively pure-PTSD" clients explode. However, as psychologist James Newman (1987) explains, "When these outbursts occur, (they are) out of character . . . generally infrequent (and carry with them) intense feelings of guilt and shame." Furthermore, such outbursts "usually cease as soon as the underlying PTSD symptoms begin to be addressed."

In contrast, clients with a dual diagnosis of PTSD and personality disorder do not suffer from the self-reproach characteristic of clients with a primary diagnosis of PTSD. Instead, these dually afflicted individuals blame others and societal institutions for their problems almost entirely. Such clients rarely evidence any introspective awareness of the destructiveness of their behaviors to themselves or others. Their explosive outbursts tend to be more frequent and "are expressed with little concern for their effects on others." Nor do they "manifest the 'fear of loss of control'" common among trauma survivors with a primary diagnosis of PTSD (Newman 1987).

The flashbacks, nightmares, and intrusive thoughts that are symptoms of PTSD may appear to resemble the visual and auditory hallucinations associated with various psychoses and, in the case of child abuse survivors, multiple personality disorder (MPD). Some cases are relatively clear cut; others are not. Even psychotic patients can suffer from PTSD and, at times, severely traumatized clients with untreated PTSD who have recently been subjected to an additional overwhelming loss or trauma may become (temporarily) psychotic.

A good clue that you are dealing with a flashback or some other PTSD symptom, rather than a psychosis, is that the auditory and visual images of PTSD sufferers are exact replays of the original event, portray events or persons closely associated with the original trauma, or contain themes or feelings reminiscent of the trauma, such as powerlessness, violence, danger, blood, being attacked or chased, chaos, natural disaster, and sudden noises. The object of attack or danger may be the client, one of the client's family members or close friends, or some other individual (or pet or object) that the client deeply values.

For example, Janet S. had a persistent flashback of opening a school locker and having dead bodies fall out. The bodies' arms were stiff and the index fingers on their hands pointed at her. The faces were blurred and indistinguishable. When she opens the locker and the bodies fall out, she "freezes" in horror. The pointed fingers, she feels, mark her as the next to die and have the power to kill her.

In the flashback, she is twenty years old, the age at which she married a man who soon began to physically abuse her and control her economically and socially.

In reality, Janet had never opened a locker full of bodies. However, she had suffered a miscarriage, which she blamed on one of her husband's beatings. Her husband would not allow her to seek medical help after the beating, even though she was bleeding profusely. Consequently, Janet could not medically verify that the beating had caused the miscarriage. Of even greater importance, however, Janet could not verify that medical attention might have saved the baby. She blamed herself for not going to a hospital after this particular beating, even though her husband had taken the car keys, her wallet, cut the telephone wires, and threatened to drown one of their other children and make it look like an accident.

Janet also blamed herself for going to work and driving while she was bleeding during another pregnancy. Yet her husband had insisted that she earn money or he would retaliate. Once again she was not allowed to seek medical help, and once again, when she miscarried, she blamed herself as well as her husband for the miscarriage.

To make matters worse, her husband told family members that it was Janet's "stupidity" in not seeking medical help that caused the miscarriages. Members from both sides of the family blamed Janet, yet she was not permitted to speak the truth because of her husband's threats to kill these very people if she revealed any of his abuses.

In light of these realities, Janet's flashback can be understood as a visualization of being blamed by her dead (miscarried) children and her fear that adult family members (who blamed her for the marital problems as well as the miscarriages) would be killed.

Coexisting mental disorders tend to be more common among survivors of long-term, repeated, or intense traumas (such as family abuse, prisoner of war, and torture experiences) than among one-time trauma survivors. In the former cases, reactions to the trauma may include not only the development of depression, borderline personality disorder, paranoid disorder, and substance abuse problems, as mentioned above, but chronic pain syndrome, psychosomatic problems, acute psychotic episodes, and psychotic disorders such as manic-depressive illness and schizophrenia (Chelser 1972; van der Kolk 1984, 1986; Herman 1992; Langer 1987; Walker 1979). As van der Kolk (1984) writes, "The precise interaction between trauma and constitutional factors, the level of personality development, cultural factors, and the ultimate expression in the form of altered affect, behavior, pain perception, and somatic functioning remains an unexplored territory."

For example, in his study of former World War II prisoners of war, Ron Langer (1987) found that only 28 percent of Pacific theater and 11 percent of European theater POWs were given a PTSD diagnosis, but most had received some other psychiatric diagnosis. "My impression," he writes, is "that the number of ex-POWs with PTSD is far greater than this, and that some of these ex-POWs who received other psychiatric diagnoses actually have PTSD."

Langer aptly notes that "PTSD is a diagnosis that is difficult to make, and one that is often missed. It is often confused with character disorders, on which it is sometimes an overlay. It is difficult to differentiate from dysthemic disorder and various anxiety disorders." He also notes that, "when PTSD has psychotic features, it is often confused with other psychotic disorders, including schizophrenia." Walker (1979) has made the same observation regarding battered wives; Herman (1992), about incest survivors; and Kinzie (1989) and Lee and Lu (1989) of torture survivors and survivors of mass violence. Consequently, as Walker and Herman both observe, in many cases the client needs to have been in treatment for several months, or longer, before the PTSD can emerge and be distinguished from other disorders.[1]

If you suspect that a client suffers from another disorder, or if he or she tells you about previous disorders, you need to assess for these disorders using the appropriate *DSM-IV* criteria. Do not rely on the assessment of previous mental health professionals. Complete your own assessment. Also, obtain a history of the other disorder to ascertain its relationship to the trauma. Did it preexist the trauma, emerge during the trauma or immediately afterwards, or present itself at some later time? Perhaps the other disorder has no relationship to the trauma at all.

Substance Abuse and Depression

As with mental disorders, some trauma survivors have dual diagnoses of PTSD and substance abuse. Within this group as well, it is important to differentiate which individuals suffer primarily from PTSD and which primarily from substance abuse.

Clients with a primary diagnosis of PTSD use their substance of choice for purposes of medicating the symptoms of PTSD. Usage tends to increase with the onset, or expected onset, of symptoms and at anniversary times. Such individuals frankly admit they have a substance abuse problem, and are aware of its negative psychological and medical costs, but feel they need it to get by.

In contrast, individuals with primary diagnoses of substance abuse deny or minimize their substance abuse problem, discount its impact on their lives, or blame others for it. These individuals are also reluctant to give up their substance in order to attend individual or group PTSD therapy. Individuals with primary diagnoses of PTSD, however, readily agree to at least try to abstain from their substance to promote the healing process.

As therapy progresses, individuals with a primary diagnosis of PTSD experience a remission or lesser need for their substance. Some become substance abuse-free. Others remain addicted, though they may report feeling less need for their substance. In contrast, individuals with a primary diagnosis of substance abuse do not experience or report any decrease or remission of their addiction once insight into trauma-related issues has begun.

In order to make the diagnosis, you need to determine whether the substance abuse began before the trauma, during the trauma or immediately afterwards, or only after other losses were experienced, for example, after the death of a child or parent or the loss of a job. The relationship between the addiction and the trauma is critical not only in formulating a diagnosis but in formulating an effective treatment plan.

Depression presents a similar, and perhaps more difficult, problem of dual diagnosis. It is perhaps the most common presenting problem of survivors of long-term trauma, (Langer 1987; Walker 1979; Herman 1992), but is itself often misdiagnosed. For example, even though the majority of ex-POWs in a Veterans

---

1. For more in-depth discussions of the problem of assessing PTSD in relation to coexisting mental disorders, see Courtois (1988) section II, Newman (1987) and Langer (1987).

Administration study were found to have received a diagnosis related to an anxiety disorder, anxiety disorders in this group have been interpreted by some as a defense against depression (Langer 1987). Substance abuse, for example, alcohol abuse and eating disorders, has also been found to be highly correlated with depression and is interpreted by many mental health professionals as a form of self-medication for the symptoms of depression (see chapter 3).

Therefore, you need to familiarize yourself with the *DSM-IV* criteria for depression and assess your clients for depression during the early stages of therapy if you see any suggestion of depressive symptoms. At this point, inquire about depressive symptoms prior to the trauma and about any history of depression, manic-depressive illness, on the other psychiatric problems in the client's family, including those of parents, siblings, grandparents, aunts, uncles, cousins, and so forth.

Even when there is no prior or family history of depression, you need to be on the lookout for depression throughout the entire course of therapy. Giving your clients a brief handout listing the most common symptoms of depression and asking them to let you know if they begin to develop any of the symptoms may be helpful in some cases. Assure your clients, however, that you will be on guard for the symptoms of depression as well. You do not want to give your clients the message that you are abdicating your responsibility as therapist. You are only inviting them to take a more active role in their mental well-being. The more active they can become in terms of self-care in any area of life, the more they can counteract the feelings of powerlessness engendered by the trauma.

Medical Problems

You should also inquire about medical problems and encourage your clients to get a complete physical examination. Pay special attention to medical problems that are the direct result of the trauma experience or secondary wounding experiences, as well as to medical problems that were exacerbated by the trauma and subsequent stress. Inquire also about major medical problems in the client's family of origin.

Stomach problems, rashes, backaches, headaches, warts, minor tumors, allergies, and susceptibility to colds and certain diseases are considered by many physicians and mental health professionals to be stress related or to have a strong psychological component. Animals subject to inescapable shock have been shown to suffer from impairments in their immune systems that increase their susceptibility to tumors and a variety of illnesses. And it is now widely accepted that the financial, psychological, and social pressures that are part of trauma and its aftermath can severely tax the body's immune system, making it more susceptible to a wide variety of medical problems.

Also keep in mind that a wide variety of trauma survivors have been subjected to head injury as part of their trauma. Such injuries are especially prevalent among abused persons, survivors of vehicular and other accidents, combat veterans, prisoners of war, and crime victims. In some cases, chronic or intermittent headaches, upper-body pains, problems with concentration, memory loss, and periods of disorientation are neither psychosomatic nor symptoms of PTSD but are the direct results of head trauma.

Even if a client received a medical examination following the trauma and it was "determined" that she or he did not suffer from any significant head injury, that diagnosis may have been erroneous. In recent years, it has been discovered that the effects of head trauma are not always immediately discernible. Physical evidence of such an injury can be minimal or undetectable at the time of the injury, with long-term aftereffects of the head injury appearing only years later.

If you suspect a client has suffered from head trauma, consider a neurological examination or psychological testing oriented toward detecting organic factors. A Bender Wechester Adult Intelligence Scale (WAIS), or some other simple screening test for organicity, might be a good beginning. A complete neurological battery might also be in order.

For any medical problems your clients have, obtain a history. Also ask your clients if their medical symptoms seem to fluctuate depending on external circumstances. For example, do their medical problems seem to intensify around the anniversary date of a traumatic incident or in particular situations? However, be sure to emphasize that you believe their medical problems and physical pains are real, that you are not implying their pain is purely psychological or "just in their head." Such statements deny the existence of what is often excruciating pain and blame sufferers for their own pain.

Self-Mutilation

Self-mutilation is not listed in the *DSM-IV* as a symptom of PTSD; however, it occurs with sufficient frequency among victims of repeated trauma, especially family abuse survivors, that it bears consideration in the diagnostic process.

Self-mutilating behaviors include burning; hitting; cutting; excessive scratching; using harsh abrasives on skin or scalp; poking sharp objects into flesh; headbanging; pulling out hair or eyebrows for noncosmetic purposes; inserting objects into the body's orifices; refusing to drink, eat, or take necessary medications, and various forms of self-surgery.

Substance abuse and eating disorders can also be viewed as forms of self-mutilation. In addition, according to David Calof (1992), who has worked extensively with self-mutilating adult survivors of childhood abuse, excessive tattooing and excessive exercise can, in many cases, be considered forms of self-mutilation—depending on the function of these behaviors for the individual involved.

Self-mutilation among abuse survivors can be interpreted in many different ways and serves different functions for different people. For some trauma survivors, self-mutilation is their way of talking, their way of telling the world "I hurt" or "I was hurt." Consequently, self-mutilation is especially prevalent among survivors who were instructed not to tell by the perpetrator of their trauma, who were abused at the preverbal level, or who simply do not have the language with which to tell their story or express their feelings about it.

Another major function of self-mutilating behavior is that it serves to contain or externalize the affect (emotions), memories, and other psychological effects generated by the trauma. If even "normal" people when under stress wring their hands, bite their fingernails, or pull their hair to alleviate tension, imagine what trauma survivors might need to do to lessen the stress. Trauma can so greatly affect individuals that the emotional and other forms of arousal it generates are managed through self-mutilation. This interpretation is based on the biochemistry of PTSD. According to van der Kolk (1989), there is a physiological basis for the feeling of relief from anxiety, numbing, and other psychic pain experienced by trauma survivors who self-mutilate. One child abuse survivor explains it in this way: "Sometimes the pain is so great I get numb. Strange as it sounds, the numbing hurts, so I cut myself. Then I feel relieved, as if I am finally alive instead of one of the walking dead."

Along these lines, self-mutilation is sometimes caused by errors in the therapeutic process. For example, a therapist might push a client to reveal or discuss incidents that arouse feelings or traumatic material that either client or therapist is not prepared to handle. The client could then attempt to manage his or her heightened feelings and heightened physiological arousal levels through self-mutilation.

Another interpretation is that self-mutilation is a form of reenactment of the trauma. In self-mutilation, the formerly abused person is in control of the abuse, as opposed to the original traumatic situation, in which someone else was in control of inflicting the harm. Incest survivors, for example, may become prostitutes because in their prostitute role they hope to wield the power they never had while being abused as children. Their sense of power, however, is illusory.

Self-mutilation can also be viewed as a form of self-punishment. Child abuse survivors commonly believe that they were abused because they were bad or inadequate. In self-mutilation, they are assuming the parent role and punishing themselves for their shortcomings.

In some cases, the intent of the self-mutilation is self-protection or some similar purpose. Even though the behavior hurts the client's body, the motivation of the client is not self-harm but saving her or himself or someone else. This can include protection of the therapist. The client's notion is, "If I hurt me enough, you won't get hurt" (Calof 1992). Such thinking is obviously not logical, but it can result from the client's having lived in a situation of captivity where the survivor decides to bear the abuse without complaint or retaliation in hopes that other loved ones or comrades will be spared. Sometimes this is a form of wishful thinking. In other instances, the perpetrator actually promises to leave others unharmed if the victim complies without protest.

Self-mutilation can also be a means of reducing rage at the perpetrator. When expressing anger is too dangerous or when the perpetrator is unavailable, the rage can be inflicted on the self instead. In the case of suicidal clients, self-mutilation may be a means of protection from further harm.

For some clients, making the body unattractive through self-mutilation serves a self-protective, rather than a self-punitive, function. Even though our culture highly values external physical attractiveness, for incest survivors and other sexual abuse survivors, physical attractiveness may feel dangerous. Such survivors may either gain weight or become unattractively thin, cut themselves, or otherwise injure their bodies in hopes of warding off sexual advances.

This is especially the case in instances where being considered attractive by the abuser was the stated reason for sexual abuse. For such individuals, being unattractive is a form of self-protection, not self-injury. To take away their form of protection (self-mutilation) without their acquiring other forms of self-protection or ways of feeling safe sexually would only increase their level of fear and anxiety. This could lead to an increase, rather than a decrease, in their PTSD symptomatology, which could result in these clients considering more drastic forms of self-mutilation.

Another possibility is that the survivor was conditioned by the perpetrator to associate pain with sexual pleasure or with a respite from abuse and even love. In violent homes, the abuse runs in cycles. A battering incident is usually followed by a "honeymoon" stage, in which the perpetrator asks the victim for forgiveness and showers her or him with love, attention, and praise. Consequently, physical pain and sights and smells associated with pain (for instance, the sight of blood), may signal to the victim that the abuse is over and that a period of positive relationship with the perpetrator, or at least a period without abuse, is forthcoming. Thus in self-mutilating, clients may be trying to attain the peace and reinforcements of the "honeymoon stage" of the battering cycle.

In my experience and according to the clinical accounts of others (Calof 1992; Courtois 1988; Herman 1992), most self-mutilating clients are ashamed of their behavior and therefore keep it secret. Consequently, as part of the intake procedure, you should ask clients if they self-mutilate.

If clients state that they don't self-mutilate, but you still suspect that they do (or might begin to in the future), you will want to give them a short talk about the prevalence and function of mutilation among trauma survivors, enumerating the various explanations discussed above. The purpose of this mini-lecture is to make it safe for clients to disclose about self-mutilation if they later begin the practice or if they are currently self-mutilating but hiding it.

Sometimes signs of self-mutilation are obvious, for example, knife cuts or cigarette burns on the arms, face, or legs. In other cases, the signs are more subtle. In my practice, I become suspicious of self-mutilation when clients seem overdressed or dressed in clothing that is inappropriate for the weather. For instance, a client of mine named Cathy, an incest survivor, always wore long wool socks to our interviews, even during the summer. When I asked why, she replied that she tended to get cold, even during the summer. I gave her a short self-mutilation talk, in which I briefly explained that self-mutilation was common among survivors of severe child abuse and that I had had previous clients who engaged in self-mutilation. I then gave an example of two clients who had used self-mutilation to cope. This brief lecture was aimed at helping the client disclose this symptom.

At the next session, I asked about self-mutilation again. At that point, she reluctantly revealed that she cut her legs. In fact, she had at the time a wound that was infected and bleeding badly, but she was too ashamed to go for medical help. I immediately sent her to a physician who I knew would not humiliate her. Had the wounds gone unattended, she might have suffered serious medical consequences.

If you have a self-mutilating client, you need to find out all you can about your client's self-abuse. As you broach the subject, however, emphasize that you understand self-mutilation is a result of the trauma, not a sign of insanity. Ask questions such as the following:

> What kinds of self-mutilation have you engaged in?
>
> How often do you self-mutilate? Do you feel there is any pattern in when or how often you hurt yourself?
>
> Do you experience relief when you hurt yourself? How else does self-mutilation help you?
>
> Are you worried about your self-mutilation? Are others, for example, your parents, friends, or spouse worried about it? Do they know, or do you do it in secret?
>
> Have you ever felt that you couldn't stop hurting yourself and that you might go on to do serious damage or even kill yourself?

You need to try to create an accepting atmosphere so that your client can feel free to talk about self-mutilation. However, you do not want to convey the message that self-mutilation is desirable or acceptable. At some point you need to convey the following:

> Many trauma survivors hurt themselves the way you do because, in its own way, hurting yourself helps you. I am not saying that self-mutilation is good for you so you should go out and hurt yourself some more. I am only saying that there are some good reasons why so many trauma survivors do what you do.
>
> Usually they hurt themselves because they haven't received any help yet and don't know any other way to deal with their feelings. But you are here to learn how to say how you feel and tell what you've been through in different, more self-loving ways than hurting yourself.

Do not keep the relationship between self-mutilation and suicide a secret from your clients. Tell them the following:

> Your hurting yourself concerns me because statistics show that people who self-mutilate are usually in so much pain that they are suicide prone. I want you to be sure and tell me about the times you hurt yourself, because they may indicate a suicidal crisis is on the way.

In asking about the self-mutilating behavior, one of your goals is to form an understanding of the functions of the self-mutilation so that you can plan an effective treatment strategy. As Calof (1992) stresses, the behavior needs to be distinguished from its function, and treatment must always be addressed to the function.

In sum, assessing and working with self-mutilating clients is extremely challenging. Not only are many of these clients unable to articulate the reasons they self-mutilate, but the same behavior may serve more than one function. For example, an incest survivor may allow herself to become obese not only to avoid sexual advances but also to punish her body for being sexual and (formerly) considered attractive. Her overeating may also be "revenge eating" in that she overeats to show her perpetrator, and the world, the full extent of her rage. A five-foot one-inch incest survivor who weighs 350 pounds is making quite a statement of rage. At the same time, she is also reenacting the trauma in that she is treating herself as unworthy of respect, just as she was treated by her abuser.

Some treatment suggestions for self-mutilating clients are discussed in chapter 6. Additional concerns for the professional dealing with these clients are addressed in chapter 11.

Effect of Former Therapists and Doctors

A history of your client's previous treatment is also essential. Ask your clients the following:

> How long were you in treatment and for what reasons?
>
> What did you feel helped and what did not help about each particular form of treatment?

Were you given any formal or informal psychological or psychiatric labels by former therapists? How do you feel about these labels?

Were you given a prognosis? How do you feel about your former therapists' assessments and predictions about your future mental health?

Gathering information about former therapies is important in working with any kind of client. However, such information is essential in working with trauma survivors, because so often they have been misdiagnosed or mislabeled. Perhaps some of their former therapists or doctors were not even aware that these clients were trauma survivors. And even if a former therapist or doctor did know that a client had a history of trauma, he or she might not have understood the full implications of the trauma on the client's mental, emotional, or physical well-being.

Formulating a Treatment Plan

To help both you and your client focus on what might seem like an overwhelming number of symptoms and problem areas, it is highly recommended that, together with the client, you formulate a treatment plan. In either the first or second session, you need to tell clients that you will be formulating a treatment plan, which you will share with them and revise to incorporate their input. The treatment plan, you must emphasize, is flexible and will be changed according to your professional judgment and their needs.

If you work for an agency or clinic, your organization may already have a protocol for outlining client treatment plans. In that case, the suggestions for formulating a treatment plan for trauma survivors presented here may or may not match those of your organization. However, they can most likely be used in conjunction with your office's protocol. Perhaps some modification of the existing protocol that would incorporate the needs of trauma survivors could be considered as well.

If your organization does not require treatment plans, or if you as a private practitioner are not in the habit of writing treatment plans, you may want to consider beginning such a procedure. It can help both you and the client focus on a limited number of specific therapeutic goals, which ultimately gives both client and counselor a sense of achievement once progress is made towards achieving those goals. Identifying therapeutic goals and working towards them will also help commence and later reinforce the empowerment phase of the healing process (see chapter 10).

Although treatment plans outline specific therapeutic goals and some means of obtaining those goals, they are not static. If a client is in counseling for a considerable period of time, his or her treatment plan will probably need to be revised several times. New treatment goals will be identified as new issues arise in therapy or as the client achieves some of her or his original goals, grows in self-understanding and self-acceptance, and gains the interest and ability to deal with new challenges.

Selecting Treatment Goals

In most cases, a treatment plan cannot be formulated until you have had about ten sessions. Before devising a treatment plan, you need to have assessed the client for PTSD and other relevant problems, for example, depression, substance abuse, and any significant medical problems. Ideally, you will have completed at least a cursory history on the client, identifying both pre- and post-trauma family, social, vocational, educational, legal, and emotional history. If the client has seen other therapists before coming to you, you need to have contacted those individuals and consulted with them regarding the client.

Most importantly, however, you need to have listened to the client enough that you can identify some of his or her major present concerns—the forces that propelled him or her to seek help in the first place. If, after ten or so sessions, you are still unclear on these matters, you need to share your confusion with the client, in a nonaccusatory manner, and ask for help in clarifying her or his major problem areas.

Some clients present seeking healing for a past trauma. However, the majority of clients I work with present problems in some area of current functioning—problems on the job or in social and intimate relationships. Whether or not they relate their present problems to the trauma, their immediate concern is in finding relief from whatever symptoms are disrupting their present lives: irritability, sleeping difficulties, extreme difficulty in socializing and maintaining long-term love relationships, or any of the many side effects of severe substance abuse. It is important not to underestimate the significance of those problems.

Management of the PTSD symptoms and related problems that trouble the client must be included in the treatment goals, for a variety of reasons. Not only does incorporating the client's concerns reempower the client, it also fosters the trust necessary to the therapeutic relationship. Even more important, with PTSD, as opposed to other diagnoses, the symptoms to a large degree *are* the problem. It can be difficult, if not impossible, to treat the underlying cause if the symptoms are not first brought under some degree of control.

Once you feel familiar enough with the client, you can begin to formulate four or five treatment objectives. If you work with a staff, you can present the case to them and obtain their feedback on these objectives as well. However, the main person with whom to share your thoughts on treatment objectives is the client.

At all points during therapy with trauma survivors, you need to give the client as many choices as possible. Remember that you are working with someone who has been disempowered by a trauma, and one of your goals is to help the client regain a sense of control over his or her life. Thus the treatment goals you present to the client should be phrased as suggestions. Ask the client for feedback, and use the treatment-planning session as a learning experience for you—as an opportunity to learn more about what is truly bothering the client.

As an example, consider a client who fears losing his job and marriage because of his outbursts of anger. Anger management needs to be on the list of treatment objectives for this client, as does a corresponding list of possible means of achieving the goal. The goal of increasing the client's skills in anger management could be met using a variety of methods, alone or in combination:

- A specified number of individual sessions oriented toward anger management

- Participation in an anger-management group or seminar

- Participation in a relaxation or desensitization program

- Reading books and pamphlets on anger management

Although these are all workable means of achieving the goal of anger management, they will not all be useful for any given client. You first have to ascertain what the client is capable of doing and then what he or she is willing to do. For example, if the client is unable or disinclined toward reading, then reading about anger management is not an appropriate approach. Similarly, if the client becomes flooded with frightening or otherwise negative images while in the state of relaxation, a relaxation-therapy approach to anger management will not be useful. You need to work with the client to agree on a method to achieve the goal and obtain the client's commitment to achieving that goal.

The Issue of Safety

Many, if not most, of the goals will be based on the client's needs and stated objectives. However, there may be objectives that you as therapist feel are important but that the client does not consider of primary significance. These objectives fall into the category of creating an emotionally and physically safe environment for the client and also need to be included in the treatment plan.

Even if the client does not agree to work toward these goals you need to make the client aware that you feel they are important. For instance, if you are working with a family abuse survivor who is still in the original abusive situation or who is currently being victimized or at risk for victimization, attaining safety needs to be a treatment goal (although it may be very difficult to achieve if the client is in denial about the abuse or tends to minimize its effects). Similarly, if you are working with a combat veteran who has chosen a life-threatening occupation or hobby, his or her physical survival needs to be part of the treatment plan. However, he or she may deny any danger.

Nevertheless, you need to include objectives related to safety because your first obligation is to keep the client alive. (There may even be legal considerations if you do not include such life-preserving objectives and methods.) Hence you might include objectives such as developing an emergency exit plan for clients in abusive or potentially abusive situations or increasing awareness of physical safety precautions for clients with dangerous jobs or hobbies. Similarly, when clients are suicidal or homicidal, you need to work with them to identify signs of potential suicide or homicide and attempt to establish a contract whereby the client promises to notify you if suicide or homicide seems imminent.

Coexisting Problems

Substance abuse and other problems that coexist with PTSD can also be life-threatening. If you have determined that a client suffers from alcoholism, drug addiction, or an eating disorder, you need to include objectives related to controlling, and ultimately eliminating, the addictive behavior. Consequently, you may need to include in the treatment plan the client's attending a twelve-step program or participating in a special rehabilitation program oriented toward her or his particular problem.

If the client is near death due to an addiction, or if during the time you have seen the client you have observed a rapid escalation of the substance abuse problem, you may need to recommend hospitalization or intensive outpatient care in addition to or instead of sessions with yourself.

Gambling can lead to financial ruin, and indiscriminate sexual activity can result in physical illness, if not death. Curbing these addictions also needs to be included in the treatment plan, whether or not the client feels it is necessary or warranted.

Along these same lines, if the client suffers from a physical problem that he or she has failed to attend to, seeking medical help for that particular problem needs to be included in the treatment plan. Similarly, if in your judgment the client has depression, manic-depressive illness, or some other psychiatric disorder that could potentially benefit from medication, seeking a psychiatric consultation on this matter also needs to be included in the treatment plan (see below).

Revising the Plan Over Time

When you ask clients about what concerns they want to work on, ask them to select two or three goals for the initial focus of your sessions. "We can't work on everything all at once—you don't want to feel overwhelmed, as you did during the trauma—so let's work on two or three goals and save the rest for later," you might say. You can then advise the client that you will review the treatment plan with him or her in three months (or at some other date) to assess what progress has been made and make any desired changes in focus.

The ultimate treatment goal is healing from the trauma. However, this goal can best be achieved when current major stresses are dealt with first. In dealing with these initial concerns, you will inevitably touch upon the trauma and thereby lay the groundwork for more intensive focus on traumatic material in later sessions.

Considering Medication

Medication is usually suggested when clients suffer from depression, manic-depressive illness, panic disorders, or other significant problems such as intermittent psychotic episodes, for example, auditory or visual hallucinations. Medication should also be considered when PTSD symptoms such as outbursts of anger, insomnia, or anxiety prohibit clients from holding down a job, staying awake or concentrating in therapy, or maintaining at least a few personal relationships.

The changes in body chemistry that can accompany chronic or severe PTSD include alterations in sympathetic arousal, in the neuroendocrine system, and in the sleep-dream cycle. In sum, chronic PTSD is a state of hyperarousal associated with excessive sympathetic activity (Barrett 1990). As discussed in chapter 3, as a result of this state of hyperarousal, current life stresses can be experienced by the trauma survivor as a repeat of the original trauma. Both physiologically and emotionally, the traumatized person may respond to everyday problems with either hyperarousal or numbing symptoms. Because these reactions are often involuntary, they are interpreted by the survivor as a sign of defectiveness and incompetency. Thus these reactions create not only self-doubts but problems in relating to other people and in job functioning.

Some medications have been found to reduce the hyperreactivity of trauma survivors. However, research on the drug treatment of PTSD has been extremely limited. Furthermore, most of the research that has been done has studied only Vietnam veterans with long-term PTSD (van der Kolk 1987). The applicability of the findings to survivors of other types of trauma has not been ascertained.

Hence any statements regarding the effectiveness of particular medications must be taken with some trepidation.

Referral to a Psychiatrist

Unless you are one yourself, you will need to refer clients to a psychiatrist if you feel medication is needed. Ideally, the psychiatrist will have some expertise not only in PTSD, but in whatever other problems a client has, for example, depression or addiction. However, given the relative newness of the PTSD diagnosis, such psychiatrists may be difficult to find. You can begin by calling clinics, agencies, and groups that handle PTSD populations, for example, Veterans Administration Medical Centers or Vet Centers, small clinics or hospital units that serve abused persons, or the local chapter of the American Psychiatric Association. Other sources of referral are the Anxiety Disorders Association of America (6000 Executive Boulevard, Suite 200, Rockville, MD 20852-3801, (301)231-9350) and the International Society for Traumatic Stress Studies (435 North Michigan Avenue, Suite 1717, Chicago, IL 60611-4067, (312)644-0828).

Clients may be reluctant to seek psychiatric help. In that case, assure them that all she or he is agreeing to do is go for a consultation. The psychiatrist may or may not recommend medication. And even if the psychiatrist does recommend medication, the clients can choose whether to follow the psychiatrist's recommendation or disregard it. You also need to explain to clients that the psychiatrist is not going to replace you as therapist. The psychiatrist is there primarily to help with the biochemical aspects of the problem, not the psychological ones.

In addition, clients need to know that medication is not a cure-all—that it is no substitute for counseling or for taking other positive steps to improve their lives. For example, you might tell them the following:

> Psychiatric medications are not "happy pills." They will not make you feel good all the time. You will still feel anger, sadness, and other feelings that are difficult to manage. However, the medication can serve to moderate these feelings so that they don't overwhelm you with their intensity.
>
> You will still need to work in therapy and on your life in general to achieve your goals. However, if there is a match between the medication and your body chemistry, you may experience some relief from the symptoms that are bothering you. But notice that I said "some relief," not necessarily total relief. For example, the medication isn't going to completely eliminate your anger or take away all of your anxiety. The best medication can do is reduce the intensity of your anger and anxiety so that you can manage them better than you are currently able.

Some clients fear that medication will turn them into "zombies." Tell clients with these fears, "If that happens, you need to tell me and also call the psychiatrist. That means your dosage is too high and needs to be adjusted. Or perhaps another medication is needed."

When clients agree to a psychiatric consultation, you can help prepare them for the interview by discussing with them the information in the handout If You Are Referred to a Psychiatrist. This handout discusses what clients can expect from the psychiatrist and presents a list of questions they may wish to ask.

Effects of Specific Medications

As of the writing of this book, the most commonly used medications for treating severe PTSD include those listed below (van der Kolk 1987; Barrett 1990; Kolb et al. 1984). However, given the research now in process, it is possible that this information may become outdated at any time. An excellent source on medication for PTSD clients is *Biological Assessment of Post-traumatic Stress Disorder*, (Giller 1990).

Furthermore, the potential positive effects of each of the drugs listed varies from one individual to the next. For example, MAO inhibitors have helped reduce nightmares in some individuals but have caused increased flashbacks in others. Each of these drugs also has side effects. Thus if your client is on psychiatric medication, you need to be aware of both the potential positive and negative effects of the medication and have a working relationship with the client's psychiatrist.

- MAO inhibitors help to reduce nightmares and improve motivation.

- Tricyclic antidepressants have an anti-panic effect.

- Benzodiazepines (Valium, Librium, Xanax) help to block anxiety and stop panic attacks, improve sleep, decrease nightmares, and may decrease use of alcohol and other drugs.

- Carbamazepine (Tegretol) helps reduce anxiety.

- Beta blockers (for instance, propranolol) block sympathetic arousal.

- Clonidine decreases startle response.

- Lithium helps alleviate depression, mood swings, and impulsivity.

If You Are Referred to a Psychiatrist

If you have a clinical depression or your PTSD symptoms are severe, your therapist may refer you to a psychiatrist who can prescribe medication. If and when you go to a psychopharmacological psychiatrist, he or she will probably do a complete medical and psychiatric workup. You should be prepared to list your symptoms, their duration and frequency, and any other observations you have about your symptoms. In addition, you have the right to expect the psychiatrist to explain your diagnosis and the medication in detail. You might want to ask the doctor these questions:

- What is my psychiatric diagnosis?
- What are the various types of medications that have been found useful for this diagnosis?
- What are the potential benefits and the possible negative side effects of each of these medications?
- Are there any initial side effects that should disappear in time, such as nervousness or extreme fatigue? If so, how long should I wait for the initial symptoms to disappear before I call the office?
- Why is this particular medication being selected over another?
- How much research has been done on this particular medication and what is the probability that this medication will be helpful?
- How long does it typically take for this medication to have an effect?
- If I were to overdose on this medication, would I die?
- Should I give myself the daily medication or should somebody else have the responsibility of giving it to me?
- What if I forget to take the medication at the prescribed time? Should I take it later in the day or wait until the next day? If I skip a day, should I double the dosage the next day, or not?
- What should I do if I vomit the pill for some reason?
- Will this medication interact with other drugs such as alcohol? If so, will the effect be harmful or possibly deadly?
- Will the drug be administered in ever-increasing doses?
- How will you [the psychiatrist] determine if the dosage needs to be changed? Will blood tests be required? If so, how often?
- Do you [the psychiatrist] have any literature on the medication that I can read?
- Can I become addicted to this medication?
- What will happen to me, physically and psychologically, if I suddenly stop the medication on my own? What if I don't tell anyone I am stopping the

medication, what are the signs others can see that will tell them that I have stopped? What should these others do to help me if I stop taking the medication?

- At what point can the medication be discontinued? Is there a point after which the body becomes immune to the effects of the medication so that it ceases to be effective?

- How long does it take for the effects of the drug to leave the body? How long after the drug is discontinued should any dietary or alcohol restraints be observed?

- If this medication does not work, what other medications might be available?

Medication needs constant monitoring. Until the right dosage is established, you may need to telephone the psychiatrist several times. You will also need to call if the negative side effects are problematic or seem to be causing more hardship than is warranted by the positive effects of the drug.

For example, if you are sluggish or extremely tired all the time, are unable to concentrate, or if you have physical symptoms such as bleeding, muscle tremors, seizures, dizzy spells, hyperventilation, dark or discolored urine, rashes, inability to urinate, constipation, loss of menstrual period, severe headaches, vomiting or nausea, loss of sex drive, or other physical difficulties, you should call the psychiatrist right away. Similarly, if you still feel suicidal, homicidal, or self-mutilating, or if you develop hallucinations, delusions, or begin to feel hyperactive or out of control, call the psychiatrist immediately. If your call is not returned promptly, call again. Do not let these side effects go unattended.

Finally, be wary of any psychiatrist who does not seem familiar with the medication, who seems to discount your concerns, or who does not return your phone calls regarding questions about the medication or problems with it. If contacting the psychiatrist is always a problem, consider changing psychiatrists. However, you might want to discuss your decision with your therapist or support group first.

Chapter 5

Groundwork for the Therapeutic Process

In general, studies indicate that PTSD is amenable to treatment. They confirm that with proper treatment, trauma survivors can overcome many of their debilitating symptoms. The approaches that have proven useful include a combination of cognitive therapy, feeling identification and expression, and stress inoculation and assertiveness training. Discussion about existential, spiritual, or moral issues related to the trauma and consciousness raising about the sociopolitical and legal context of the trauma have also been shown to be helpful.

This is not to suggest that trauma survivors are all alike. You cannot, for example, put all your trauma-survivor clients in the same group and expect to have an effective group process. Child abuse survivors, crime victims, survivors of auto accidents, and combat veterans are all trauma survivors, but their issues can differ radically.

It bears repeating that there are important differences between one-time trauma survivors, such as a mugging victim, and persons who have been repeatedly victimized over a long period of time, for instance, child abuse survivors. That said, however, there are several fundamentals that underlie the treatment of any case of PTSD:

- Increasing clients' sense of control over their lives, beginning with their bodies, minds, and emotions. This goal can be achieved by familiarizing clients with the symptoms of PTSD and the reasons for those symptoms and by aiding them in learning coping skills such as anger and stress management. Some clients will also need to tend to neglected medical problems and to learn the rudiments of self care, for example, proper nutritional and sleeping habits.

- Increasing the clients' sense of safety in their work, home, and living environments by helping them identify areas of potential danger or victimization and take active steps toward self-protection.

- Helping clients to identify the trauma and the secondary wounding experiences and symptoms that resulted from the trauma and to reframe these experiences and behaviors in less self-blaming ways.

- Helping clients see how their current life struggles have been affected by the trauma and its aftereffects.

- Supporting clients through the necessary grieving process.

- Supporting clients as they attempt to form meaningful goals and connections with other people.

In addition trauma survivors come for help not only with the trauma, but with other problems as well. Like other clients, trauma survivors have areas of deficiency and conflict (Kluft 1992a). Most certainly trauma, especially severe trauma, exacerbates any preexisting deficiencies and conflicts. For example, an individual who was relatively nonassertive before the trauma may become still more passive as a result of the trauma. Not only the trauma, but these preexisting areas of deficiency and conflict must be identified; for if they created emotional pain or placed limits on the client's growth prior to the trauma, they are probably continuing to do so in the present.

This statement is not meant to imply that preexisting problems caused either the trauma or the client's PTSD or other reactions to the trauma, but rather that trauma is only one aspect of an individual's concerns. The exceptions to this generality are survivors of long-term trauma, such as child abuse, concentration camp or torture experiences, and mass violence. Here the traumatic experience can easily, and understandably, dominate the personality. In such cases, most other concerns may pale before the impact of the trauma.

Richard Kluft (1991) points out four general therapeutic goals for all kinds of clients. These goals are especially relevant for PTSD sufferers, who typically suffer from considerable anxiety and numerous fears about themselves (for example, fears about their ability to control their emotions and behavior). These fears severely limit their ability to interact with people, identify goals for themselves, and take action toward meeting those goals. Kluft's goals are as follows:

- To "increase the range of affect considered acceptable." For example, a combat veteran learns that it is okay, he can still consider himself a man, if he cries, is afraid, or allows himself to be tender towards others.

- To "increase the amount of anxiety which can be tolerated without feeling the need to do something." For instance, a car accident survivor learns to be able to tolerate longer and longer car rides.

- To "increase the range of available defenses and, wherever possible, trade in primitive defenses for more sophisticated ones." For example, an adult survivor of child abuse learns to tell her family when she needs time to herself, rather than making up excuses or telling lies in order to have the quiet she needs.

- To "decrease self-deception." For instance, a client comes to the realization that he has limitations that he must respect.

A Collaborative Model

Establishing Groundrules

In almost all forms of psychotherapy or counseling, the counselor-client relationship is important. Without a satisfactory therapeutic alliance, few positive results can be expected. Our clients need to bond with us, at least to some degree, in order to self-disclose and to subsequently take risks and grow. However, in working with trauma survivors, especially abuse survivors, combat veterans, and others whose trauma involved direct disruption or distortion of intimate human relationships, the therapeutic relationship takes on special significance.

The importance of your relationship to any particular client is a direct function of the extent to which that client's trauma involved losing trust in specific human beings or in human beings in general. Therefore, in most cases, relationship factors will be more critical in working with victims of family violence than in working with survivors of many other types of trauma.

In particular, if your client was neglected or abused by a parent or caretaker, you need to distinguish your role from that person's. For example, in working with clients who were neglected or abused by a parent, and who you see becoming overly dependent on you, it may be important to distinguish your role as a nurturing force in their lives from their wish for an all-giving, ever-present parent. You need to make it clear to them that you can never be the protective, caring parent they lacked, while also acknowledging that it is perfectly understandable and normal for them to desire to have such a parent and to wish at times that you could be that parent. For example, you could say this:

> Do you sometimes wish I could be the mother (father) you
> never had and yet needed so desperately? I can't be. But I can
> help you learn to value yourself enough so that you will want
> to take better care of yourself than you do now. I can also
> help you find ways of taking care of the child inside you that
> never really had anyone who consistently cared for her (him).
>
>   I cannot be with you all the time, as you might want me to
> be. I cannot be there when the pain hits, when the memories
> come back, or when you have PTSD attacks. But I can help
> teach you how to nurture yourself and take the best possible
> care of yourself under these circumstances.

Establishing boundaries like this is particularly important in working with trauma survivors, because typically their physical and psychological boundaries have been violated at least once, if not many times. As discussed in chapter 2, traumatic situations are situations in which there is no way out or in which all options are undesirable. As Herman (1992) repeatedly stresses, trauma can only exist in conditions of captivity. In traumatic situations, certain boundaries entrap the victim: enforced economic or psychological dependency, the threat of violence and bodily harm, barbed wire, the body of an airplane or automobile. At the same time, there is chaos and disorder. Even in prisoner-of-war or domestic violence situations, in which perpetrators tend to establish strict rules (and horrendous penalties for breaking them), the perpetrators often change their own rules or enforce them arbitrarily. In sum, in traumatic situations there are many boundaries yet at the same time none at all. Implied boundaries of humanity and mutual respect, for example, are violated by whatever cruelties are imposed on the victims.

Consequently, in therapy it is critical that the boundaries chosen serve the goal of healing and that the therapist be consistent in adhering to whatever boundaries are established. This is especially important in working with family violence survivors, prisoners of war, and other individuals who have been held captive for a period of time. Establishing boundaries, however, does not mean you act in an authoritarian manner. But neither can you—simply because your client has suffered much—adopt an overly permissive stance in which anything goes. Courtois (1988) recommends "a stance of openness to and acceptance of the client":

> Although the therapist might studiously maintain the neutrality associated with some therapeutic orientations, it is advisable that s/he be active and open in engaging the client. The nonresponsive abstinent therapist is often perceived as judgmental and unavailable. A warm, caring, but not over-indulgent therapist provides the interpersonal environment conducive to disclosure and examination.

The more you can clarify your role to the client, the easier it will be for both of you. Let your clients know what you can and will do for them and what you cannot or will not do. For example, are you available for extra sessions? Do you accept phone calls between sessions? Will you go to court or write letters on your clients' behalf? If so, under what circumstances and with what restrictions or procedures?

You may wish to give clients the option of ending sessions early, getting up and walking around, or going outside for a walk if they become too agitated. Some clients are so restless or hyperalert they can only tolerate twenty- to thirty-minute sessions. These options should be stated ahead of time.

There needs to be an outside time limit to your sessions as well. Extending the therapy session is generally not advisable, because some clients become over-stimulated. (Though this may be mitigated if the possibility is established beforehand.) They may feel anxious because you have changed the predefined boundaries of the session. Some clients may even feel guilty because they assume they are tiring you or don't deserve the extra time.

Money issues also need to be explicitly discussed. You do not want your clients to feel they are being "surprise attacked" as they were during the trauma. For instance, do you charge for time on the phone? If so, how much? Do you charge more when your sessions go over the prescribed time limit? If so, how much?

You also need to be clear about the scope of the therapy. For example, you might contract with the client to meet a specific goal within a certain time frame. Alternatively, you might contract for an open-ended therapy process with periodic evaluation sessions. During these evaluation sessions, you and the client will evaluate the progress made so far and decide whether or not to continue with therapy, take a break, or terminate it altogether.

For some types of trauma survivors, especially family abuse survivors, war survivors, and others who have been severely traumatized, consider the possibility of conducting therapy in stages. In some cases, there are simply too many traumatic episodes or the traumas are of such horrendous proportions that continuous therapy focused on trauma issues may be overwhelming or even detrimental to the client.

These "horror story" cases may need to proceed slowly, allowing the impact of one traumatic episode to be absorbed before going on to deal with yet another tragedy. Such clients may need, or want, to take a time-limited, mutually agreed-upon break from the pain and effort involved in therapy. For some clients, however, taking a break is the prelude to their never returning. Only you can decide if suggesting a break will mean a client might never return. If you feel the client may lose the motivation to return, you can suggest an extremely short break of one or two weeks. Alternatively, you can agree to continue to meet but focus on present-day or other nontrauma concerns as a form of "break."

A related point concerns your availability. Do not attempt to work with trauma survivors unless you will be available long enough to complete the work at hand. For example, it is not fair to your client, or to yourself, to begin working with a trauma survivor who may need three or four years of counseling when you know you will be available only three or four months.

Likewise, if you are working on a trauma unit where therapy is time-limited, be sure you will be available for the course of the treatment. For example, if you work on a three-month unit, it is important that you be committed for the three-month period unless other arrangements are made. For clients for whom abandonment is a major issue—such as survivors of child abuse, combat veterans with years of untreated PTSD, and multiple-trauma survivors—you may need to consult with colleagues or a supervisor about the match between the needs of your work and your ability to make a commitment, if you have plans to change jobs, leave town, or otherwise stop your trauma work.

At all times, you need to expect and demand appropriate behavior. You need not tolerate abuse in any form, emotional or physical. Although much has been written about therapists seeking sexual relations with clients, the opposite can also be true. Some clients, especially clients with histories of sexual abuse, may offer themselves sexually. Their offer may be a means of testing you—to see if you will maintain professional boundaries—or it may have other purposes.

Other clients may be interested in a physical relationship with you because of your status or perhaps simply because they truly are physically attracted to you. Yet dual relationships with clients are forbidden in the code of ethics for all mental health professionals. Your clients need to be informed of these and other limitations on your relationship, such as any policies about accepting gifts.

Gaining Clients' Trust

Some clients remember their trauma in vivid detail; others have only partial recall. Still others have only a vague sense that "something terrible" happened, but have total or almost total amnesia about the particulars of the event or series of events. If clients are turning to you for help in remembering, they must feel safe with you before the memories can begin to unfold. They must also feel safe, or relatively safe, in other areas of life. If a client is under economic stress, for example, or the stress of caring for a severely ill family member, the memories may stay in partial or total repression because there is simply not enough psychic energy available to cope with the external and internal stresses that disclosure of the memories brings about.

Some clients will trust you immediately. It will seem as if they can't wait to share with you the memories they have kept to themselves all these years. Telling you is like the lifting of a great burden, and they will find immediate relief in this important cathartic process. On the other hand, some clients may be more cautious. They may test you before sharing their most upsetting or shaming traumatic memories. They may first share their relatively benign experiences or experiences they think you will judge less harshly, and then watch carefully for your reaction. Are you horrified? Are you blaming? Do you get upset?

Causing an authority figure to become upset may be problematic for abuse survivors, who often learn to placate such figures in order to avoid abuse. On the other hand, upsetting an authority figure may provide satisfaction to survivors who wish to retaliate against authority figures, whom they feel have injured them physically, psychologically, or both.

Clients may not be fully aware that they are watching for your reaction to their stories. In many cases, this testing whether it is safe for them to disclose more personal details is unconscious. A combat veteran might begin by describing a bloody firefight. If you seem to tolerate that description, he might then go on to describe the deaths of civilians during battle. If you pass that test, he may begin to trust enough to tell about greater horrors, such as the sadistic mutilations and murders so common during war.

Similarly, an abused woman might share with you that her husband has once again shoved her down the stairs. While she relates her story, she watches your face intently to see if you are condemning her for continuing to live with such a brutish man. If you pass the test, she may dare to tell you about weekly spankings or other, worse forms of abuse. If you are still are able to maintain empathic listening and true lack of condemnation, she may trust you enough to tell you more.

For example, Ginnie's husband sexually abused her by inserting objects into her vagina and anus and making her get down on all fours and bark like a dog. He also paid other men to have sex with her while he watched, and then he would beat her savagely for "cheating on him."

Ginnie couldn't leave her husband because he had threatened their children when she talked about leaving. To prove he would carry out his threats, he inflicted minor injuries on the children. He threatened to kill them and then commit suicide if she called child protective services. When Ginnie approached the police, they told her they could do nothing until he acted on one of his threats.

And to add to her burden, Ginnie was unable to tell her therapist what was happening. "I could never tell my therapist the whole truth," Ginnie said. "She was a very nice lady, but if I even talked about my husband shoving me, she'd wrinkle her forehead and look like she was going to vomit. I didn't want to make her feel bad, so I never told her about the other things my husband did to me." Until Ginnie found a therapist who knew enough about domestic violence to realize that most abused people are not masochists but are simply trapped, Ginnie had no one with whom to share the enormity of her pain.

Believing the Client

Keep in mind that, in addition to being repressed, memories of trauma can easily be distorted by fear and panic, by temporary or partial amnesia, or by the fight-flight-freeze reactions and the resulting perceptual distortions. All these phenomena are involuntary reactions to trauma. Furthermore, traumatic incidents—war, crime, natural disaster—are themselves confused and chaotic. Such events often occur without warning; those involved have no time to overcome their shock or get a thorough and accurate description of what is actually happening.

Memories of family violence are influenced by the confusion and chaos of the violence, but also by the abuser's deliberate lies or inconsistent behavior. To complicate matters, abusers are seldom purely monsters. They can be loving people one day and virtual beasts the next, for a variety of reasons.

Furthermore, as chapter 8 "Uncovering the Trauma" will explain in greater detail, childhood trauma survivors often suffer from sequencing errors in their recall. Usually events are rearranged so that they can conclude they were at fault, which preserves the illusion of a protective caring parent or caregiver on whom they can rely. There may also be distortions due to the effects of drug or alcohol abuse. Given such conditions, it is no wonder that trauma survivors are often somewhat confused about what really happened.

Ultimately, what matters is what the client believes occurred, not what you believe. Thus it is important, from the beginning of your sessions, that you establish that you are not the judge of whether or not an event actually took place or whether memories are 100-percent accurate. What matters is what the client thinks and feels.

In order to believe clients' accounts of trauma, you need to suspend any preconceived notions you have about what is possible or impossible in human experience. As simple as this may sound, it may be difficult to do so. Some of the experiences endured by human beings on this earth are virtually unbelievable. However, if you do not believe your clients, they may sense your doubt and never fully trust you.

As Bruce Goderez (1986), director of a PTSD inpatient unit says, "It is important for the clinician and counselor to be willing to be made a fool." In other words, it is better that you believe a client who is lying or distorting the truth than to disbelieve a hurting trauma survivor who may never seek help again if your attitude is one of disbelief or disdain. Even if that client were to continue in therapy, he or she might never truly be able to share with any therapist. As a result, the healing process could be stunted or might not occur at all.

A vicious cycle can result, in which the therapist interprets the client's lack of progress in therapy as a confirmation of suspicions that the client was lying, exaggerating, or using the trauma as an excuse for his or her symptoms or other problems. The therapist remains unaware that the client's lack of progress, in part, reflects an inability to bond with the therapist due to lack of trust.

Note: It's a good idea to seek outside consultation if you and your client reach such a "stuck point." Stuck points occur when therapeutic progress has ceased or when the therapeutic relationship appears to be breaking down. If you find it impossible to believe a client, refer the client to another therapist or agency.

Given a trusting therapeutic relationship, as the healing process progresses, clients may be able to clear up their memories and remember forgotten elements of the trauma. With your assistance, they can complete the picture and possibly rectify any errors in their initial views. Do not be surprised, however, if instead of a more sedate, less gruesome, or less heartbreaking version of the incident, the new, more accurate account contains more horror and emotional pain than the original.

Treating the Client with Respect

Your eighteen-year-old incest survivor is engaging in prostitution; your fifty-two-year-old World War II veteran is camping out in his backyard, coming in to the house only to shower, eat, and beat his eternally loyal wife; and your thirty-year-old child abuse survivor is still burning himself with cigarettes and plotting to blow up old buildings. How do you maintain a neutral attitude toward your clients' dysfunctional, morally questionable, or otherwise destructive behaviors?

The answer is, you can't. As Herman (1992) so eloquently spells out, survivors whose trauma involved a violation of their human rights—for example, some concentration camp survivors and formerly battered children—pose a moral dilemma to therapists just as they do to other people. It is impossible to be morally neutral on issues such as torture and child abuse, which is one reason such survivors are often shunned and rejected.

Similarly, it is difficult, if not impossible, for therapists to stay neutral when they observe their clients breaking the law or violating themselves or others. Here you must make a distinction between behavior that is illegal and behavior that may be technically legal but is disrespectful or deleterious either to the client or to others.

Illegal behaviors need to be confronted immediately and directly. In some cases—for example, child abuse or the intention to murder someone—you are called upon to report your client to the authorities. (You need to tell clients in the initial interview that the law requires such reporting.) Abuse of an adult does not require that you report it to authorities. However, it is criminal and punishable by law.

Behavior which is legal, but destructive, for example, self-mutilation, poses a different set of challenges. As discussed in chapter 4, in working with trauma survivors, especially war and abuse survivors, you are likely to encounter a number of clients who engage in self-abuse. As Kluft (1992b) observes, therapists tend to take one of two positions towards self-abuse: that it is the client's responsibility, not theirs, and that therefore they will stay uninvolved, or that such behavior is an affront to the individual and to the therapy, and that therefore they will do everything in their power to stop it. Many therapists vacillate between these positions, naturally or by force of events. For example, it is impossible to maintain the former position when the one's client is in the emergency room as the result of self-mutilation or makes a serious suicide attempt. Similarly, it is difficult to maintain the latter position when numerous attempts to assist the client end in failure.

Kluft stresses that it is difficult to be dispassionate when you have a client who is an "accident about to happen" but that it is also difficult to maintain a balance between having enough distance in order to be helpful without losing your empathic bond with the client. Furthermore, since therapists are people, not saints, they will inevitably become angry and exasperated with self-mutilating clients at times, including alcoholics and other addicted individuals.

However, it is not necessary that the client be informed of your frustration at every turn, and even when you are angry with or weary of the client, this does not mean you treat him or her disrespectfully. However clients present themselves in therapy, and whether you tend toward the relatively detached mode or the more involved mode with your self-mutilating clients, treating them with respect is an absolute must.

Remember that no matter how character disordered, borderline, manipulative, paranoid, or neurotically dependent certain clients can be, they are trauma survivors, and as trauma survivors they have suffered numerous losses and enormous emotional pain. If they haven't felt the pain yet, someday they may. If they never feel the pain, then they will suffer the pain of their life-restricting defenses or addictions. Thus the rule to follow is that if you find yourself repelled by a particular client, refer that client to another therapist or agency.

Avoiding Blame-the-Victim Attitudes

In working with stigmatized clients, for instance, incest survivors, battering victims, and other clients who have endured humiliation as a part of the trauma or secondary wounding experiences, it is absolutely critical that you avoid any questions or interpretations that imply blame. As Christine Courtois (1988), who has worked extensively with incest survivors, writes, "Whatever the technique used, the therapist must keep in mind that a shamed client is being treated. The therapist must take care to be very respectful and avoid behaviors or techniques which reinforce the client's sense of unworthiness."

In particular, it is important to view your trauma survivor clients as victims, not willing participants. Trauma survivors are simply people who become trapped in destructive circumstances for reasons beyond their control. They are not people who consciously or unconsciously designed, provoked, or enjoyed their own torment.

It may happen though that you, as a knowledgeable therapist, assess a client as having self-destructive components to his or her personality. In that case, even if you are correct, and though you are well-intentioned, such an interpretation will probably be more harmful to your client than helpful. If your client is indeed self-negating or self-abusive, he or she probably already feels intense self-hatred, shame, and guilt. Your interpretation will only affirm the client's idea of "I'm so worthless and stupid that I don't even love myself." If you are incorrect in your assessment, then you are, unfairly, blaming the victim.

Before you draw any conclusions about your clients, you need to listen to their stories again and again, and you need to ask questions, questions, and more questions. Unless and until you are informed about the particulars of the specific trauma, you can easily misinterpret placating behavior, provocation, and other seemingly enabling, willing-participant, or masochistic behaviors of your clients. Until you are informed, you will fail to see how these behaviors might have functioned as survival mechanisms or might reflect the regression that can occur when physical or emotional survival is at stake.

Most likely your clients already feel ashamed, embarrassed, or guilty about having been involved in the trauma. They may already be superconscious of what they perceive to be their voluntary, or semivoluntary, participation in their own abuse or victimization. Perhaps their role in the trauma has already been described to them by family members, previous therapists, or twelve-step program friends or sponsors as indicative of some form of negative personality trait or of an unwillingness to grow up and take responsibility for themselves. They don't need to hear that blaming message from you as well.

Letting the Client Set the Pace

During trauma, individuals are rendered powerless; they also tend to become overwhelmed emotionally. In subsequent secondary wounding experiences, their emotional and other reactions to the trauma are either ignored, discounted, or denied outright, by peers, family members, or individuals in authority positions. Your task is to minimize the traumatization inherent to PTSD therapy by doing all you can to avoid recreating such conditions in your sessions. In other words, because trauma survivors are people who have been "shoved around a lot"—literally, figuratively, or both—you do not want to shove them around in therapy. They cannot control the therapy, but you need to allow them as many choices as possible within the therapeutic context.

You need to honor your client's defenses. Neither you nor your client gain anything by your pressing, either overtly or subtly, for certain emotional material before she or he is ready. Even if you are certain the client is capable of dealing with certain core issues that would speed up the recovery process, you must not press the issue—it is the client's decision, not yours, and that decision must be respected. It is not necessary for clients to push through from the least traumatic incident to the most traumatic incident like a steamroller until the ultimate end is reached. Clients need to proceed at rates that are comfortable for them, not for you.

For example, Albert J., a combat veteran, had been diagnosed as having both PTSD and alcohol addiction. He went to a PTSD group, but found he "couldn't handle it." Alcoholics Anonymous however, helped him achieve sobriety within a few months. Then, after two years of sobriety, Albert began having insomnia, intrusive thoughts, and other PTSD symptoms, yet he still refused to even consider counseling regarding his war experiences.

Around the anniversary of an important battle, he came to me seeking help. He couldn't stop thinking about the war, and he had started to think about drinking again. He was even driving around to liquor stores, fighting the urge to walk in and buy the same brand he used to drink. So far, he had been able to restrain himself, but he knew he was weakening. Nevertheless, he still refused help concerning his war issues. "I know I'm dealing with a two-headed monster—alcohol and war trauma—but I can only handle one," Albert said.

I was tempted to say, "But you have to deal with your war experiences sometime. The fact that you want to drink again after having made such wonderful progress in AA should be proof enough that you can't run forever. Look at you, unless you're the exception to the rule, you're bound to slip into the alcohol again. Can't you see, you have no choice but to deal with the trauma." But I said nothing of the kind. Instead I congratulated him on his sobriety, which was no mean achievement given his family history of alcoholism, and on being sufficiently in touch with himself not to deal with war issues until he felt ready. He came asking for support in maintaining sobriety, and that is what I would help him with. When, if ever, he wanted to talk about the war, I would try to be of assistance with that issue as well. In time (his, not mine) Albert did finally decide to grapple with his combat memories.

Make it clear to your clients at the outset that you will listen to whatever they desire to share, but they do not have to answer your questions about the trauma or any other matter if they choose not to. You can assist them by always asking them if they are willing to discuss a particular topic. For example, instead of asking a fire survivor what it felt like to have her art work destroyed, you could ask, "Do you want to talk about how you felt when you saw your years of effort in ashes?"

At all times, refrain from statements such as the following:

> You really need to tell me more about . . .

> You came to me for healing from your trauma. Therefore you must give me more information about . . .

> I can't do my job if you won't tell me . . .

> You'll never get better unless you talk about . . .

> Why are you resisting me? I am only trying to help you. You need to be more cooperative. Is this how you treated your other therapists?

Instead, talk to clients along these lines:

> As a child you were told never to tell, but here it is safe to
> share. I am not ordering you to talk about what happened,
> nor suggesting that you have to, but I am inviting you to do
> so, if you want to. You can accept this invitation now or later
> or never.
>
> Maybe you don't feel ready right now, but if and when you
> do, you can share with me what happened when . . .
>
> At some point, you may want to tell somebody what
> happened. I am willing to listen. But if it happens that you
> talk with someone else, be sure that person is supportive and
> knows something about trauma.

If you feel the need to give the client further permission to share, you can make an invitation such as the one that follows. However, you need to avoid any statements which are—or sound—demanding, forceful or like ultimatums:

> In listening to you for several sessions now, it seems to me
> that (the particular incident) was pivotal in your experience.
> We have discussed this incident briefly, but in my professional
> opinion, it needs more attention. In my view, this incident was
> so critical that it changed your life.
>
> As you know, there are no guarantees, but, in general, the
> more people can talk, write, or draw pictures about the events
> that traumatized them, the less they need to replay those
> events mentally or work them out unconsciously through
> dreams or flashbacks (or whatever your client's reexperiencing
> symptoms might be).
>
> If you someday want to deal with this incident, I am
> available. And if and when that happens, remember that we
> can deal with the incident a little bit at a time. If you become
> uncomfortable as we are discussing it, we can stop at any time.
>
> However, if you choose never to deal with it, that's okay
> too. It does not mean you won't make progress or that you
> are a bad person. We can still work together on whatever
> other aspects of the trauma concern you. It just limits how
> deep we can go.
>
> Are you following me? How did you feel about what I said?

A final point to keep in mind is that clients may intuitively know when it's time for them to stop attending sessions and apply the energy formerly spent in therapy on practicing some of the skills they have learned and developing areas of their lives that have been suffering due to their depression, limiting self-concept, or PTSD symptoms. Any achievements made outside of therapy, along with the application of skills, will bolster clients' self-esteem and can eventually make them better able to progress in a therapeutic setting.

When at a future point a given client feels ready to dig deeper, he or she may return to you for help or perhaps—due to a change in location, insurance company, or other factors—begin work with a new therapist. This does not mean your contribution was not important. You helped them through one leg of their journey. Without your help, they would not be able to move on to the next stage of recovery.

Attending to Clients' Feelings

With all clients, but especially with clients who are trauma survivors, you need to periodically inquire about their emotional reaction to the therapy session, either to the topic being discussed or to one of your interventions. You also need to pay careful attention to verbal and nonverbal cues that your clients might be overstimulated, confused, angry, ashamed, or otherwise emotionally overwhelmed. If you see a client staring into space, looking blank, or starting to fall asleep, ask how he or she is feeling: "How are you feeling? Do we need to talk about it?" For clients who are in numbing, pinpointing how they feel at the moment is extremely therapeutic.

With some clients you may have to start at square one. That is, you will have to explain what a feeling is, how a feeling differs from a thought, and the names of various feelings. Instruction on feelings (and other topics) is far from a waste of time. Even though you are not dealing directly with the trauma at that moment, in teaching them how to identify their feelings, you are giving clients a valuable skill. (Chapter 9, "Feelings Work," addresses this topic.) Identifying feelings is particularly important with clients who were abused or neglected as children, since typically the parents of such children do not encourage them to identify and express their emotions.

Feelings experienced during therapy can provide an insight into your clients' reactions to the trauma and their general mode of interpersonal relating. If they are silent about their negative or uncomfortable feelings during the therapy session, this may be the exact position they assumed in their family of origin, during the trauma, or during secondary wounding experiences. Remaining silent may or may not have been functional in these situations. However, silencing feelings is obviously destructive to therapeutic processes, as well as to intimate relationships in the outside world.

Encourage your clients to express their negative and uncomfortable feelings to you, especially their anger and frustration, even if it involves you. Assure them you will not reject them for such sharing. Although you should not tolerate verbal abuse, you need to be willing to listen to negative feedback about the therapy or the therapeutic process. In fact, such information is absolutely essential.

Domestic Violence Survivors: Special Concerns

Domestic violence victims, in particular incest survivors and battered women, often suffer from blame-the-victim attitudes on the part of therapists (Walker 1979; Courtois 1988; Savina 1987; Quinna-Holland 1979; Herman 1992). Battered children (infants to elementary school age) and abused senior citizens, although also victims of domestic violence, escape some of the stigma heaped upon teenage and adult family violence victims because they are more obviously physically unable to protect themselves.

In contrast, battered women (who constitute more than 95 percent of battered adults) and incest survivors (especially adolescents) have been perceived by therapists and the general public as somehow responsible for or contributing to their fate. Such attitudes can be largely attributed to ignorance of the dynamics and sociopolitical setting of family violence and sexual abuse. Sexism is also involved, since most of the victims are female, as is the often enigmatic loyalty and attachment some victims display towards their abuser.

To an outside observer who is unaware of the underlying processes in an abusive home, it may legitimately appear that certain clients participated in, enabled, set up, or unconsciously desired their victimization experiences. For instance, in some cases it might seem that the abused spouse or child "asked for" the abuse as a form of attention from the abuser, particularly when the abuser bestows special favors or gifts on the victims. Therapists who spend enormous amounts of energy working with families in which there is wife abuse often see that, despite their best efforts, the husband continues to batter his wife and the wife, although she may leave her abuser, eventually returns to him. After three or four such cycles, these therapists often throw up their hands in disgust, saying, "They must like it. He likes going to jail and she likes getting hit. Freud was right. Women are just masochists. There is no other explanation."

However, there are other explanations. For example, the emotional attachment victims feel toward their abusers is frequently the result of *traumatic bonding*—the phenomenon responsible for Patty Hearst's attachment to her kidnappers and Hedda Nussbaum's to her batterer. Although such attachments seem unbelievably irrational to the outside observer, they make perfect "trauma sense" (van der Kolk 1989, 1990a).

Statistically, incest and child abuse survivors of both sexes have higher rates of retraumatization through battering and rape than never-abused persons. These victimizations in later life by people other than the original abuser, also may seem to indicate masochistic tendencies. However, there are several other possible explanations for this fact:

- The low self-esteem of childhood abuse survivors may prevent them from defending themselves.

- The anxiety, guilt, and depression abuse survivors feel as a result of being traumatized may make them a target for exploitative or malicious personalities.

- The lack of love and affirmation in childhood may make abuse survivors more vulnerable to persons who, at least initially, offer them affection.

- The original trauma may cause psychological and biochemical alterations that impair the victim's ability to sense danger and defend against it or otherwise set the stage for further exploitation (van der Kolk 1989, 1990a).

Knowledge such as the above is essential not only to your own understanding of and compassion for your clients but also so that you can help them put their experiences and feelings in perspective. Most of all, it can help reduce the tremendous self-blame and shame involved in being a victim of domestic violence.

It is hard for someone who has never been brutalized by a family member to comprehend the shame involved. To be in a situation where one is repeatedly brutalized because there is no way out or every way out is fraught with danger or conflict, is not only demoralizing but shaming, and leads to a level of self-abasement unknown to victims of natural catastrophes, vehicular accidents, and robberies.

In today's world, domestic violence survivors, like other survivors, are influenced by talk shows and "pop" psychologists in the media who speak freely of concepts such as "codependency" and "love addiction." Such labels are not only technically ambiguous, they are stigmatizing. Many people have used these labels to punish rather than free themselves (the latter being the original intention of these concepts' authors). Domestic violence survivors are particularly vulnerable to such labels and to the input of others. In working with them, you will have to counteract the negative and simplistic analyses of the battering situation proffered by the media (and perhaps former therapists), substituting a more complex view that takes into account sociopolitical realities and a more personal view that includes the psychological, economic, and other means by which your client became entrapped.

Perhaps those who hold the strongest blame-the-victim attitudes towards family abuse survivors are the survivors themselves. If you are to be effective, you will need to be informed. For example, if you are to help such clients understand why they are or were in a battering relationship, you need to be aware that threats of violence toward the victim, other family members, or pets are common in abusive homes, as is the tendency for victims to repress these threats. If you have this awareness, you can at least ask clients if such threats were made. Your questions may jog their memory and help put their life situation in perspective.

Similarly, clients might be discounting or overlooking the social isolation, emotional abuse, and economic controls they endured or could be misinterpreting their forced dependency on the abuser as "codependency" or as a "love addiction" in the most pejorative sense of those words. They may also be overestimating their power in the abusive situation in many other ways. It is important that you don't do this as well, and that you educate, educate, educate to the best of your ability.

Didactic Interventions

In classical psychoanalytic therapy, the therapist is, in the words of psychiatrist, psychologist, and psychoanalyst Richard Kluft, "technically neutral." This does not mean that the therapist does not care about the client, but rather that the therapist perceives his or her role as one of remaining relatively silent. The purpose of this stance is that the therapist not interfere with the clients' airing of their concerns and to give them the opportunity to eventually identify their core childhood conflicts. These childhood conflicts, the classical theory holds, are the root of many, if not most, of the clients present-day concerns (Kluft 1992b).

Such an approach is not useful for trauma survivors, who, especially if they suffered long-term or childhood trauma, need to learn communication and coping skills. A large amount of the work you will do with your clients involves teaching them about trauma and trauma reactions, PTSD and its symptomalogy, and ways to deal with symptoms and current stressors. If the client also suffers from depression or a substance abuse problem (which includes eating disorders), continual education on these illnesses and ways of coping with them are also needed.

Orienting Clients to PTSD Therapy

Either in an introductory session or at some early stage in therapy, the nature of the healing process needs to be clearly delineated for the client. Clients need to be informed about and prepared for the following aspects of PTSD therapy:

- Their need to inform you of the times when the material being discussed in therapy becomes overwhelming, overstimulating, or too painful to handle.

- The emotional impossibility of constantly working on the most painful aspects of the trauma and its aftermath in every session, both for the client and for you.

- The possibility of placing trauma work on hold when necessary, including the possibility of taking short "vacations" from therapy or of lightening up some sessions by dealing with topics other than the trauma.

- The absolute necessity of telephoning or otherwise contacting you or some other responsible party when they feel suicidal, homicidal, drawn toward self-mutilation, or out of touch with reality.

- What constitutes progress or recovery for trauma survivors.

- The possible persistence of certain symptoms, especially sleep disorders, regardless of the level of healing.

- The fact that some symptoms persist does not mean they are doomed to a life without love, sex, meaningful work, or inner peace. Many effective compromises can be reached between trauma survivors and their nontraumatized family members, employers, coworkers, and others.

Any unrealistic expectations about therapy, such as that you have a magic wand that can make all their hurts go away and stay away forever, need to be addressed. Equally unrealistic negative expectations, such as that there is no hope for the future and no relief from PTSD symptoms, also need to be addressed (see "Countering Hopelessness" later in the chapter).

Educating Clients About PTSD

If you were a physician treating diabetes, you would teach your patients about diabetes. You would let them know the full range of symptoms and possible outcomes of the disease. You would also clearly outline the variety of controls available. As a mental health professional treating trauma survivors, you need to do the same. You need to educate your clients about the origin, symptoms, and cyclical nature of PTSD and the nature of PTSD therapy. You would need to cover the following points:

- Therapy can initiate a period of intense emotions, mood swings, and temporary diminishment of the ability to work and relate to others, since the client's energies are focused on unresolved issues having to do with the trauma.

- Therapy can, in some instances, increase the frequency and intensity of PTSD symptoms, and any depression or substance abuse problems, as the survivor confronts repressed memories and emotions.

- Emotionally intense periods may be followed by the respite of numbing, since it is difficult to live in a state of emotional intensity for long periods of time.

- Substance abuse can serve to stimulate the survivor during numbing phases as well as to soothe and calm the survivor during the intrusive phases of the PTSD cycle.

- Traumatic situations give rise to mindsets—such as all-or-nothing think-ing—that are entirely appropriate and useful for surviving life-or-death situations. However, these mindsets may not be universally useful in pres-ent-day nontraumatic circumstances. The task of therapy is to help the survivor decide in which current life situations traumatic mindsets are useful and in which they are not.

- Therapy can help clients identify the ways PTSD affects present relation-ships, job functioning, and self-esteem.

The PTSD self-assessment questionnaire presented in chapter 4 can be used in many ways, one of which is to use the time you spend on the questionnaire as a means of explaining to your client the meaning and origin of PTSD symptoms.

Education about the trauma also needs to be trauma-specific. For example, rape victims need to learn about the social, medical, and legal aspects of rape. Similarly, combat veterans need information about the stresses of war and abused children need to learn about the dynamics of child abuse.

In addition, education about PTSD and the trauma in question needs to be ongoing. Even though your clients may already have seen a video, read a hand-out or book, or listened to your didactic sessions on PTSD and their trauma, the information needs to be reiterated throughout treatment.

The importance of continually providing the client with the information about PTSD and their particular trauma cannot be overemphasized, especially when dealing with family violence, rape, and other stigmatized clients, including com-bat veterans. As Courtois (1988) has said, "repeated exposure to this information is necessary because it contradicts (what survivors learned previously, and it) may not be immediately comprehensible or applicable." Furthermore, in cases where the victimization was chronic or occurred at a preverbal level, most sur-vivors had their reality negated so frequently that they feel they are going crazy or losing their minds. New material contradicting the old, although initially incomprehensible, is nevertheless very relieving since it validates and depatholo-gizes emotions. Some clients explain that their rational self understands and ac-cepts new conceptualizations even though they do not "compute" on an emotional level. Over time and with repetition, the information becomes more emotionally congruent and is assimilated and used.

Inevitably, some clients will have mixed reactions to the new information. Even though they sought your help, your help has brought about an awareness that has shattered the illusion that "It really didn't happen" or "It wasn't that bad" or "It didn't really bother me" or "I'm not really that scarred." The reve-lations you work so hard to provide may cost them not only their innocence but any conscious or unconscious hope that in the end there would be a happy end-ing or that they would at least be justly compensated for their losses. Conse-quently, you, to whom they first might have turned as a savior, might become a villain in their eyes. The degree and likelihood of this depend on the extent of the client's victimization and his or her support system.

Framing Clients' Problems in Terms of the Trauma

Throughout the therapy, when it is psychologically true, you need to frame the client's problems in terms of the trauma. For instance, if a client is describing a current problem with a relationship, you need to inquire if, in the client's view, the trauma or a secondary wounding experience has contributed to the problem.

You never want to put words in a client's mouth. However, if you feel fairly certain that the trauma or its aftermath has influenced the problem at hand, you can suggest to the client that prior work with trauma survivors indicates that this is often, but not always, the case. The following example will illustrate some of the uses, and difficulties, of reframing.

Joanne began stealing food at age seven, several months after her mother began taking her to bed with her and in other ways making Joanne a "little adult." Joanne not only served her mother's physical and emotional needs but replaced her mother as cook and babysitter for younger siblings. Joanne's father encouraged the relationship because it freed him from meeting his wife's needs.

As incestuous fathers are toward their child-victims, Joanne's mother was extremely jealous of Joanne's outside involvements and tried to impede or dominate Joanne's relationships with other girls and women. In elementary and junior high, Joanne was not permitted to socialize much with peers or to attend school social functions, and her family roles occupied much of her free time. In response, she continued to steal food and clothing, symbolizing her unmet needs for nurturance and protection.

She ate most of the food and returned the clothing for cash, with which she bought more food. At fourteen she was double her ideal weight, and by age sixteen she had discovered bulimia. As her bulimia progressed, the number of binge-purge cycles per day grew, until sometimes Joanne would binge and purge ten times a day or more. As with alcohol or drug addiction, where over time more and more alcohol or drugs are needed to achieve the desired emotional state, Joanne also needed increasing amounts of food to cope with her victimization. She therefore had to steal more.

Joanne was "eating to" her family dynamics, for example, her guilt about her incestuous relationship with her mother, her anger at her social and other deprivations, and her unmet dependency needs. However, Joanne was also eating to the guilt of eating (binging and purging) and the guilt of stealing. The more guilt she felt about her feelings, the more she ate to punish herself. Yet the fatter she got, and the more out of control her bulimia became, the worse she felt about herself and the more she needed to eat to confirm her "badness." Stealing was necessary to continue the binges, which further exacerbated her guilt.

At age seventeen, she ran away from her home with a man twice her age. He encouraged her to continue stealing—for him. He used the money for drugs, and Joanne tried her hand at cocaine, marijuana, and other such drugs. Eventually she was caught stealing, so at age nineteen she had a police record.

Only after ten years of therapy did Joanne stop calling herself a "low-life food junkie who would sell her children down the river for a piece of sugar." Ten years, not ten sessions, were required for her to appreciate, and respect, the life-preserving survival functions of two of her greatest areas of shame: stealing and binging and purging.

Her therapist continually asked, "And how did you used to feel after you overate (or stole)? And what function do you think your being fat served in the family? What did it do for your mother? For your father? What did it not do? How about your brothers—did your eating and stealing habits affect them? If so, how did that serve the survival of the family? If you hadn't binged and purged and stolen, what might you have done? Then what do you think would have happened to you? To your mother? To your father? To other family members?"

Through asking such questions, offering data about the high incidence of eating disorders among sexually abused girls, and educating Joanne about the caretaking functions of many incest survivors, the therapist was able to cast a more benign light on Joanne's addictions, without necessarily applauding them.

You need to continue framing problems in terms of the trauma so that the client can see the connection between the trauma and subsequent symptoms and behavior. It is necessary to repeat your framing statements throughout the course of therapy in order to counteract the deeply ingrained tendency many clients have to blame or debase themselves. Consequently, you want to reframe your client's symptoms in neutral, functional terms. Although it may seem redundant, most clients need to hear repeatedly that their symptoms are not defects but the remnants of survival mechanisms or ways of coping with emotions generated by the trauma.

For example, if you were Joanne's therapist, you would point out to her that overeating served as an expression of her anger and as a way to calm herself after being sexually overstimulated, but not sexually fulfilled, by her mother. If Joanne had expressed her anger, she would have been given away to another family, or so she was told repeatedly. If she had not been her mother's caretaker, her parents might have divorced. She could not have done much else with her sexual energy but use food to subdue it because she was not allowed to go out: Her father had threatened to kill her if he saw her on a date, and would certainly have at least punished and humiliated her verbally. The only other alternative would have been drugs or alcohol, for which she had no money and which would have been no better than her eating disorder.

Stress to your clients that although many of their survival mechanisms may be highly undesirable today, originally these behaviors arose to help them survive a highly undesirable set of life conditions. For example, dissociation is commonly viewed as a negative symptom by both clients and therapists. However, dissociation for the trauma survivor often originally served the purpose of allowing that individual to function:

> Dissociating serves many purposes. It provides a way out of the intolerable and psychologically incongruous situation. It erects memory barriers (amnesia) to keep painful events and memories out of awareness, it functions as an analgesic to prevent feeling pain, it allows escape from experiencing the event and from responsibility/guilt. Over time, it commonly changes from being functional (a survival skill) to being dysfunctional and getting in the individual's way (a symptom). (Courtois 1988)

Obviously, not all of a client's symptoms can be attributed to the trauma. Careful work on your part will be necessary to determine which symptoms are related to the trauma or secondary wounding and which are not. It cannot be overemphasized that reframing symptoms as coping mechanisms or as responses to abuse or other life-threatening situations is *not* intended to extend to all maladaptive symptoms. Neither should your positive reframing interventions be misconstrued by the client as condoning or encouraging the use of highly destructive behaviors such as self-mutilation or substance abuse. The purpose of reframing symptoms is simply to reduce the client's self-blame and guilt. Once these feelings are reduced, perhaps the client will no longer need the symptoms for purposes of self-punishment.

The above suggestions regarding framing apply primarily to clients with a primary diagnosis of PTSD uncomplicated by a dual diagnosis of personality disorder or substance abuse. If clients also have a personality or character disorder, an addiction, or some other disorder that includes antisocial or antagonistic behavior, you will need to alter your approach considerably. Although you may still need and want to make such clients aware of the connection between the trauma and their behavior, you do not want the trauma to become an excuse for antisocial or other negative behavior.

Furthermore, clients with dual diagnoses who externalize their anger in a destructive manner do not need help reducing irrational guilts surrounding trauma issues as do relatively pure PTSD cases. Instead, they need help seeing the self-defeating aspects of their current behavior and the ways in which their behavior negatively affects others. Such clients need to take increased responsibility for their behavior and learn how to control their anger, not express it. In contrast, the relatively pure PTSD usually presents with suppressed rage, and the therapeutic task is to bring that rage to the surface and teach the client to express it in a prosocial or otherwise constructive manner (Newman 1987).

Correcting Cognitive Distortions

Reframing the trauma and correcting cognitive distortions are forms of cognitive therapy. The basic assumption of cognitive therapy is that if you change the way a person thinks, you can change how the person feels. For example, cognitive theory postulates that by helping clients reframe their trauma-related symptoms in neutral or functional terms instead of personally pejorative ones, you will improve the way clients feel about themselves. The result of their improved self-esteem, will be that they spend less time and energy in self-abasement and more time and energy in pursuit of their goals and relationships and thus eventually experience greater success in these areas, increasing their sense of mastery and life satisfaction.

The objectives of correcting cognitive distortions are similar. The goal is not only to correct distorted thinking but to improve client self-esteem and increased functionality in the world, which will lead to further positive action, and so forth.

However, cognitive therapy has its limitations. Even experts in the field, such as Catherine Fine (1991), stress that while straight thinking can help improve a client's emotional state, it can only do so on some levels. "Cognitive therapy," she states, "is not the whole answer, but it does help clients get control over themselves. . . ." Cognitive therapy can help diminish some of the negative, draining feelings related to the trauma. However, even if all cognitive distortions are corrected, the survivor will still have to deal with uncomfortable painful feelings that cannot be "thought away."

Fine stresses that, when working on cognitive distortions, therapists need to ask themselves the following basic questions:

- Which cognitive distortions prevent the client from getting the most involved in and the most satisfaction from their lives?

- Which cognitive distortions disrupt and complicate the client's life?

- Which ideas, while they distort reality, help clients stabilize themselves?

Fine also suggests the following principles for helping to correct cognitive distortions. (The same principles can be applied to your attempts to reframe the trauma.)

In order that the client not feel attacked, you need to question the client's distortions in a "gentle, nonaccusatory" manner. For example, rather than challenging the client's ideas directly, speak in terms of being confused or concerned, or ask for more information.

Other ways of challenging cognitive distortions without directly attacking the client's ideas are to ask clients to identify the origin of their symptom or thought, and let them challenge it themselves, or to present examples of the harm cognitive distortions can create.

As always, tell clients what you are doing. Let them know that your role includes challenging their ideas, from time to time, when you suspect they may be making assumptions that are not accurate or helpful today, although they may have been relevant and helpful during the trauma.

Do not overwhelm the client. Work on one distortion at a time, and go slowly. You do not want to challenge too many cognitive distortions at once, no matter how subtle your method, because some of these ideas serve to stabilize the client.

Finally, Fine recommends, do not use paradoxical intent; do not allow the client to be left to roaming fantasies; and point out to clients when they are catastrophizing or overgeneralizing.

Suppose you have a client, a formerly abused child, who presents both idealized views of his abuser as a wonderful caretaker and horrible stories of torture at the hands of the same individual. The wrong approach is to make statements such as, "You just can't accept that he wasn't a wonderful father, can you? Can't you see how cruel and exploitative he was?" or "Are your dependency needs so great that you need to hold on to this fantasy of a good father when, in reality, he was a brute?" or "It's really true, isn't it, victims do fall in love with and defend their victimizers."

Instead, you would want to say, "I'm confused. Last week you were telling me about the time your father tied you up and punched you for two hours. And this week you are telling me that you don't have enough money to buy this same person the kind of lavish birthday gift he deserves for being such a wonderful parent. I'm having trouble putting the two pictures of the same person together. Can you help me out?"

Although entire therapy programs have been built around the idea of confronting clients with "the truth . . . the raw truth," in dealing with trauma survivors (especially long-term multiple-trauma survivors), you must keep in mind that when you challenge their cognitive distortions, you are also dismantling their defenses—the very same defenses that have helped them survive thus far.

It is wise to treat gently what has thus far been the client's life preserver. Your goal, as therapist, is to help the client build new, less rigid, more growth-producing, and reality-based defenses. But until these develop, it is wise to refrain from all-out attack. Not only is it unethical to take away an individual's defenses until he or she has built up others, but it is counterproductive therapeutically.

Too much pressure applied prematurely can have several results: The client may resist you, and with very little therapeutic interaction will occur. The client may terminate therapy. Or the client may accept your challenge and discard the defenses associated with the distortion. However, being left defenseless may also leave the client extremely vulnerable to self-destructive, aggressive, or psychotic behavior in response to stress, including a return to or escalation of any substance abuse problem. In particular, harsh confrontations with clients with dissociative disorders can be extremely dangerous. If you remove the dissociative defenses all at once, these clients will most definitely become emotionally overwhelmed. Some may even decompensate.

In sum, in dealing with trauma survivors, unless you are extremely familiar with the client and are certain that direct confrontation will not lead to negative effects, it is better to ask judicious questions than to make evaluative or other kinds of comments. When all else fails say, "I don't understand that. Please tell me more." If a client is particularly argumentative or resistant to your interventions, you might want to examine the trust level between you and the client. You might want to ask, "Is there a possibility you might not trust me on this? I wouldn't be surprised if you didn't trust me. From what you've shared with me about your life, many people have let you down, so it is only natural that you are careful about whom you trust."

Four common cognitive distortions that typically arise as the result of trauma include the following (Alford, Malhone, and Fielstein 1988; Glover 1988):

- Intolerance of mistakes in others and in the self—"I can't make any mistakes. Neither can anyone else. All mistakes are deadly."

- Denial of personal difficulties—"I'm okay. I have no problems."

- All-or-nothing thinking—"It's either black or white. There are no in betweens in life."

- Continuation of survival tactics—"If I stop doing what saved my life (or sanity) during the trauma, disaster will surely befall me or my loved ones."

Intolerance of Mistakes

During certain traumatic events (combat, fires, floods, family violence) and in certain occupations that involve injury and death (nursing, rescue work, firefighting, police work), mistakes are anathema. Even the tiniest error can result in death or injury to another person or to oneself. If your clients have been in such a situation, they have likely seen how the mistakes of others caused needless deaths, injuries, and other losses. As a result, they can develop a mindset of "no mistakes allowed."

The same mindset can develop during secondary wounding experiences, in which clients may have felt that if they made even the slightest mistake they would be denied help or mistreated by authorities or others. Or perhaps they attributed the denial, discounting, or other secondary wounding experiences they had to "mistakes" made in how they presented themselves or how they handled interactions with others.

This mindset can easily lead to perfectionist values. They may demand perfect performance of themselves, others, or both. Expecting others to be perfect, however, inevitably leads to disappointment and conflict in their relationships. If they also expect themselves to be perfect, they will undoubtedly suffer from endless heartache, low self-esteem, and even depression.

The following is a list of "shoulds" that commonly creates problems for people, even nontraumatized people (McKay and Fanning 1987). For trauma survivors, these perfectionist shoulds impose yet another weight on an already burdened psyche. You may want to share this list with your clients, orally, or on paper.

I should be the epitome of generosity and unselfishness.

I should be the perfect lover, friend, parent, teacher, student, spouse.

I should be able to find a quick solution to every problem.

I should never feel hurt. I should always feel happy and serene.

I should be completely competent.

I should know, understand, and foresee everything.

I should never feel certain emotions such as anger or jealousy.

I should never make mistakes.

I should be totally self-reliant.

I should never be afraid.

I should have achievements that bring me status, wealth, and power.

I should always be busy: to relax is to waste my time and my life.

I should be able to protect my children from all pain.

I should not take time just for my own pleasure.

If applicable, you can ask your client the following questions:

Were any of these shoulds a necessity during the trauma?

Are any of these shoulds a necessity now?

Which of these shoulds are important to try to live up to in order to meet your present-day needs?

Which of these shoulds help motivate you to meet your goals, and which are sticks with which you beat yourself?

Are these shoulds truly *your* shoulds, or are they shoulds imposed on you by others: parents, spouse, children, and so on?

Which shoulds would you like to keep? Which would you like to discard?

You need to emphasize that, unlike in the traumatic situation, the client has more choices now.

Denial of Personal Difficulties

Certain occupations, for instance, medicine, police work, combat duty, and rescue work, emphasize the necessity for solid thinking, quick action, and endurance, both physical and psychological. There is little room for expression of emotions or for personal weaknesses. Hence, from firefighters to combat soldiers, those who are involved in life-or-death situations tend to keep their personal difficulties to themselves. The legitimate fear of such workers is that if they are emotionally honest they may be seen as cowards, weaklings, incompetents, or otherwise unfit.

Victims of crime, childhood abuse, battering, and natural catastrophes may also deny personal problems for fear of being seen as weak or defective because of their experiences. In order to avoid this stigma, some trauma survivors put on a macho or stoic facade. It makes absolute sense for clients not to share their personal difficulties with individuals who are or were apt to denigrate them. However, problems arise in the present, in intimate relationships and during the healing process, when the client persists in denying personal pain, conflicts, and other psychological or physical symptoms.

You need to point out to your clients that denial of personal problems can lead to psychological symptoms, addictive behavior, psychosomatic symptoms, or worse. Emphasize that they owe it to themselves to find at least a few people that they can trust enough to share with openly, besides yourself.

Clients may be afraid to take the risk of sharing with friends or relatives. However, they need to be encouraged to take a few limited risks. You could suggest to clients that they make a list of people they feel might be supportive. Clients should not begin their efforts to reach out by sharing their most intimate secrets or the most vulnerable parts of themselves. Instead, they need to "test the waters" first and start out by sharing one of the least intense or least threatening personal problems with the person they feel would be the most supportive—on a trial basis. If the person cannot be supportive, because he or she does not have the time to listen, does not understand, or is rejecting or hostile, the client need not approach that person again and should try someone else.

Encourage your clients to take a long range, rather than a short range, view of their situation. If they take a few emotional risks now, they can save themselves long-term scars. The same goes for professional help. Money spent now can save larger amounts in the future, should their trauma wounds develop into serious psychiatric problems due to lack of adequate attention now.

For example, I have told the following to individuals who have addiction problems and are hesitant to consider a rehabilitation program or twelve-step program meetings:

> If you had cancer and your doctor told you to come for chemotherapy or some other treatment, you'd be there in a minute. You wouldn't question whether you needed the treatment or not. You wouldn't care how much the treatment cost, how long you had to wait in line for it, how far it was from your home, or how inconvenient it was for your schedule. It wouldn't even matter whether you liked the doctor's personality. You'd be at the appointment, on time, with your checkbook ready, grateful that treatment existed and ready to do whatever the doctor told you.
>
> May I suggest that this problem is potentially as harmful as cancer? Some people who have suffered through horrible experiences similar to yours, who have not sought help, have gone into hiding. Some stay with their family or in their relationship but are lonely and suffer intensely, not only from their PTSD and other problems but from shouldering the entire weight of their pain alone. Consequently, they feel deprived in the present, which causes them to focus on the past even more than they would ordinarily.
>
> These lives of isolation can lead to so much anger and pain that to escape reality the person considers suicide, or even homicide, or evolves a life that revolves around an addiction or some delusions.
>
> I've seen this happen to some very intelligent, gifted people, and I don't want to see that happen to you. But it can happen to you, just as it can to anyone else—just like a small tumor of cancer can grow to envelop the entire body—if you don't take emotional care of yourself.

All-or-Nothing Thinking

For some clients, life is either all bad and hopeless or a bowl of cherries with endless possibilities. For example, they might see themselves as total failures or total successes, and make few allowances for partial successes or partial failures.

Clients who were traumatized during childhood or adolescence, may be especially prone to such all-or-nothing thinking, especially if they also suffer from depression. Absolutist thinking is especially strong among survivors who, due to the characteristics of the traumatic event, learned to trust some people almost entirely and some people not at all. Consequently it may be difficult for these survivors today to learn that different levels of trust are appropriate for different people.

In a variation on this, it has been suggested that some trauma survivors view other people as falling into four rigid categories: persecutor, fellow victim, indifferent bystander, or rescuer (Herman 1992). You might want to ask your clients if, on some level, they categorize people in such a manner. You might also want to examine with your clients those areas where they apply absolutist thinking to themselves. Is the all-or-nothing thinking restricted to certain areas of their lives, or does it encompass many areas of their lives? If it is restricted to certain areas, examine those areas of their life that they view in absolutist terms. For example, if being swindled by a corrupt attorney was one of their secondary wounding experiences, do they now view all attorneys as thieves? Alternatively, if they were assisted by Asians during the trauma, do they now view all Asians as beyond reproach?

Continuation of Survival Tactics

Anger and aggression are often soldiers' survival tactics. In contrast, domestic violence survivors tend to increase their chances of staying safe by being passive and obedient. Incest survivors may learn to minimize harm to themselves by flirting or acting coy or seductive or by manipulating their abuser to harm someone else in the family. Survivors of a wide variety of traumas may have learned to dissociate from their body or the experience in order to cope.

As discussed, such survival tactics may have saved your clients' lives during the trauma. They may even have helped your clients obtain what they needed during secondary wounding experiences. Today, however, some of your client's survival tactics may be impinging on their happiness. This does not mean they will readily let go of them.

You can try to help clients identify their survival tactics and explore with them the function these tactics served during the trauma and afterwards. However, identifying these tactics may be difficult, because they may be so ingrained that they seem more like personality traits than survival tactics. This is especially true of family abuse survivors and others who have been severely traumatized.

When clients cannot identify their survival tactics the first time you introduce the concept, assure them that they might in the future, as their awareness grows. As these tactics come to be clearly defined by clients, you may want to have clients consider whether these tactics help or hinder their everyday functioning and the pursuit of their life goals. Equally, if not more, important, you need to have clients articulate the fears they associate with not using these tactics.

Do not assume all of the clients' fears and concerns about letting go of a survival tactic are unfounded. Although some are relics of the past, other fears may be realistic and worthy of respect.

Teaching Coping Skills

Trauma survivors often have recurring problems with anger and with stress management. For those clients who have a backlog of unresolved anger regarding the trauma or secondary wounding experiences, current anger-provoking experiences can easily become infused with anger that rightfully belongs to the trauma. In addition, overwork (role overload) and other stresses can easily lead to anger because any type of overload is reminiscent of the original traumatic situation.

Research has shown that trauma survivors are more vulnerable and reactive to stress than nontraumatized individuals. And when trauma survivors encounter present-day stressors, and once again become overwhelmed or dysfunctional, their negative self-image is confirmed.

On the positive side, given adequate support and adequate training in stress-management skills, clients can improve their ability to handle subsequent stresses, which subsequently improves their self-image and self-confidence. However, if an individual has been severely traumatized, has suffered a permanent or major medical or financial loss as a result of the trauma, or has been subject to a series of retraumatization experiences as a result of the first trauma, improvement in stress management skills may still fall short of making that person truly effective at work, at home, and in the social sphere. Despite all the individual's efforts, he or she may still be obviously less functional than his or her siblings, coworkers, and other contemporaries.

You can reinforce such clients for the strides they have made, but if they are aware of their areas of relative dysfunction you also need to support them as they grieve their limitations, especially those limitations that may never be truly overcome. Do not add insult to injury by sugarcoating these people's very real losses. Only if they feel you are with them in their sorrow do you have a chance of showing them what perhaps might be done to make their life a little better. However, if they feel you are ignoring or discounting their pain—pain grounded in truth they must bear daily, that there are areas in which they are irreparably damaged—they may dismiss any suggestions you have for positive change as "Pollyanna thinking."

Elderly clients are another category for which change may be difficult in some areas, if not impossible, due to the physical changes of advancing age. Recent research suggests that some traumatized individuals who were able to avoid PTSD symptoms as young adults or middle-aged persons may find themselves beset with PTSD symptoms in their later years:

> As trauma survivors age, the risk of experiencing physical and
> cognitive impairments due to advancing age and diminished
> health increases. In particular, neuropsychological impairments
> that lead to a disinhibition of affect, behavior, and memories,
> may uniquely affect survivors of trauma and contribute to
> delayed PTSD. (Cassiday and Lyons 1992)

Severely or multiply traumatized clients, as well as elderly clients, quite possibly have central nervous system alternations due to trauma. Consequently, they have an even greater need for anger and stress management skills than most. Furthermore, these clients tend to be more sensitive to social rejection, more intolerant of noise and other irritating stimuli, and less capable of anger control. Their catecholamine depletions, for example, predispose them to all-or-nothing responses to other people and life situations, as well as to outbursts of rage.

These clients will also need more help in improving their self-care skills and more encouragement toward self-nurturance.

True PTSD clients are aware of their propensity for rage. This awareness often leads them to withdraw from others. Social withdrawal, they reason, will minimize the chances of their becoming agitated and losing control of their anger. PTSD clients also have a propensity for depression or depressive episodes, and at such times often want to hide from others or be alone. They fear they are not enjoyable company and do not have the energy, or perhaps even the inclination, to pretend that they are fine. They may also be disinclined to be open about their depression or other sad feelings for fear of being rejected or viewed disparagingly by others.

However, the loneliness that stems from this self-imposed isolation creates its own anger and depression—the very emotional states it was intended to avoid. A vicious cycle can develop whereby withdrawing from others in order to avoid anger leads to the pain of loneliness and feelings of being abandoned by others and betrayed by life. These feelings lead in turn to more anger. The same dynamic can hold true for depressive episodes. The individual stays home alone when feeling depressed, but the lack of stimulation, companionship, and support serves to create further depression.

Trauma survivors need to learn and practice anger-management skills so that they do not respond aggressively, or alternatively by passively shutting down, when they become frustrated or angry. (Some trauma survivors—for example, some combat veterans—simply walk away from confrontations. They fear that if they become the slightest bit annoyed they will lash out verbally or even physically, as they were trained to do in the military.)

Assertiveness skills are often useful, especially for clients abused as children. In most cases, in their family of origin these clients functioned as a rescuer or caretaker for one or more dysfunctional parents. Consequently, they may have never learned how to ask for their needs to be met. Such clients first need to feel they are entitled to have their needs met, and second they need to be able to identify these needs. One of your tasks as a therapist is to assist clients in these areas.

Reinforcing Clients' Strengths

Whenever possible, you need to reinforce your clients' strengths and courage. It takes courage for clients to talk about their traumas: in self-disclosing they risk rejection, blame, and disbelief. Talking about the trauma can resurrect pain, anger, grief, confusion, and other extremely uncomfortable emotional and mental states. Therefore, you need to reinforce their sharing with statements such as the following:

> Thank you for trusting me enough to tell me about . . .

> It takes courage to share what you have just shared. I really admire you for that.

> Is it difficult (painful, sad) for you to share what happened with me? I know that it would be for me. Please know that whenever you begin to tell me about a traumatic incident and you become too anxious, sad, angry, or in any way uncomfortable, you can stop at any time.

In contrast, the following statements are nonaffirming and discourage self-disclosure:

Aren't you exaggerating somewhat?

Could it be that you are mistaken about . . . ?

Are you telling me the truth?

Did you ever hear voices or see visions when you were a child? Is anyone in your family a schizophrenic?

Emphatic comments are also helpful. For example, you could say:

I feel so sad [angry] for you.

How unfair!

How did you survive all that?

How exhausting! What fortitude you had!

I'm impressed. How did you go through all that and keep your sense of humor [keep on working full time, take such good care of your children, hold onto your sanity].

Of all the personal narratives you are likely to hear, those of domestic violence victims may sound the most outrageously fabricated. Not uncommonly, abuse survivors are aware that their stories sound like sado-masochistic soap operas and consequently remain silent. Chances are that when they shared their accounts in the past, their reality was negated by others. Such stigmatized clients benefit greatly when the therapist validates their reality.

As stated before, trauma survivors often harbor considerable self-blame and guilt regarding actions or inactions on their part that they feel contributed to the trauma or to its negative outcomes. To counter the self-blame and guilt, clients can be asked to identify the positive qualities they displayed during their time of extreme stress. The following handout, Identifying Your Strengths, can be used as a written homework assignment or you can ask clients the questions in session.

Countering Hopelessness

You will also need to counteract the sense of doom that frequently plagues PTSD sufferers. Especially in working with multiple-trauma and family abuse survivors, you will need to continually encourage every small step they take toward recovery. Your support is absolutely crucial in countering three attitudes frequently held by trauma survivors:

- That they are incurable "nut cases"

- That they will never be free of the memories and the associated low self-esteem, self-hatred, shame, and guilt

- That the most they can expect out of life is to simply endure their PTSD symptoms

"If I can just go to the grave without killing myself, or someone else, I'll be doing good," an adult survivor of childhood physical abuse once shared in therapy. The same sentiment has been expressed by combat veterans, incest survivors, and individuals who have lost family members to crime, fires, floods, and tornadoes.

In some instances, this sense of hopelessness has been confirmed by psychiatric diagnoses that carry negative connotations (such as borderline personality,

Identifying Your Strengths

Part I

For each of the traumas you experienced, identify those thoughts and actions on your part about which you feel some pride. Don't worry about seeming conceited. Just make a list of all the positive qualities you can think of.

You may want to begin as follows: "As a result of the way I acted and felt during the trauma, I now see myself as . . ." Consider the following list of possibilities:

- Brave

- Clever, intelligent, or resourceful

- Righteous

- More moral

- Praiseworthy

- Emotionally strong

- Physically strong

What are some of the other positive qualities that were evident during the traumatic event? List these as well.

Part II

How did it feel to list your positive qualities? Did you feel you were boasting or immodest? Do you think it is egotistical to take pride in yourself? If you were raised on the virtues of humility and modesty, you may feel that it's wrong to think well of yourself. If that is the case, bear in mind that reminding yourself frequently of the strength, endurance, integrity, and intelligence you showed during the trauma is one of the few ways you have of countering the negative, self-blaming thoughts you may harbor inside.

"But what if I can't think of any way in which I acted positively?" you might say. If that's the case, don't be devastated by your admission. Many trauma survivors feel as you do. Perhaps as you move further along in the healing process, you will be able to take more pride in how you acted and felt during the incident that changed your life. Do not beat yourself up if you can't complete this particular exercise. Simply consider the possibility that you have strengths, and then move on.

If you can't think of any ways you were strong during the trauma, after you have looked at the trauma more closely later on in therapy, you may see things differently and feel differently as well.

character disorder, or schizophrenia) and by mental health professionals who have told survivors that they will never get better. However, in my experience, trauma survivors who have been told by psychiatrists, psychologists, social workers, and others that they are incurable are clients who never had the opportunity to benefit from any solid healing effort. Since these clients have never really dealt with the trauma in counseling, there is no basis for proclaiming them incurable. I have, unfortunately, seen individuals who have been so traumatized that indeed the prognosis for recovery is *slim*. However, slim does not mean hopeless.

Case Example

Paul's case illustrates some of the difficulties in working with some PTSD-afflicted clients. The day of his first appointment, Paul walked in the door and immediately sneered. "You can't help me. Nobody can. Look, the chair you have for me is too small. You planned it that way, didn't you? Trying to get rid of me already. I know you therapists. You can't fool me." Paul weighed more than 350 pounds and reeked of body odor and alcohol. As he continued to talk, he repeatedly lashed out about my status as doctor, the Mercedes he felt certain I had parked outside, and my unscarred face. His own face bore several scars, obvious remnants of knife wounds.

In a hostile tone, Paul revealed that he had been regularly beaten by both parents as far back as he could remember. Also, during adolescence he had been the object of numerous unprovoked racial attacks. At first he had not tried to fight back. But surrendering to the bullies attacking him only seemed to escalate the abuse. When he then fought back, Paul's mother, who for religious reasons, didn't believe in fighting beat Paul with a belt. When he didn't fight back, his father called him a sissy and beat Paul with a stick to "toughen him up" and "make him a man."

When Paul was seventeen, he ran away from home, found a job as a clerk, and eventually opened his own business. He drank occasionally, but he was not an alcoholic. When he married, there were a few marital problems, but basically marriage provided Paul with the emotional stability and affection he had never had as a child.

Seven years later, however, Paul's two children were killed in an automobile accident. Soon afterwards, his wife left him. And a few years later, shortly after Paul had remarried, his new wife died of cancer.

By this time, Paul had become an alcoholic. He was also a diabetic and a heart patient. But when the alcohol failed to drown his pain and anger, he began binge eating. Paul fantasized about hanging himself, but instead he was committing slow suicide with food and alcohol. Yet a part of him must have wanted to live. Something propelled him to seek help and kept him showing up for appointments.

Paul was not easy to work with. Not only was his appearance offensive, but for several sessions he took obvious pleasure in insulting me. I needed to set strict boundaries on his verbal abusiveness, yet it was not my job to make him socially acceptable. Rather, my job was to help him understand why he needed to present himself in such an antisocial manner.

In order to do my job, however, I had to continually remind myself that the man before me had endured many traumas, hopefully more than I would ever experience myself. Although Paul was not my favorite client, he still deserved to be treated with dignity and respect.

At our second session, I assured Paul that I was used to angry people and that his anger would not scare me or cause me to abandon him. However, if he could begin to get at the hurt and grief behind the anger, he might begin to feel better. But Paul was not ready to deal with pain. All he knew was anger and bitterness. The first sessions were mainly cathartic renditions of how unfair life had been to him and how talking to therapists like me was a waste of time. His manner was not one to elicit empathy. Yet empathy was what I gave him and eventually he responded favorably.

After about two months of counseling, Paul stopped complaining and began talking about his abusive childhood and the grief he felt about losing his children and two wives. His drinking and compulsive eating abated, but did not disappear. He began to bathe and take better care of himself physically. Around the fourth month of counseling, Paul finally began to grieve. He wept for his present loneliness and for the mother he never had. He wept for the wives and children he had lost. But most of all, he wept for himself, for the ways he had abused his body. Much to my disappointment, however, after this emotional breakthrough, he decided to terminate his weekly sessions.

Initially Paul's case was difficult because he was so hostile and attacking. Also, I had no text to guide me. In lieu of one, I clung to the following principles:

- Respect clients as trauma survivors.

- Listen to them without unnecessarily challenging them or internally dismissing them as "hopeless cases" or "trouble-making malingers."

- Do not blame them for their own pain.

- Set boundaries on verbal abusiveness and other problem behaviors.

- Affirm the good in them.

- Help them set tangible, achievable goals for themselves.

- Give them hope for a better life.

- Assist them in reclaiming their lives.

If you have clients who, like Paul, present with hostility and antisocial traits, who provoke you to challenge them, or who test your patience, you may secretly wish they would move out of town or find a new therapist. As offensive as such clients might be, however, give them a chance. If you are consistent in your approach, respectful of them, yet establish clear boundaries for yourself, they may well respond.

Not only with difficult clients, but with all clients, whenever possible and appropriate, attempt to include information about trauma into your responses. You do not want to engage in a lecture or long discussion of a certain point, but repeating the definition of trauma, citing the relationship between PTSD and substance abuse, or noting that large numbers of trauma survivors tend to react or feel in certain ways helps the client normalize PTSD symptoms and provide an apppropriate framework for the symptoms.

Chapter 6

Symptom Management

One of the major goals of PTSD therapy is to restore to the survivor the sense of control and mastery that was lost as a result of the trauma. While the terms *control* and *mastery* are often assumed to refer to external objects and events, for PTSD sufferers control and mastery begin with the self—with the body, the mind, and the emotions.

The "hell" of being a trauma survivor (to quote a client) is not so much having gone through a trauma, with its attendant losses and fears, but continuing to pay for being traumatized with symptoms that make the survivor unable to plan ahead. "You never know how you are going to feel: if you are going to have a flashback, if you're going to be up all night with nightmares, if your psychosomatic rash is going to break out, if you're going to be hyper or numb, and on and on and on. People learn not to count on you, and even worse you learn not to count on yourself."

Self-control and self-mastery are seldom complete or perfect, even among nontraumatized persons under the best conditions. Who among us can claim to be in total control of his or her anger, sexuality, impatience, and anxiety at all times? With PTSD sufferers, however, especially those with severe symptoms, mastery over the self is eroded by symptoms such as intrusive thoughts, irritability, depression, and physiological hyperarousal.

Not only can such symptoms make it extremely difficult, if not impossible, to do everyday things, such as sitting through a family dinner or getting a good night's sleep, but they are stigmatizing. Few PTSD sufferers take pride in these symptoms: For most, their symptoms are a source of considerable anxiety, emotional pain, and low self-esteem. Most of the survivors I have seen, for example, do their utmost to hide their symptoms from others (sometimes even their therapist), for fear of negative judgment and rejection.

The more your clients can regain some control over their physical and psychological reactivity, the more "normal" they will feel. In essence, they will feel safe within themselves. This sense of safety then needs to be extended to the immediate environment—home, workplace, and so on. Indeed, according to Herman (1992), without this sense of safety, attempting the rest of the healing process is almost useless. Similarly, emotional catharsis is of limited utility, if in their daily lives clients cannot exert some control over their symptoms and are not taking steps to make their lives as danger-free as possible.

Symptoms vary in frequency, intensity, and duration from one client to the next. In general, the more frequent and intense the symptom, the more disruptive it is. However, this is not always the case; you will have to ask the client. A client can, for example, become habituated to a certain symptom and may have made creative adaptations so that he or she can continue to function despite its relative frequency. For another individual, the same frequency of the same symptom may make his or her vocational or personal life extremely unmanageable. For example, one survivor with insomnia may have learned to use sleeplessness to work a second job or pursue a hobby, whereas another survivor with insomnia may find sleeplessness makes working or maintaining familial relationships almost impossible.

As part of your assessment and treatment planning with the client, you need to determine which symptoms are the most painful, humiliating, or debilitating for the client. Working with the client, the symptoms can then be loosely ranked. Finally, you assist the client to bring the most problematic symptoms under increased control.

In presenting the various methods of symptom management in this chapter to clients, you can utilize the presentation technique developed by Baker and Salston (1992). They ask clients to imagine a toolbox which they can carry with them and pull out when they need it. Clients can design the toolbox any way they wish. In the box they can place the tools they learn from therapy, but also tools of their own invention. They can also discard tools which others have suggested, but which are not useful for them.

However, clients need to remember that the box contains tools, not magic wands. There might be situations where they feel as if they are going to lose control of themselves, yet the tools in their toolbox are not applicable. At such times, they can repeat a self-designed series of statements that grounds them in the here and now. For example, they could tell themselves, "I feel like I'm losing control and I am frightened. But I need to remember that it is only anxiety [fear, panic, rage, grief]. I don't have to act on these feelings. They come from the past, from when I was in danger. But now is now, not then, and I can certainly figure out something to do to calm myself down."

Clients need to understand that the therapeutic goal is increased manageability of symptoms, not their disappearance. They will not be able to erase their symptoms or achieve total control over them. Rather, what the healing process can promise is a reduction in the frequency and intensity of symptoms. Some symptoms may diminish to the point of being negligible, but the timetable for this degree of healing is unknown. The more severe the trauma and the greater the number of secondary wounding experiences or other revictimizations, the smaller the support system and other resources, the more time that will be required to achieve this level of healing.

This chapter will provide you with some interventions that can prove useful in helping clients manage some of their most problematic symptoms, such as anger, flashbacks, and insomnia. The interventions are not cures but suggestions that have the potential to increase client control over these problems.

Self-Care and Safety

PTSD symptoms can only be regulated under conditions of relative safety (both in the therapy session and in the outside world). The threat or presence of danger in the present will exacerbate trauma-related symptoms because a major condition of the original trauma—fear of injury or death—continues to exist. Thus clients need to ensure their self-care and safety to lay the groundwork for coping with trigger situations, anger, flashbacks, and other PTSD and related symptoms. Chapter 5 provides guidelines on creating a safe environment for the client in your sessions. The following sections focus on creating physical safety with respect to the client's self and external world.

Physical Self-Care

Self-care has physical, emotional, and, for some clients, spiritual dimensions. Many trauma survivors, especially family abuse survivors and others who have endured long-term or severe trauma, neglect their physical selves. Indeed, neglect can be considered a form of self-mutilation (Calof 1992). As part of your work with the client then, you need to identify those areas in which the client is not attending to needs for nutrition, rest, recreation, and care of medical problems. In particular, crisis work with trauma survivors involves encouraging them to seek medical attention for any injuries sustained during the trauma and to follow through on that advice.

Some areas of lack of self-care may predate the trauma; other areas needing self-care may be the result of the trauma. In either case, you need to determine whether any lack of self-care is the result of ignorance, low self-esteem, survivor guilt, or some other psychological issue. Some clients, for example, simply need to be made aware that one of their behaviors or physical ailments is a problem and to be directed to proper sources of help. Others are well aware of their problem areas, but refuse to take appropriate action due to survivor guilt or some other problem. As mental health professionals, we are called upon first and foremost to preserve life and to do no harm. If a client has a medical problem we feel needs attention, we are obligated to inform the client that she or he needs a medical consultation.

Be on the lookout for trauma-related medical problems that clients refuse either to acknowledge or to bring to a physician's attention as part of their general denial of the trauma. For example, Jerry C. had hand tremors, which he related to "nerves." He refused to see a physician about the tremors, even though they severely limited his vocational options and affected his social life. The tremors began after a severe industrial accident, which was followed by the murder of a family member. Yet he declined the invitation to talk about the accident or the murder. For Jerry to go to a doctor would mean facing the reality of his hand tremors, which would mean facing the reality of the losses brought about by the trauma.

Conversely, some clients are preoccupied with their medical problems. When this is the case, you need to explore with them the real costs of the problem—the financial costs involved and so on. This line of inquiry should not be misinterpreted by clients as your suggesting that they overestimate the effect of the medical problem. Rather your questions should reflect a genuine effort to obtain a fuller picture of the client's life.

Using this framework, you may also want to explore any symbolic meaning attached to the medical problem and other ways it may have special significance.

For example, some incest survivors who were abused before the age of five or six have underdeveloped or overdeveloped (shrunken or enlarged) genitalia. Lack of development can be seen as a "fear" of growing up, perhaps to be further abused; whereas overdevelopment may have occurred due to all the sexual stimulation received. Either way, the significance of the problem to the client needs to be explored. In addition, the client's medical problem may have other kinds of psychological meaning unique to the client.

For instance, Mike S., a child abuse survivor, developed hypoglycemia as a result of chronic stress. Hypoglycemia is a relatively emotionally neutral condition. However, in Mike's family of origin, his father (the abuser) frequently mocked a homosexual relative who had hypoglycemia. Therefore, for Mike, having acquired hypoglycemia was hardly an emotionally neutral problem. For him to admit that he had the condition and seek help for it was tantamount to admitting he was a homosexual (which he was not) and earning his father's intense disapproval and ridicule, which he associated with being beaten.

For other clients, focusing on their medical problems is a way to avoid dealing with the emotional aftermath of the trauma.

We cannot force a client to seek medical help. However, we can repeat the suggestion that medical attention is needed, as well as explore the reasons for the client not seeking help. Sometimes when the reasons for not seeking help are discussed, the client becomes more willing to see a physician.

Loretta T., for example, suffered from extreme headaches, which suggested that she needed to see a neurologist. Three times she agreed to at least talk to her general practitioner about her headaches, but each time she failed to follow through. I was careful not to sound angry, blaming, or scolding, when I asked Loretta what the difficulty was.

She burst into tears. She was afraid that the headaches meant she had problems with her eyes, and she confessed that in fact at times her vision became blurred and she could barely see. She secretly feared she was going blind and that if that was the case, she would be unable to pursue her career in music. Yet music was her only solace. She feared she would be unable to bear the memories of her trauma and would lose her mind if she couldn't continue to compose and play with her small band. She was afraid going to see a physician would prove her fears a reality.

I empathized with her dilemma. Her emotional pain was difficult enough to bear now. Without music, her suffering would be almost intolerable. "That's right. I won't be able to stand it and I'll have to kill myself," she blurted out.

It was then time to bring Loretta out of the world of fear and imagined future catastrophes and back to the reality of concrete options. "You are so scared, aren't you? I'd be scared too, if my eyesight became blurry. But I'd be more scared if I didn't know what was wrong with my eyes. Blurry vision doesn't necessarily mean imminent blindness, just as having an irregular heartbeat doesn't mean it's time to plan the funeral.

"You may have a serious vision problem, but right now, we don't have enough information to support that fear. In the first place, your headaches may or may not be related to your vision problems. In the second place, your vision problems remain undiagnosed. Since I am not a physician, I can't even make a guess as to what the problem is. However, I know that every vision problem doesn't automatically lead to blindness and that the longer you let a problem go by unattended, the greater the probability it will get worse.

"Right now, by not seeing a doctor, you are out of control of the situation. If you see a doctor, you may have a minor problem, in which case you have very little to worry about, and you will eliminate all the anxiety you are suffering now about what the problem is.

"On the other hand, if your fears are true, and you do have a serious problem, there may be things you can do to help yourself. But if you don't see a doctor, you won't be able to do anything to arrest the problem. Of course, there is always the horrible possibility that you are going blind, and that there is nothing you or medical science can do about it, but that's only one possibility, and for now you don't know that this is the case. As it stands, you are giving up all your chances to do something to help yourself, and maybe save your eyes, by refusing to go. Even if the worst is true, some aspects of music don't require sight. There may also be aids for blind musicians of which you and I are unaware, but which could be sought out."

Note: It is important that you document your efforts to encourage the client to obtain needed medical treatment, in case an illness, injury, or death occurs as a result of physical self-neglect. You do not want to be blamed (or sued) by relatives or others for not advising or encouraging the client to seek medical help when it was so obviously necessary. If the client is seeing a physician or psychiatrist, obtain permission from the client to speak to these professionals and be appraised of the client's physical problems and progress.

Creating a Safe External Environment

As with medical problems or other self-neglect, if a client is living in an unsafe environment, it needs to be pointed out. Safety includes not only taking precautions to minimize being a victim of crime, but safety in terms of obtaining and maintaining financial security. However, if the client is still in an abusive household, such safety may be impossible to create. At any moment, the client may be injured or even killed.

With such clients, legal remedies such as restraining orders, need to be explored. Sessions need to be arranged with a local abused-persons center so that the legal and other options available are known to the client. However, do not expect that legal and police remedies will necessarily solve the problem. For example, in some areas, abusive men who harass or beat their former girlfriends or wives cannot be arrested unless a police officer witnesses the harassment or abuse. Such laws offer only minimal protection to abused women.

Men can also be battered. For abused persons still living with the abuser, regardless of their sex, it is necessary to formulate an emergency escape plan. For example, the client needs to be aware of available shelters and other assistance, have a car (and its keys) or other means of transportation available, as well as a suitcase, some cash, and other necessities for a quick getaway.

If you equate this escape plan with a separation or divorce, your client may not accept it, because typically abused women want to preserve the relationship, only without the violence (Walker 1979). Instead, the plan should be presented as a temporary measure designed to ensure safety for all. Battering victims can be persuaded of the necessity for such a plan by making a statement such as, "Hopefully, you will never need to run for your life. However, if you feel the situation is becoming dangerous, leave immediately. Trust your intuition. After all this time, you can sense when he might explode.

"Don't wait to be 100-percent sure that a beating or some other horrible incident will take place—it's better to be safe than sorry. Leave when you become frightened. Remember, this does not mean you are leaving him for good. You need to tell him that also: that you are leaving to stay safe.

"Leaving temporarily instead of being beaten just means you are keeping yourself safe so that he can continue to have a partner, your children a mother, and you yourself. You are also doing him a favor, because if he hurts you he may be arrested or he may feel so bad about his behavior that he may hurt himself. By keeping yourself safe, you are not only helping yourself, you are helping everyone in the family, including him."

The emergency plan should go into effect if the client feels her life is being threatened or if violent threats are made. If she has children, they need to be made aware of the plan also.

In general, clients are helped in creating a safer world first by identifying the areas in which they can exert more control toward their own betterment, and second, by identifying and trying to find ways of overcoming obstacles to achieving this control. For example, money may be an issue, in which case you might want to explore possible assistance through social services, crime victim's assistance programs, and so on.

In some cases, however, outside money will not be available, and a client may have to greatly change her or his living situation in order to create a safer environment. For example, an abused woman, child, or elderly person will have to move away from the abuser and accept a reduced standard of living. Or such an individual may need to sacrifice other aspects of the financial support of the abuser, for example, funds for college, medical bills, art lessons, in return for freedom from abuse. In such cases, you can support the choices of your clients when they are life-preserving and ego-enhancing.

To help create an emotionally supportive environment, the client's significant others and family members could be brought in for consultation—but only if these individuals, in the client's view, can truly be supportive. Family members and friends can learn about PTSD and voice concerns about their relationship with the trauma survivor.

In addition, you may want to review with your clients their current support system (or lack thereof) and help them either develop or expand the number of people in their life to whom they can turn for emotional support. In some situations, for example, twelve-step programs and certain kinds of therapy groups, clients also have the opportunity to return that support, which is empowering in itself.

Trigger Reactions

As explained in chapter 3, PTSD is not only a psychological phenomenon but a biochemical one. The human brain remembers everything; its memory cells store information about every event that occurs to a person, especially unusual events such as traumas. The physiological response to trauma and secondary wounding experiences causes the senses to be particularly alert. Consequently, these experiences tend to make a greater impact on the brain and are stored in the memory tracts more vividly and deeply than ordinary events. In addition, traumatic incidents can be stored in unconscious or subconscious memories as a protective mechanism.

Perhaps one of the worst parts of being a trauma survivor occurs when the adrenals are aroused by an event in the present that reminds the survivor of a past event. Long-term memory tracts, in which memories of the traumatic event and secondary wounding experiences are stored, tend to be activated, and the survivor then experiences feelings associated with the past event. These present-day events are often called triggers, because they trigger the emotions associated with the trauma. Even if the client does not recall the traumatic event when confronted with an individual, object, smell, or situation that is reminiscent of the trauma, the feelings and physiological reactions attendant to the trauma may be resurrected.

The results of triggers include increased nightmares, flashbacks, anxiety, rage reactions, and other PTSD symptoms. Because the brain does not know the difference between a real threat and one stored in the mind, when the adrenals are set off by a trigger, clients may feel as angry, threatened or confused as they did during or after the original event.

Triggers can work with conscious, unconscious, or semiconscious memories. For example, in situations of family violence, even if their abuser is dead and their memories of the abuse are hazy, abuse survivors can have increased PTSD symptoms in response to being in a room similar to the room in which they were abused (for example, in shape and color) or in response to other reminders of the abuse (for example, the kind of food they were made to prepare after being injured). Reactions to these triggers can be intense, even though the triggers do not pose any real threat in the present.

It is sufficiently painful and distressing for clients to respond to triggers with emotions and symptoms that are uncomfortable or create problems. If clients are also unaware of their triggers, and thus do not understand their reactions, they can become bewildered or even frightened by their responses. Since they do not understand why they have so rapidly become angry, numb, disoriented, paranoid, hyperaroused, or defensive, they can easily conclude that they are "abnormal," "crazy," "weird," or "psycho."

During the trauma, they could not control their situation. Now, away from the trauma, they once again have that feeling of being not in control—this time of themselves. Not feeling safe within oneself is a frightening experience. Therapy can help clients identify their triggers and anticipate some of their reactions to these triggers. Clients can then take steps toward modifying their reactions to the triggers and, over time, build a new "history" in their brain. For example, a client who was carjacked may forever automatically react with fear, hyperalertness, and other PTSD symptoms to men who resemble the carjacker; however she can learn not to respond to her automatic reaction and instead to process and modulate it so that she feels more in control of herself.

Recognizing Triggers

Anniversary dates, people, places, objects, and even emotional situations that remind the survivor of the original trauma can serve as triggers. Combat veterans, for example, may experience increased PTSD symptoms in months of the year during which they were engaged in heavy combat; these are called anniversary reactions. Reminders of secondary wounding experiences and present day stresses can also be triggers, even if they are not similar to the trauma—for example, an increase in work load, a financial or vocational loss, the illness or death of a family member. As van der Kolk (1988a) points out, individuals often adapt to a trauma, but traumatized individuals, especially those who were traumatized repeatedly or intensely, are forever extremely reactive to subsequent stress and loss. Furthermore, biochemical factors are involved in this hyperactivity to subsequent stress.

Nonconsequential aspects of the trauma, as well as more charged ones, can serve as triggers. For example, if a rape victim was attacked by someone who had just eaten pizza, the survivor may forever respond negatively to the smell of garlic and may be sexually nonresponsive to partners who smell of that seasoning. In addition, media presentations relevant to the client's trauma, or any kind of trauma, may serve as triggers. Simply talking to others about their trauma, or listening to others talk about theirs, can also serve as a trigger for clients.

As part of the healing process, clients will need at some point to write about, talk about, or draw pictures of the trauma. However, you need to prepare your clients for the fact that most likely they will react to such disclosure with confusion, anger, or—even more painful—a profound sadness. Even once the healing process is complete, clients may still feel that way when they share their stories. This is as it should be. Something terrible happened to them. They can learn to live with it, but they cannot, and should not, wipe it away entirely. Along with the rest of their life experiences, it makes them who they are.

The first step in helping clients cope with triggers is to help them identify their triggers. You can use the Identifying Your Triggers handout either as a homework assignment or you can work on this exercise together with the client in your session. In the former case, you would need to review it with your client face to face both before and after she or he has completed it.

As part of your assessment of the client, you wrote down descriptions of the client's traumatic experiences and any secondary wounding experiences that followed. If you used the PTSD self-assessment questionnaire in chapter 4, the client may have recorded descriptions of these events, including physical and sensory details. If you have that level of detail to work with, you and the client can now go back and identify those aspects of the trauma and secondary wounding experiences that may be serving as triggers for the client in the present. If you do not, if the client had difficulty remembering the trauma during the assessment procedure and has had difficulty remembering the trauma in subsequent sessions, you can still complete this "trigger chart" exercise now, to the degree possible. However, you will also want to return to it after some of the client's memories of the trauma and its aftermath have returned, especially after having completed some of the work outlined in chapter 8, "Uncovering the Trauma."

Note: It may or may not be advisable for clients to share their trigger chart with families and friends. If these individuals will most likely be supportive of the client, sharing the trigger chart may be an invaluable aid in improving the client's relationship with them. However, if the client anticipates, or you suspect, that the client will be mocked or the triggers trivialized, then it is best not to share the chart. Discretion will be necessary, and the client should talk with you before sharing his or her trigger chart with significant others.

Techniques for Coping with Triggers

As much as you and your clients might prefer it, the world cannot be arranged so that all trigger situations can be avoided. There simply are and will be situations reminiscent of the trauma with which trauma survivors will have to cope or else pay extremely high prices.

Indeed, some trauma survivors do choose to withdraw, rather than face, triggers and trigger situations. For example, some combat veterans live as virtual

Identifying Your Triggers

At this point you will make a "trigger chart," which can be invaluable to you first in identifying, and later in anticipating, situations in which you might react as if the trauma were recurring.

Give a piece of paper the heading "Trigger Chart" and draw three columns. Label the first column "Trigger," the second "My Reactions," and the third "Traumatic Memory," as shown in the example.

In the first column, list those times or instances when you feel the adrenaline rush to fight or run, or where you shut down or go numb—emotionally, physically, or both. Examples of triggers include smells, sights, sounds, people, or objects that remind you of the trauma or of events associated with the trauma. Anniversaries of traumatic events can also be triggers, as can current stresses, such as the following:

- Interpersonal difficulties at home or at work

- Any kind of work or emotional overload

- Financial or medical problems (including premenstrual syndrome)

- Increased crime or other problems in your neighborhood

- Witnessing or being involved in a current trauma

In your second column, indicate your reactions to each trigger situation. You may react differently in different situations. Possible responses include these:

- Anger or rage

- Isolating yourself or overworking

- Self-condemnation

- Increased cravings for food, alcohol, or drugs

- Increased flashbacks

- Self-mutilation

- Depression

- Self-hatred

- Suicidal or homicidal thoughts

- Increased physical pain (headaches, backaches)

- Activation of a chronic medical condition (such as increased blood sugar if you are diabetic, increased blood pressure if you suffer from hypertension, recurrence of urinary tract infections if you are prone to bladder problems)

In the third column, try to connect the trigger to the original traumatic event, to a secondary wounding experience, or to an event associated with these experiences. If you cannot remember the original events, do not be overly concerned. The main point of completing this chart is to help you understand and anticipate when you might be triggered. This understanding is the first step toward change and control.

Trigger Chart Examples

Trigger
Car trips, confinement in vehicles or rooms.

My Reactions
Sweating, nausea, panic, followed by intense anger. Then numbing and depression for about two days.

Traumatic Memory
When my abuser was being prosecuted, I was taken to the courthouse over and over. It was two hours from home, and when I got there they didn't believe me. It kept getting more complicated, and each time they treated me worse.

Trigger
Someone, an authority figure, tells me to do something in a disrespectful, rough, or impersonal voice.

My Reactions
Anger, desire to fight back, desire to run away instead of hitting the person or having to hide my rage.

Traumatic Memory
It reminds me of taking orders from that C.O. who sent us all out to be killed so he could look good.

Trigger
Red dresses.

My Reactions
Fear, anxiety, repulsion. If I can, I avoid people wearing red dresses. If I can't, and someone approaches me, I break into a sweat. I also start feeling guilty, as if I'm causing her to attack me.

Traumatic Memory
I was wearing a red dress when I was raped.

hermits in forested areas of our country, and some trauma survivors barely leave their homes or other "safe places." This self-imposed isolation can lead to suicidal depressions or other disorders, not to mention the misery of chronic loneliness. In such cases, what began as an attempt to feel safe resulted in a self-defeating endeavor. In cases where needed medical help has not been received due to fear of leaving home or a "safe place," or because doctors, hospitals, or medical examinations are triggers, survivors have actually died.

These examples may be extreme, but they illustrate what can happen when the anxiety aroused in anticipation of a trigger results in avoidance behavior. If one of the goals of PTSD therapy is increased reconnection to life in the present (and reduced involvement with the trauma), then your work in teaching or improving clients' coping skills in managing triggers is of supreme importance. Even if you never get to the later, more dramatic stages of healing (where the trauma is remembered, reconstructed, and so on), if you assist clients in better managing their present life, with its inevitable trigger situations, you have completed a significant piece of professional work.

One group of coping techniques consists of deep breathing and relaxation techniques, which have been used for a variety of anxiety disorders and others. These include calming breath exercises, deep breathing exercises, and any of the varieties of progressive muscle relaxation exercises typically used in relaxation or desensitization programs. Physical exercise, such as walking, aerobics, swimming, and tennis are other ways of reducing tension and anxiety surrounding trigger situations. Clients can use any of these methods before or after they confront a trigger situation or both. In some cases, these techniques can even be used during the situation.

Specific instructions for each of these coping techniques can be found in any number of books. Once you have decided on specific exercises, you may want to record the directions on an audiocassette to expedite your early practice sessions, or you may wish to obtain some of the professionally made tapes available for certain exercises, such as progressive muscle relaxation.

Note: Some such tapes are designed to be played while the listener sleeps. These tapes have not been proven to be particularly effective, nor are they helpful for clients who have trouble sleeping.

Cautions

Before using deep breathing or muscle relaxation therapies or doing any kind of imagery work, ask the client what occurs when he or she sits still or attempts to meditate. If the client states, or you suspect, that when quiet he or she becomes flooded with traumatic memories, such exercises are to be avoided at all costs. Even with clients who appear to have no such difficulties, you need to try out the relaxation or imagery technique in your office, observing their reactions and asking them for feedback before you send them out on their own with instructions to practice and use the technique.

Some kinds of trauma survivors, for example, those who have been physically or sexually abused or were injured in war, car accidents, and other such situations, may have physical limitations that preclude physical exercise or make exercise dangerous. With these clients in particular, but with any client, it is wise to have a physician's approval before any exercise program is attempted.

Other coping techniques, such as writing about the trigger, planning ahead, and asking others for help, have much less potential for backfiring and can be used in conjunction with exercise and relaxation techniques and imagery.

Planning Ahead

Your task is to work with the client to find out what works—not what *should* work according to some theory, but what actually works—to help the individual client through the particular problem situation. (Some techniques work better for some people and some triggers than for others. For example, one client may find writing about one kind of trigger extremely helpful, whereas for another person or another trigger, two hours of jogging is necessary.) The goal here is functional: for the client to be able to endure the trigger without self-injury or injury to others. Hopefully, with each attempt to face a trigger, rather than avoiding it, your client will experience increased success at managing the symptoms or emotions the trigger seems to predictably elicit. With each successful experience, your client will gain increased confidence and therefore become more able to take further risks and become increasingly involved in the present.

Planning ahead for the anticipated trigger situations is critical. Part of the planning can include the client responding to the following questions as a homework assignment, to be shared with you in a session. Or you can ask the client the following questions (Vernon and Kilpatrick 1983) in a session that by pre-agreement, is devoted to planning for the trigger event. Have the client respond to these questions:

What is it that I will have to do? (What is the situation, thing or person that I will be facing?)

How have I reacted to similar situations (things or people) in the past?

Did anything bad happen?

What is the likelihood of something bad happening again?

If something bad happens, what can I do?

How can I ask others to help me?

Who would I ask for help? Who would I not ask for assistance? (What is the situation, thing, or person that I will be facing?)

As you work on this assignment with the client, point out any gruesome or unrealistic fantasies she or he may have. One way to handle these highly improbable projections in a way that respects the client's fears is to ask the client to assign a numerical probability to these fantasies' actually occurring. In my experience, when clients are given a chance to think about this question, they realize their fears have a minimal chance of recurring.

For example, John L.'s social life was severely limited by the fact that he was afraid to go to the movies for fear there would be a fire in the movie house. John had been in a fire as a child, in which one of his parents and two cousins had died. When I asked John what he thought were the real chances of his worst fear coming true, he assigned a probability of 5 percent. Since neither of us had any data on the rates of fires in theatres, John agreed to go to the library to see if he could find any statistics on the rates of fires in movie houses and other locations.

Whenever possible, incorporate reliable information into your sessions to counteract unrealistic fears. In addition, keep reminding clients that whatever feelings or bodily sensations they have during the trigger are "okay." In fact, feelings such as dread and anxiety, and bodily sensations such as hyperalertness, are to be expected because having such reactions to a situation is what makes a trigger a trigger.

The goal is to manage the trigger event, not necessarily to enjoy it or to have no negative feelings or sensations about it. Perhaps someday a trigger situation will be emotionally and physically neutral for your client. But for now, triggers pose difficult challenges. Stress to clients that facing a trigger is hard work and takes much courage. They need to applaud themselves for continuing to try when giving up and just retreating from the situation can seem so much easier.

At all times, clients need to remember that they are going through the agony of facing a trigger situation for some important reason. Either the reason is survival, for instance to maintain a job, or the reason is to achieve a self-chosen goal, for example, increased involvement with family. Such a goal may require participation in a trigger-laden family event.

Some therapists have been known to suggest to clients that they need to endure a particular trigger event in order to "prove" that they have overcome the past and developed mastery over their PTSD. In my view, such a suggestion places unnecessary pressure on and creates unnecessary pain and anxiety for people who are already anxious and burdened enough. In fact, my usual suggestion is that, when it is possible and not too costly, clients should follow their natural inclination and avoid trigger events and situations. However, since this is not always possible, and since many clients have life goals that require managing a variety of trigger situations, clients need to learn to cope with painful trigger events. To tell clients that they need to purposely go look for a trigger situation to overcome just to prove that they are "overcomers" serves little purpose. It may also be detrimental if they find they cannot manage the trigger situation well.

On the other hand, if the client decides to prove to herself or himself that she or he can handle a certain situation just for the sake of handling it, then you, as therapist, should be supportive of the client's goal. In these situations, the idea comes from the client, not the therapist. You can, however, help clients determine if they are somehow setting themselves up for failure by trying to overcome impossible odds or taking too much on too soon. As the next section explains in more detail, it is best to start working on managing triggers by tackling the least stressful trigger first.

Working on a Trigger

You want the client's first experiences with coping with a trigger to be a success, not a failure. Therefore, it is best to begin working on triggers by selecting a trigger that the client (not you) identifies as being one of the easiest to manage. The first step in selecting a trigger to work on is to label each of the triggers listed in the client's trigger chart as belonging to one of four categories:

1. Triggers the client feels might be the easiest to endure

2. Triggers the client feels might be manageable after a few more months of healing

3. Triggers the client feels he or she might be able to confront in a few years

4. Triggers the client plans to avoid for the rest of his or her life

Have the client select a trigger from category 1 (triggers the client feels might be the easiest to endure) with which to start, then ask the client to describe in detail his or her reactions to this trigger in the past. Pay special attention to the symptoms the client reports and the specific fears he or she voices regarding the symptom. Such information will form the basis of your selection of coping methods.

After you have listened to the client's account of his or her history with the trigger, ask the client why he or she wants to face the trigger again. Why not simply avoid it? At this point clients will probably state that they want to achieve some important goal. Stress to them that it is therefore their choice to face the trigger. The agony involved in facing a trigger isn't their choice, in that they cannot control the unpleasant associations of a trigger, but going through the agony has a self-chosen purpose.

You can then work with clients on the questions listed above, under "Planning Ahead" and discuss the various coping mechanisms available, (exercise, deep breathing, and so on). Select those that suit the client and the situation.

After this preparatory work is completed and the client has actually faced the trigger situation, spend time discussing what occurred: what methods seemed more helpful than others, where progress was made, what areas need more work, and what was gained by facing the trigger.

Depending on the client's experience in coping with the trigger, you may want to stop trigger work for a while—for example, if the client reports that the experience was too stressful—or you may want to consider choosing another trigger situation to work on. Start with another trigger from category 1, the relatively easy category.

After you have attempted to work with all the triggers listed in category 1 and when the client is ready (not when you think the client should be ready), you and the client may want to tackle situations in category 2, and then in category 3.

Remember that coping with triggers is psychological, mental, and often physical work. Any kind of change, even positive change, can create a temporary increase in stress. If the client is already under considerable stress, you may want to wait to tackle the extremely difficult task of trying to overcome a trigger until the client's life is less full of pressures. Although it is important for clients to challenge themselves and not let the past inhibit their lives in the present, it is also important that clients be kind and not overtax themselves.

Anger

PTSD is formally classified as an anxiety disorder, but informally it has been called a sadness or an anger disorder. Indeed, unresolved anger and grief regarding the trauma can touch every aspect of a survivor's life, especially if the survivor has long-term or ever-present reminders of the trauma, for example, a lost or impaired limb or body function, a lost loved one, or diminished religious faith. Typically, anger surrounds the losses involved with trauma and secondary wounding experiences.

Survivors are often angry for the following reasons, among others:

- That the trauma occurred at all

- That the trauma happened to them

- That they or others were injured or that others died

- That certain secondary wounding experiences followed

- That they still bear psychological and spiritual scars, if not economic and physical scars as well

- That there is no way to erase the trauma and restore to themselves the sense of innocence, immunity from harm, and faith in the goodness of life they had prior to the trauma

- That therapy, healing, or recovery is so much work: so emotionally painful, time-consuming, financially expensive

Survivors of man-made trauma can also be angry that they, not their attacker or abuser are the ones who must undergo the time and expense of therapy and who continue to suffer deeply, not only from the emotional and physical scars of having been injured but from the scars of the coping mechanisms they employed to survive the trauma. For example, survivors who abused their bodies with food, alcohol, or drugs can bear serious financial, vocational, social, psychological, and health costs related to their addiction.

In most programs for recovering from substance abuse, it is acknowledged that there is a grieving period during which the former addict grieves the time, money, opportunities, and physical health lost to the addiction. During this grieving period there is anger at the perpetrator or situation that gave rise to the need for the addiction as a numbing or soothing agent. However, there can also be tremendous anger at the self, for becoming an addict. Even though addiction might have been life-preserving at the time of the trauma, survivors frequently disparage themselves for their dependence on a substance. Even if they do not berate themselves, others do so. Furthermore, in the case of illegal drugs, addiction may have resulted in a criminal record also, which further stigmatizes the survivor.

The angers that result from injustices associated with the trauma and secondary wounding experiences can be considered forms of righteous indignation or rage. This type of anger can lead to the angry outbursts or rage reactions that are typical in PTSD. Angry outbursts, which range from verbal tirades to the destruction of property and physical assault on others, are usually the result not only of leftover righteous anger, but of that indignation in combination with a number of other factors, including clinical depression; flashbacks, nightmares, and other reliving experiences; accumulated stress; poor self-care due to ignorance or the desire to punish oneself; and biochemical alterations due to the trauma.

In addition, clients may never have been taught how to manage minor angers in their formative years. Anger may have been taboo in their homes, or, alternatively, the expression of anger through verbal or physical abuse may have been a normal part of their family life. Such clients are hardly prepared for handling the deep angers associated with many kinds of trauma.

Anger as a Problem

Anger can pose a major impediment to the two major goals of PTSD therapy; empowerment and reconnection with others and with society (Herman 1992). The sad truth is that trauma-related anger, acknowledged or unacknowledged, expressed or unexpressed, can color every aspect of clients' lives: their work or school performance, their daily habits, and most of all, their self-esteem and relationships with others. Anything that might prove frustrating will have the additional charge of unresolved anger related to the trauma. This can result in the client experiencing the old familiar feelings of being out of control, and the attendant fears and anxiety. Clients are often aware that their responses are out of proportion to the current situation, which only serves to decrease their perhaps already damaged self-esteem and sense of intrapsychic safety.

If clients are in touch with their anger, and vent it indiscriminately, they often alienate others: intimates, family members, social acquaintances, coworkers, employers, and so forth. Given survivors' history of trauma, the intensity of their reactions is perfectly understandable. But most of the world is not understanding of, and shuns or avoids, angry people. Even those individuals who care deeply about the survivor, even those who have taken the time and trouble to learn about PTSD, can be taxed almost to the breaking point by the irritability, rage reactions, and many other forms of anger experienced by the trauma survivor.

On the other hand, if clients are not in touch with their anger, and they turn their anger inward on themselves, they may suffer from depression, psychosomatic pains, or self-mutilating behavior (including substance abuse). Such clients may also alienate others, but for different reasons than the vocally angry client. When people are depressed, self-abusive, addicted, or in chronic pain, they may be seen as weak, needy or deficient by others or may be otherwise stigmatized. In addition, conditions such as depression and addiction can pose formidable handicaps for survivors in terms of acting toward achieving their goals. Some even feel as if they are not entitled to have goals.

Clients who are vocal about their anger may be difficult to tolerate at times. Yet at least they know they are angry, and, having experienced the fears associated with being out of control of their anger (which may be the reason they sought your help in the first place), they may be eager to learn anger management methods and ways of channelling their anger in constructive ways.

On the other hand, clients who are unaware of their anger, or who minimize it or turn it inward on themselves, need help first in unearthing their anger and then in managing and directing it. Even before they uncover their anger, however, such clients may need to be taught, or at least made aware of, anger management techniques. One reason some of these clients keep their anger suppressed is they fear that once it emerges it will be too volatile to be handled. Thus, you need to assure clients that, with your help, they can deal with their anger in doses, rather than all of it at once, and that there are ways of containing anger so that it does not become explosive. Explaining this, and then showing them how it can be done, often helps clients begin to own and gradually unleash the anger that may have stymied their growth for years. Keep in mind, however, that the therapeutic task of helping clients who have spent years denying their anger (or expressing it indirectly through depression, psychosomatic pains, or self-mutilation) to finally own that anger, can be tediously slow and may require much skill and patience on your part.

As a result of the healing process, some clients will be able to divest themselves of much of their trauma-related anger. Some clients will not be so fortunate; the healing process may help them understand their anger, and perhaps even reduce it to one degree or another, but, for whatever reasons, for certain trauma survivors the anger never really dies.

All survivors will need anger management skills at one point or another during the healing process. However, for that unknown percentage of trauma survivors for whom trauma-related anger may remain a life-long problem, these skills may mean survival. If they cannot control their anger at work, they may lose their job—and with that job, their life structure, their role in society, their family, their home, and their dignity. If they cannot control their anger in relationships, they may lose the love, affection, and respect of others—all of which are critical to healing the wounds left by the trauma.

Heading Off Anger

Trauma-related anger can be exacerbated by present stresses and lack of self-care. You need to inform your clients of these points and determine which life stresses, if any, are contributing to your client's anger. You might say something like the following:

> As a trauma survivor, your rage may become so intense that you feel like you are going to explode. You need to take that feeling seriously.
>
> It is not unheard of for trauma survivors, especially child abuse survivors and combat veterans, to lash out and seriously hurt themselves or others. Murders, suicides, self-mutilations, and substance abuse binges (which often set the stage for murder and suicide) can occur when a survivor reaches the point of feeling "I'm so angry I can't stand it anymore."
>
> If you find yourself at the explosion point frequently, you need to examine your life carefully. Are some of your basic needs not being met? You may be overextending yourself in one or more areas of your life. Is there any possibility that as a result of the trauma you have developed a self-denying or self-punitive lifestyle? Are you, to any extent, overcompensating for low self-esteem born of trauma or of trauma-related self-blame or survivor guilt by trying too hard or giving too much at work or at home?
>
> Has overcompensating or overworking in one or more areas of your life resulted in emotional deprivation or other unfulfilled needs? Given that anger can be a means of reducing stress, is your anger a coping mechanism for the pressures of your life? Are there any ways to reduce those pressures so that you are less stressed and as a result less angry?
>
> Frequent explosions or near explosions suggest one of three possibilities: either you are in a situation of great stress or you have a nonfunctional lifestyle or you have considerable unresolved anger regarding the past. If one or more of these is the case with you, then you need to give yourself the support necessary to deal with these issues.

Present anger may be the result of ongoing victimization. Depending on the nature of the victimization being experienced by the client, the client or you may need to contact authorities, lobby for legal changes, organize support groups and other efforts with similar survivors, or in some other effective way, fight back.

Substance abuse can also exacerbate anger. This includes not only alcohol and other commonly abused drugs but also, if to a lesser extent, nicotine, caffeine, and even sugar. Alcohol produces a temporary high, which is usually followed by a period of irritability. Similarly, nicotine and caffeine often function as stimulants, but only temporarily. Eventually, these substances lead to a "downer" fraught with irritability.

As part of their self-care, encourage your clients to pursue hobbies and leisure activities they find enjoyable and to develop new interests. If you are using a plan that incorporates "working breaks" from trauma work, you might want to use one of these sessions to discuss ways the client could reduce stress and enjoy life more. For many clients (and others) enjoying oneself is a neglected skill.

Preparing Clients for Anger Management Work

In preparing clients for anger management work, you need to make certain that clients can distinguish the feeling of being angry from angry acts. You cannot stress the following enough to your clients that:

- They have a right to be angry.

- Feeling angry does not need to lead to acts of aggression.

- Anger is a normal, human emotion which, although it can be acted on destructively, is often instructive in that it can in many instances (not all) be a signal that they are not living in ways that meet their basic needs. (Some of these needs may be physical, others psychological. For example, common causes of anger are inadequate sleep and poor nutrition.)

Clients also need to be told that although they have a right to be angry, their task is to deal with their anger nondestructively and hopefully to eventually channel their anger in positive directions.

You also need to take a history of how clients have handled anger in the past and how anger was handled in their family of origin, their present family, and other significant people in their lives. Clients may have erroneous assumptions about anger or have received contradictory messages about anger. For example, clients may have been told that if they expressed anger they would be punished by God or beaten by their fathers. On the other hand, male clients may have been told that not acting aggressively on their anger would show they were "sissy" or homosexual. In contrast, female clients may have been told that merely expressing anger would indicate that they were unfeminine and would make them undesirable to men.

First, clients need to explore their fears and attitudes about having anger, and then those about expressing anger, before anger management work can begin. Your role will be to collect inaccurate attitudes toward anger and to point out the variety of nondestructive ways of expressing anger that are available to them. Clients who come from violent families can be reinforced for breaking the chain of violence, which may otherwise have extended for several generations.

You also need to make it clear that anger management is not the same as eliminating, reducing, or getting at the roots of chronic anger. Rather, anger management techniques are simply means of controlling anger so that whatever situation they are in becomes manageable.

For example, Andrea had a problem being kept waiting. As a child, her alcoholic parents often left her waiting places because they had simply forgotten her or to punish her for some alleged misbehavior. Often they were inebriated when they picked her up and beat her upon their return home. Obviously, for Andrea, being kept waiting was closely associated with being abandoned and physically abused.

Before coming to therapy, Andrea used to feel depressed, even suicidal, when she was kept waiting, especially if the person she was waiting for was emotionally important to her. Thanks to several years of counseling, Andrea came to own her anger. But she then began to fly into rages when kept waiting.

Rages, however, are not appropriate reactions to being kept waiting ten or fifteen minutes by a business associate, a child, or a friend. For example, Andrea once broke all the pencils on a receptionist's desk and smashed mirrors in the ladies' room while waiting for an important business associate. Another time Andrea threw a vacuum cleaner at her ten-year-old son because he was late. She also tore up a blouse given to her by a friend when that friend was late for a movie date.

Andrea was deeply ashamed of her behavior, but felt she "couldn't help it." Andrea hated her anger and wished to purge herself of it, but wishing that her anger would go away did not make it so. She lived in fear of her anger and went to great lengths to avoid situations she felt might ignite her rage. But it was impossible for her to arrange her life to avoid all triggers, and when her anger would inevitably rise to the surface, she would feel helpless and out of control of herself. At times, she felt suicidal, because her rage at being kept waiting (or in response to other triggers) was now compounded by her anger at herself for reacting with rage.

Some of the anger management techniques described below helped Andrea control her anger so that she did not endanger her business and other endeavors and her family relationships. However, healing the root of her rage required grieving—for the childhood and parental protection and nurturance she had been denied (grieving is discussed in chapter 9). The more Andrea grieved, the more her anger changed in quality. She still became angry when kept waiting or when encountering other triggers associated with her past, but her anger was subdued by a deep sadness for all that she had endured and lost.

At times, she still becomes enraged, but only for a moment, for she knows that underneath the rage are losses no angry outburst can cure. In therapy she has learned not only to respect her losses by grieving for them but to value herself enough to set goals. She knows that she was "robbed" or "cheated" in the past in many ways. However, she is determined not to let her anger about her past rob her of what is available to her in the present.

The following sections present ways of managing anger that are potentially useful for clients who become so angry that they fear they might "explode" or who have actually exploded and lashed out at property, pets, people, or their own bodies. The following suggestions, however, are just that: suggestions. Some will be more helpful than others. You may want to expose the client to several of these methods and then, together with the client, decide which methods might be helpful. The client would then use only the methods that work for him or her and disregard the rest.

Cautions

If a client suffers from clinical depression, chemical imbalances, or severe homicidal or suicidal thoughts or tendencies, the anger management suggestions offered here are insufficient. Additional help, for example, medication, psychiatric care, or inpatient hospitalization, may be needed.

Venting

Do not advise your clients to vent their anger indiscriminately. Releasing the full force of their anger toward people who are the object of their rage, or toward others just because they happen to be around, will seldom bring about better communication or help your clients obtain their desired goals (unless one of their goals is to alienate certain people). In most cases, when people hear or see an angry person, they hear the anger rather than what the person is saying. They also often become frightened or defensive and may tend to "tune out" or disparage the client.

Unrestrained venting is best saved for the client's therapist, therapy group members, twelve-step program friends, and others who can tolerate intense feelings. Warn your clients that venting with people other than these can lead to escalating verbal or physical fights. Displays of anger rarely bring about long-term solutions to problems, especially in the area of relationships, including work relationships.

"The boundaries for safe and legitimate anger are simple," writes Carol Staudacher (1987):

> First your anger should not be directed at someone who will predictably retaliate with greater anger and aggression. You will only escalate your own frustration and anger when you try to defend yourself. This does not mean (you should) pick on people who can't defend themselves. It means ... don't inflate the cause for your anger by antagonizing someone who may use verbal or physical tactics which will intensify your rage and anguish.
>
> Second, your accusations or revelations should not be directed toward someone who could suffer unjustly from them. That is, it would not be appropriate to be accusatory toward your mate who was driving the car in which your child was killed. It would, however, be appropriate to focus and channel your anger toward a judicial system which allowed your daughter's assailant to be released from prison.
>
> In summary, nothing is gained by exerting anger which has at its base cruelty, or by publicly venting anger which could provoke cruelty toward yourself.

Staudacher goes on to suggest two questions you might want to ask your clients:

> Is your anger lending you energy or taking it away?
>
> Are you using your anger, or it is using you?

If clients need to vent, screaming or yelling alone, at home or in a car, will harm no one. In addition, there are other ways of venting, for example, talking to someone uninvolved about their anger (rather than directing the anger at the person), writing about their anger, speaking the anger into a tape recorder, or drawing a picture about the anger are other ways of venting. Afterwards, the client can throw away the writing or picture or erase the tape. Clients who have a higher power or being to whom they pray can tell that entity how angry they are.

Clients can also use musical instruments or pots and pans to make noise, hit pillows, stomp their feet, push against walls, cut or tear up telephone books, or engage in physical exercise. In general, it is not wise to advise clients to hit a punching bag or anything resembling a person. Injuring pets, going hunting, or injuring or killing other living things, even plants, is not encouraged.

Some clients find that muscle relaxation, deep breathing, and other soothing practices, for example, sitting in a sauna or hot tub, helps to dissipate their anger. For others these methods may release suicidal, homicidal, sadistic, or other aggressive fantasies or otherwise make clients frightened. Advise clients that if these or any other anger management technique causes such a reaction, they should stop the technique and find a supportive person to talk to, such as yourself, a twelve-step program member, or a caring friend. If necessary, the client could also go to the emergency room of a nearby hospital.

Taking Time Out

Time-outs are another effective way to manage anger, if they are structured and executed properly (McKay, Rogers, and McKay 1989; Deschner 1984). Directions to clients for managing anger through time-outs are provided in the Time-out Guidelines handout. You will want to familiarize yourself with these guidelines as well.

Looking at Anger Objectively

Another technique that may be helpful to clients in managing their anger is to keep an "anger diary," noting the people, places, and situations that make them angry in the present. Then, in your sessions you and the client can examine those entries. You can ask them the following questions:

What was it that really made you mad?

Were there any other feelings present besides anger? For example, were you also sad, lonely, disappointed, fatigued, or stressed-out by your job?

Which angry episodes are related, to one degree or another, to the trauma or your secondary wounding experiences?

Are there any positive actions you can take to meet your needs or stand up for yourself?

After a while, clients could also begin writing answers to these questions in their anger diary on their own.

When Anger Hurts (McKay, Rogers, and McKay 1989) offers additional information about anger and anger management techniques. A wide variety of topics are covered. There are also many practical suggestions and exercises for handling anger-provoking situations, including handling angry, irrational people.

Case Example

The case of Roy C. illustrates the connection of anger and grief, the use of anger as a defense of grief, and the adrenaline surges and catecholamine depletions that lead to aggressive acts in some clients.

Time-out Guidelines

Imagine the intensity of your anger as ranging from 0 to 10, with no anger being 0, mild irritation, 2, and near-murderous rage, 10. The midpoint of the scale, 5, is where adrenaline tends to take over and you can no longer think. It may take only a few undesirable occurrences or frustrations before you find yourself hovering at that dangerous 9 or 10 level on the scale, ready to snap.

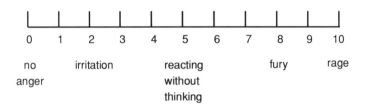

You can save yourself (and others) considerable heartache if you can catch yourself before you reach the danger point. Using these guidelines, you can learn to monitor your anger level. If you can deal with your angry feelings at the lower levels—for example, at 2 or 3, or at least before you reach the midpoint of the scale—you may be able to diffuse it. Once you reach levels of 5 and above, however, you are approaching the brink. When you become that angry, you lose the capacity to listen to others or to your rational self.

One way to arrest your anger before it reaches the danger point is through "time-outs." When you're really angry it is difficult to think rationally. At such times, consider calling a time-out. Leave the room or the immediate situation and do something else, preferably something physical such as walking or other exercise. Wait until the intense anger has subsided before you take action on the situation at hand. Give yourself whatever time you need to center yourself. Once you have centered yourself, you will be able to think about your goal in the situation before you decide on a plan of action.

If you live with other people, it is best to let them know in advance about your possible need for time-outs or any other strategy you might have for coping with your anger. For example, you could say something like the following:

> I have a problem with anger. Sometimes I become so angry I can't think rationally. My anger level is so high I'm afraid I'll say or do something I don't mean. When this happens, I need some time to myself to calm down.
>
> I need your help for this. What I plan to do is to take a time-out. I'll simply leave the room and go off by myself to do whatever I need to bring down my anger level. If I walk away from you, it doesn't mean I'm rejecting you or refusing to deal

with whatever issue we are talking about. It just means I can't handle it at that moment.

You are not the problem. My anger is the problem. I'm trying to cope with it as best I can. But I do know that if I try to talk with you when I'm overflowing with anger, my anger will make our discussion totally unproductive. If you ever need a time-out, you can take one too.

Some trauma survivors have an "anger room" in their home. No one else is allowed in this room. This room is theirs. There they can write, rest, read, relax, or do whatever they need to do to calm themselves. In this room, they can be assured of privacy in order to deal with their anger the best they can. The following was the experience of Betty, the wife of a child abuse survivor:

At first I objected to Tom's anger room. Why should he have a whole room for himself in our little house, when I didn't even have a desk for myself? When he told me he didn't ever want me in that room, I nearly hit the roof. After all, it was my house too. Then he bought weights and an exercise bike, and I was furious. They seemed like unnecessary expenses.

I couldn't understand why he still had all that anger. After all, he'd been in counseling for over two years, talking about being abused until he was blue in the face. He was angry when he started counseling, but the counseling only made him angrier. I was angry that I had to deal with his anger and that it wasn't going to go away overnight. But finally I just had to accept that Tom had this mountain of anger inside of him and there was nothing I could do about it.

Sometimes he would go into his anger room for hours at a time, lifting weights. I resented the time it took away from the family, but obviously Tom needed that room. He spent less time with the family, but when he was with us, he was really with us, not trying to fight his anger. Before, he'd try to be calm, but he wasn't. Even the children could tell that he was trying hard not to erupt into a tirade.

Now when Tom goes in his anger room, I'm glad. Better that the weights get his rage than that he vent it on me or one of the children.

Calling a Time-out

To announce a time-out to your partner, spouse, family member, friend, or whomever, you could say, "I'm getting angry, so angry I can't think straight. I'd like to call a time-out." However, sometimes telling someone you are angry is a trigger for *their* defensiveness or retaliatory anger. Because of this, it is suggested that you and your family member or friend develop a nonverbal means of communicating the need for a time-out. For example, a letter "T" could be made with the hands to signal the need for a time-out.

You need to take responsibility for your own anger and behavior—but not for the other person's. Even if he or she is obviously angry, refrain from saying, "You're so angry, we need a time-out" or "If you keep that up, I'm going to burst." Make any statements in terms of "I." Better yet, wait until after the time-out has cooled your temper and you have had a chance to think before you make *any* statements.

Timing Time-outs

You and your partner need to agree on a duration for the time-out in advance. Generally an hour to an hour and a half is recommended. If you don't agree on a time span in advance, then the time-out can easily be interpreted by the other person as a personal rejection, as your way of not dealing with the problem at hand, or as some other form of escapism. You need to show up at the agreed time and tell your partner whether you are willing or able to talk about the issues at hand. Similarly, the person who is left behind should also be there and not try to escape the situation by being somewhere else at the scheduled reunion time.

During the Time-out

During the time-out, you can do whatever you've decided upon with your therapist. Most likely some of the alternatives discussed in session include doing something physical to reduce your bodily tension. For example, you could take a walk, go running, or take a hot bath. You might also find relief in writing down your thoughts or sharing them with a friend. Or you might want to practice relaxation exercises if you find these helpful.

Do *not* drive, drink, drug, or binge eat. Also, try not to use the hour to make a list of everything that is "wrong" with the other person. Focus on calming yourself, using the methods that work for you, whether it's jogging or lying in bed.

Practicing Time-outs

You may want to practice time-outs when you aren't angry. You may also want to make a contract with your partner regarding time-outs. The following form is a suggestion.

Sabotaging Time-outs

Time-outs can become a weapon, rather than a peace-keeping tool. If you don't come back when you agreed you would, if you consistently use time-outs to avoid dealing with painful or difficult problems, or if you return from time-outs so inebriated or high that you cannot spend time talking with your partner, you will not be achieving the purposes of a time-out. You will only be further alienating your partner and exacerbating the situation, thus defeating the purpose of the time-out.

Time-out Contract

When I realize that my or my partner's anger is rising, I will give a "T" signal for a time-out and leave at once. I will not hit or kick anything, and I will not slam the door. I will return after no longer than (one hour or whatever time is agreed to). I will exercise to use up the anger energy, and I will not drink or use drugs while I am away. I will try not to focus on resentments.

If my partner gives a "T" signal and leaves, I will return the sign and let my partner go without a hassle, no matter what is going on. I will not drink or use drugs while my partner is away, and I will avoid focusing on resentments.

When my partner and I meet at the agreed-on-time, I will share with my partner what I was able to understand during the time-out about the causes of my anger, which will most likely include that I either was expecting too much, had not communicated clearly enough, was upset by matters outside our relationship, or was tired, hungry, or feeling ill.

I will also need to "own" (admit to) my error in responding with anger to my partner for situations in the world or the negative state of my physical or emotional health, which were not related to my partner's behavior or attitude.

On the other hand, if my partner did disappoint me, mislead me, mistreat me, or in some other way act in a manner that would anger almost anyone in a similar situation (or which in the past has almost always elicited my anger), then I need to share this observation with my partner as well.

Basically, I need to say, "My contributions to our conflict are . . . yet, in my view, you contributed by . . ."

Name _____   Date _____

Name _____   Date _____

Roy, a combat veteran, becomes extremely agitated if he spots dead animals in the road; they remind him too much of the dead children he saw during his war. At times the bloodied animals fill him with such grief that he must pull his car over to the side of the road.

But he never cries. Instead he becomes so filled with rage, he wants to smash his car into the cars which seem to glide over the dead animals so blithely. On occasion he has done so, and has assaulted the drivers who ran over the animals.

Roy is a multiple-trauma survivor. He is not only a combat veteran, but a veteran of ten years of extensive child abuse and three muggings, during which he was also severely beaten. His anger in the past, fueled by adrenaline reactions, military training, and his life as an abused child, has resulted in his serving several prison terms. He hates his rage, for it has left him a lonely man. But he feels that at times it is difficult, if not impossible, to control it.

When he says, "I can't help it," he is probably not a character-disordered sociopath trying to make excuses for his antisocial behavior. Rather he may be observing a truth about himself. He is in the high-risk category for having neurotransmitter irregularities, with consequent difficulty in modulating his emotions. In addition, given his background as an abused child and in the military, he had no role models for expressing anger nondestructively.

If you have a client, male or female, like Roy, you may wonder whether the client is "conning" you when he or she states that his or her rage reactions are involuntary and uncontrollable or is the unhappy result of inadequate training in anger and anger management, combined with the biochemical effects of prolonged or severe untreated trauma. One way to determine the client's sincerity is to observe the client's behavior and his attitude toward his behavior.

Roy, for example, often cancels appointments, social engagements, and any other activity that requires him to leave his home when he feels in a vulnerable state and senses that he might "go bezerk" if he encounters a trigger. His fears of losing control are so real and so strong, even he has canceled out of those few events that bring him joy. Consequently, his spotty therapy attendance record cannot be interpreted as resistance to therapy in the psychoanalytic sense, nor can it be seen as an unwillingness to be healed.

Roy is deeply ashamed of his proclivity for rageful outbursts. He does not boast about them as would a character-disordered client, for example Roy would like nothing more than to be able to drive a car, attend family and social events, keep appointments, and go about his life without fearing his aggression. But although medication has helped Roy to some degree, he still suffers. Consequently, there are still many times he stays in his home to keep others safe.

Because of this behavior, Roy's statements about the uncontrollable nature of his rage are much more believable than statements made by clients who make few, if any, efforts to protect others from their rage (and themselves from triggers), and who refuse to even consider a psychiatric consultation for medication.

Counseling Roy presents a challenge, because it is difficult to offer him hope that someday he will be able to lead a "normal life." The truth is that because he has suffered so much trauma for so long, beginning at such a young age, he may be psychologically and biologically altered in such a way that many of his symptoms will remain with him forever. Unfortunately, his activities and relationships will be constrained and limited by his legitimate fear of his anger and the fact that at this time medication can only offer limited relief for his aggression and other PTSD symptoms.

Instead of offering Roy and other clients like him false promises, you need to give them an especially empathic ear when they talk about their sufferings and frequently reassure them that their most pressing and debilitating symptoms are totally understandable in the context of their experiences. Such clients need to have their losses, and their anger, articulated and acknowledged, and to have their small gains applauded.

Reexperiencing Phenomena

Flashbacks, nightmares, and intrusive thoughts are reexperiencing symptoms. They form the core of criterion B of the *DSM-IV* definition of PTSD. Basically, a flashback is a sudden vivid recollection of the traumatic event accompanied by a strong emotion. During a flashback, individuals do not lose consciousness, but do temporarily leave the present and find themselves back in the past. They may see scenes of the trauma, smell its smells, and hear its sounds. Furthermore, they may simply be watching the flashback as if it were a movie, or they may also act as if they are in the original traumatic situation. They may be conscious of present reality, or they may be oblivious to it. Or they may alternate between being conscious of the present and the past.

Flashbacks may also be unconscious. In conscious flashbacks, individuals experience vivid images of the traumatic events and can later report what they have seen, even if they lost consciousness of the present during or after the flashback (Blank 1985). In contrast, during unconscious flashbacks individuals engage in behavior motivated by some memory of the traumatic event, but are not aware of a memory of the specific traumatic event motivating their behavior and do not make the association between the trauma and their present behavior.

Flashbacks are common among a wide variety of trauma survivors, from combat veterans and survivors of concentration camps to rape and incest survivors. Flashbacks are more likely to occur among people who have endured multiple traumas or repeated traumas over time than among victims of one-time traumas. However, some survivors of one-time traumas do have flashbacks, as do some individuals who work with the injured or dying, for example, nurses, doctors, and police officers.

Flashbacks usually last anywhere from a few seconds to a few minutes. If they last more than an hour and the individual finds himself or herself in a different place with no memory of how he or she got there, most likely more than a flashback is involved. The individual was probably in a state of dissociation or under the influence of alcohol or drugs (possibly prescribed medications in inappropriate doses or in an unprescribed combination). The cumulative effect of years of substance abuse may also be involved.

Flashbacks are always visual, but may contain voices and other sounds as well. Some severely traumatized individuals suffer flashbacks in the form of recurring auditory hallucinations. These may involve hearing frightening or loud noises, sounds that indicate an upcoming "attack" or danger, or screams, moans, and other sounds of someone in distress. In the case of survivors of child abuse, the voice may be that of a child.

Other forms of reexperiencing the trauma include intrusive (unwanted, unplanned) images or thoughts of the traumatic event and the sudden reexperiencing of certain intense feelings that do not seem clearly related to any particular memory of the traumatic event or any current, readily identifiable trigger. Yet these feelings, which include irritability, panic, rage, and grief, can be seen as residues of the intense feelings aroused by the trauma. They may also indicate repressed emotions about the trauma. Nightmares, whether more or less exact replays of the trauma or more symbolic representations, are also forms of reexperience since they recreate the emotional impact of the original event.

Special Concerns

You may have difficulty identifying flashbacks, distinguishing them from other phenomena, or helping clients cope with them because, as a profession, we do not know much about flashbacks. According to some observers, flashbacks have not been studied because they are both disturbing and easily dismissed as an aberration or a psychotic or semipsychotic symptom. Consequently, flashbacks have remained an undesirable subject for scientific study and even of clinical analysis (Herman 1992; Blank 1985). To date no studies on flashbacks other than on clinical anecdotal reports and studies of the effectiveness of various medications in helping to reduce the frequency and intensity of flashbacks have been performed.[1]

Your attitude must not be judgmental, nor voyeuristic. Although the popular media often portray flashbacks and nightmares as sensational or dramatic events, for your clients who are subject to these phenomena, flashbacks and nightmares are disruptive, if not terrifying. All too often, these symptoms are the source of considerable loneliness, self-disparagement, and other forms of misery. This point cannot be overemphasized.

Some clients isolate themselves or severely restrict their lives so as to be assured of being in a safe place should one of these reexperiencing phenomenon occur. Some even limit their social and intimate relationships for fear that their symptoms will embarrass or humiliate themselves or their family members, out of concern that others may become frightened or feel threatened, or because they fear they will not be able to handle the situation they are in while simultaneously coping with the flashback or intrusive memory.

In working with veterans with PTSD, I have observed a common pattern: A veteran will leave home temporarily, for a few hours up to several days, when he feels the intrusive phase of PTSD beginning or suffers any of the reexperiencing symptoms. Several men I have worked with have even separated permanently from women they loved deeply after one or two instances of finding themselves mistaking their wife for an enemy in a flashback or reliving combat in their sleep. A few of these men actually struck their wives during flashbacks or nightmares. Most, however, never attacked their partner; they were just afraid that someday they would. For example, Bob L. found himself sitting upright in the middle of the night looking around the room for enemy attackers. "What if I mistook my wife or kids for the enemy and caused them harm?" he wondered. On this basis, he divorced his wife and lived alone for twenty years.

---

1. Arthur Blank (1985) has suggested that flashbacks were not studied in the Vietnam veteran population because of the therapeutic community's conflicts about war: "Flashbacks . . . [are] a sudden access into consciousness of dissociated . . . experiences and related affects, fantasies, and impulses. And along with the few veterans who engage in dramatic actions in response to flashbacks, there are many others who experience intrusive imagery of war events privately, without public notice . . . Although [flashbacks] sometimes gain extensive media exposure, neither the public nor private episodes have been elucidated in the clinical literature. A few writers have mentioned the phenomenon in passing (2-4). This absence of study of flashbacks is perhaps an example of our general national denial of war and its psychological consequences for participants."

The preceding example may seem extreme, and perhaps it is. Perhaps it is only those who drastically restrict their lives who seek help at counseling centers and clinics. There are no statistics or studies on survivors to indicate how common such responses to symptoms are or how the symptoms affect interpersonal relationships, vocational choices, or lifestyles. Yet we do know that help-seeking sexual abuse and domestic violence survivors report suffering from increased intrusive images, flashbacks, and nightmares when they become involved in intimate relationships. And, as a result of these symptoms, as well as the fears and general feelings of inadequacy stemming from the abuse, a proportion of these abuse survivors either refrain from developing close relationships or end them once they reach a certain level of intimacy (Courtois 1988; Lew 1988).

You may also have difficulty helping clients with their reexperiencing symptoms if they are unable or unwilling to talk about them. Clients may be so afraid of their flashbacks, nightmares, and intrusive memories (because the content is so horrifying or personally painful) that they do not wish to share them. Do not press these clients for details. As with the original trauma, you can, however, invite them to share their flashbacks or nightmares, or a portion of them. For example, you could say, "If you want to talk about the flashback with me, I'm willing to listen. But if you'd rather not, that is fine too. Or you may choose to tell me about it at a later date, or to tell me only parts of it."

Client Education

Although flashbacks, frequent nightmares, and intrusive images of horrific events are not common or "normal" in the general population, it is perfectly normal for trauma survivors to have such experiences, especially under three conditions: if they were repeatedly traumatized or revictimized after the original trauma, if they did not receive help with the trauma soon after it occurred, or if their major coping mechanism for the trauma was repression or denial. To help your clients heal, you need to help them see reexperiencing symptoms, like other PTSD symptoms, as signs of unfinished work in integrating the trauma into their lives, rather than as signs of insanity. You might, for example, offer the following analogy:

> After all you have been through, having flashbacks or nightmares, is normal. You could think of your flashbacks and nightmares as being like what happens when you eat so much that you can't digest it all at once. You feel sick to your stomach for a while, then you keep burping and tasting it.
>
> The same way eating too much at one sitting overloads your digestive system, trauma overloads your coping system. By definition, a trauma is an experience that people cannot "digest"—emotionally, physically, and spiritually. If they could handle it, it wouldn't really be traumatic. So the trauma is still there, bubbling up at times and making you sick. The undigested parts of the trauma cause nightmares, flashbacks, intrusive thoughts, and other symptoms, which are like burps.
>
> And, if the flashbacks and nightmares are just leftovers or burps, they are nothing to be feared. The flashbacks and nightmares do not cause the trauma to happen again, and you are not actually in the trauma.

I know that simply telling you these things won't take away all your fear and concern, especially your concern that you are going to be saddled with these nightmares and flashbacks for the rest of your life. And even though, as we sit here talking, you understand that a flashback isn't the same as the trauma, when you're having the flashback it feels real—you feel as if you're back in it and that you or someone you love could die or be hurt at any moment.

Some clients ask for a list of things to do to make the flashbacks go away, but there is no sure-fire list. Our profession doesn't know enough about flashbacks, nightmares, and intrusive thoughts to generate such a list. However, we have found that there is healing in the telling. The more you talk about your symptoms and memories and what they mean to you, the less need your unconscious mind will have to repeat or deal with the trauma through nightmares, flashbacks, and so on. By talking about the trauma, writing about it, or expressing yourself creatively through music, art, or dance, the less need there will be for the trauma to break forth in the form of flashbacks, nightmares, and intrusive thoughts.

Note: If your client suffers or has suffered from an eating disorder, before using this metaphor you might ask if she or he would find an analogy to over-eating offensive or painful.

In dealing with flashbacks, nightmares, intrusive thoughts, as well as other distressing PTSD symptoms, such as numbing, dissociation, anxiety attacks, and sleep problems, you are dealing not only with the symptoms themselves, but with clients' feelings about their symptoms. Initially, clients tend to negatively judge themselves for having PTSD symptoms and may experience considerable anxiety, shame, or guilt as a result. Until they become familiar with the symptoms and dynamics of PTSD and reach a certain level of awareness and acceptance of their own particular constellation of symptoms, they may tend to view their sufferings as signs of personal deficiency, incompetence, or in some cases even immorality. As mentioned above, another common reaction is fear, or even terror.

Fear arises not only in response to the specific horrors in the content of flashback, nightmare, or intrusive thought but in response to the often unpredictable nature of these reexperiencing phenomena. In general, reexperiencing phenomena, like other PTSD symptoms, tend to occur more frequently and more intensely during times of current stress, personal loss, and around anniversaries of the trauma and in response to trigger events or other stimuli. By identifying their triggers, clients can learn when to expect increased reexperiencing of the trauma.

However, symptoms sometimes emerge "out of the blue," at times or places not obviously related to any trigger events or stimuli. The sudden and often unexpected appearance of the symptoms can make clients feel out of control of their mental and emotional life, their senses, and their behavior. This feeling can create anxiety or panic and reinforces the helplessness survivors experienced during the original traumatic event.

Compiling a trigger chart can alleviate the uncertainty to some extent, by making the emergence of reexperiencing and other PTSD symptoms predictable. However, it would be misleading, if not damaging, to give clients the notion that they will be able to predict the occurrence of all flashbacks and other symptoms. Mastery in this area is limited, and suggesting otherwise to clients will ultimately intensify already existing feelings of despair and powerlessness.

Safety Issues

It is impossible to predict whether or not a flashback will lead to harm, either for clients or those around them at the time of the flashback. Certain dangers do exist. For example, flashbacks can occur while a client is driving a vehicle, causing the vehicle to go off the road or go at unsafe speeds. If flashbacks occur while the person is cooking, climbing stairs, doing house repairs or construction work, operating machinery, performing surgery or other medical treatments, or during a wide variety of other activities, there is definite danger to both the survivor and others.

Ideally flashbacks would be predictable, and safeguards such as not driving, not going to work, or seeking a retreat to avoid harm could be used. However, flashbacks can occur without warning, in response to a trigger the survivor is not aware of as a trigger, to a trigger that manifests itself unpredictably, or as a delayed response to a recognized trigger or to accumulated life stresses. These possibilities for serious injuries underscore the importance of identifying triggers and self-care for survivors.

Clients should be informed of the advisability of telling the people they live with and see often about their flashbacks, nightmares, and so on. These family members and friends may be able to help by keeping clients from hurting themselves and telling them where they really are. Alternatively, if the client fears he or she might hurt others during the episode, those others need to be told so that they can stay away or seek assistance.

In some cases, alcohol or another drug (such as PCP) seems to trigger flashbacks in which survivors endanger themselves. Therefore, clients need to be made aware of the serious inadvisability of attempting to self-medicate for their reexperiencing symptoms.

Stopping Intrusive Thoughts

Baker (Baker and Salston 1992) suggests the following technique for helping to control intrusive thoughts of the trauma. Ask clients to think of one thought they cannot control, which, when they tell it to go away, does not. Emphasize that this is an unwanted thought. Even though others might be telling your clients to "just stop thinking about it," they cannot.

After they have shared their selected intrusive thought with you, clients are to place a rubber band around one wrist. To be effective, the rubber band must be worn at all times. Otherwise they may not have it when the thought intrudes.

When the intrusive thought comes into their mind, they are to snap the rubber band. At the moment of the snap, the thought is gone, because they are feeling and concentrating on the sting of the snap. At that moment, they decide whether or not to continue thinking the thought. If they can stop the thought at this point, that is wonderful. However, if they cannot stop it, then they need to give themselves permission to be miserable for a certain amount of time, for example, three or five minutes. The length of the time is not as important as the fact that the time is specified.

When the thought comes again, clients are to again snap the rubber band and focus on choosing whether or not to continue thinking the intrusive thought. If the thought persists, clients are to once again give themselves permission to be miserable for a specified period of time, then try to focus on the choice again.

Clients are to keep up the procedure until the intrusive thought dissipates. In Baker's experience, the clients' wrists may be red for several days, but usually the technique dissipates an intrusive thought within a week.

If the client is a self-mutilator, however, snapping a rubber band may not be a useful method to stop the thought. Snapping fingers or clapping hands may be an alternative. However, such behaviors are often noticed by others and may create embarrassment for the client. Yet they are preferable to the rubber band technique which causes some physical discomfort and thus simulates more severe self-mutilation.

Above all, emphasize to clients that they need to be consistent in practicing this technique. If they are inconsistent, then they may in fact increase the frequency of the intrusive thought.

Defusing Nightmares

According to Freud, flashbacks, nightmares, and other reexperiencing phenomena are a means of draining off excess energy generated by the trauma.

One theory about reexperiencing phenomena holds that once a living organism has undergone a life-threatening event, it is biologically registered that the life-threatening experience may recur. So as a means of survival, the mind replays the scenes over and over, scanning for ways of protecting the organism should the life-threatening event recur (Freedy et al. 1992). A couple of coping techniques use repetition in a similar way to deal with nightmares.

Baker and Salston (1992) suggest that clients write out any nightmares they can remember in as much detail as possible. You can also have them keep pen and paper or an audiotape recorder next to the bed so that they can record their nightmares immediately on waking, so they won't be forgotten.

Then later, in sessions with you, clients can rewrite their nightmares so that they are less helpless. The nightmares cannot be rewritten or revised in a highly unrealistic manner; that would not be effective. For example, if a client whose son was murdered is having nightmares about the murder, and in them he kills himself or his son's pets, the client should not be instructed to or permitted to rewrite his nightmare so that his son isn't killed or miraculously rises from the dead. However, he can be helped into a more positive version so that at the end of the nightmare, he dreams about catching the murderer or seeing the murderer convicted rather than killing himself or the animals.

Similarly, rape victims can rewrite their nightmares not so that they are not raped, but so that, at one point or another, they are less helpless or their attacker's power is somewhat diminished. For example, they could envision their rapist in diapers or wetting his pants. If they die in the nightmare, the could instead envision themselves screaming and shouting, taking themselves on a dream vacation, or joining a speak-out or some other political movement against rape. The purpose of such rewrite suggestions is not to sugarcoat the victims' traumatic memories, but rather to help victims realize that just because attackers were "all-powerful" (or relatively all-powerful) during the attack, they are not all-powerful now and were not immune to harm, human reactions, limitations, and so forth even during the attack. Obviously if the client is in a situation where an abuser or attacker is still at large and there is danger of revictimization, rewriting dreams so as to disempower the abuser or attacker and empower the victim should not be done. Rather the focus of your work should be on the reality contained in the dream and what can be done to reduce the very real danger.

Bear in mind that this technique of rewriting nightmares may not be helpful to all clients. Some may be offended by it, feeling (with some validity) that rewriting the nightmare with a "happy ending" of sorts diminishes the horror of their experiences and trivializes their pain. Not all PTSD therapists are proponents of this rewriting technique, either. One objection to this technique is that it can foster a sense of denial in terms of the client accepting his or her victimization and other forms of helplessness resulting from the trauma and reexperienced in the nightmares.

Another technique, for handling recurring nightmares, is less controversial and less problematic theoretically than the above technique. This technique is designed to help strip recurring dreams of their power by "beating them to death" through exposure and repetition.

Clients are instructed to prepare for the dream by writing it out, talking about it to someone, and in other ways acknowledging that it is likely to recur (Baker and Salston 1992). Then, each night before going to bed, they are to write the dream out again and preferably talk about it with someone. They should also write it out each time it occurs, even several times per night.

Also have these clients write a brief self-affirming script, which they are to repeat to themselves when they wake up from nightmares. For example, the statement could read, "I am here now, not in the trauma. The worst is not about to happen. I am safe. I do not have to be afraid."

In addition, they are to help themselves get a restful night's sleep by not watching violent movies prior to bedtime, avoiding caffeine and other stimulants, engaging in relaxing activities, and so forth, as described in the following section.

Insomnia and Other Sleeping Problems

Sleeping problems are perhaps the most persistent of PTSD symptoms. Even when significant progress has been made in healing, insomnia, nightmares, and other sleeping problems may persist. Nevertheless, the sleeping problems that plague many PTSD sufferers can potentially be alleviated, to some degree at least, by increasing the client's understanding of their sleeping problems; by improving the client's current sleeping environment, when possible, by removing or reducing trigger elements and creating an atmosphere which is more psychologically conducive to sleep; and by improving general sleep practices. A psychiatric consultation for medication to assist with sleeping problems can be considered in addition to (not instead of) these methods. However, there is no medication yet that facilitates completely normal sleep.

Keep in mind, however, that even following all the suggestions given here (or elsewhere) to help clients with sleeping problems will not guarantee them a good night's sleep. There are clients who, after ten years of therapy and with the help of extremely potent sleep medication, still suffer from sleeping problems.

Increasing Understanding of Sleeping Problems

As discussed above, understanding the nature of and reasons for their PTSD symptoms helps to decrease clients' anxiety. This holds true for nightmares and nighttime intrusive thoughts, as well as other sleep problems, and the decreased anxiety itself can contribute to better sleep. You may also want to remind clients that their nightmares, insomnia, and other sleeping problems, although highly anxiety provoking, draining, and emotionally painful, are not lethal. Be careful, however, to empathize with the difficulties these people encounter in sleeping. Your client may be suffering the effects of sleep deprivation in addition to PTSD and other problems such as an eating disorder or alcohol addiction. For example, you might say something like this:

> Most people take sleeping for granted, but week after week you struggle just to get to sleep (or to stay asleep, to get back to sleep after nightmares, or whatever the problem is). If I were you, I'd give a fortune just for a good night's rest. Frankly, I don't see how you do as well as you do without the benefit of sleep. The way you describe the agony of just lying there, tired, wanting to sleep, knowing you need sleep to do what you have to do the next day, and not being able to (or being afraid that if you sleep a nightmare will come or whatever the sleeping problem) sounds like torture. And you have this problem on a daily basis (or whatever the general frequency of the problem is).
>
> You've stated many times that not sleeping is hell for you. It would be for almost anyone. But I need to remind you that even though sleeplessness is miserable, it won't kill you. Not sleeping can make you irritable, depressed, and sad, and can waste your days, but you won't die from it.
>
> Don't misunderstand me. Sleep deprivation is a serious matter. It can lead to all kinds of problems, for example, a clinical depression or a problems with violence or substance abuse, any of which can ultimately cause you serious harm or even death. That's why we have to do all we can to improve your sleep.
>
> Even if you never sleep the way you did before the trauma, and you may never sleep as well as some other people, there are probably a few things we can do to improve the chances of your sleeping well, not the least of which is your being here talking about your thoughts and feelings. All this talking and sharing will ultimately help you in all areas of life, even sleeping.

Improving the Sleeping Environment

Ask your clients if any of their traumatic experiences occurred at night, while they were resting or in a resting position, or while they were in a bedroom, dressed for bed, and so on. If so, then one or more aspects of going to sleep might be functioning as triggers. You can attempt to modify the impact of the specific triggers involved by using the interventions described earlier in this chapter in the section on triggers. Once again, you will need to begin with interventions that both you and the client feel have some possibility of being successful. Do not simply tell clients what to do; involve them as much as possible in the choice of intervention tactics.

You can begin to delineate which interventions might be most beneficial by asking the client what has worked and what hasn't worked in the past. Your clients may have already attempted muscle relaxation, for example, and found it extremely helpful, or not helpful at all. They may also have tried self-destructive means of going to sleep: drinking to the point of intoxication, binge eating, or using opium or some other drug. On the basis of the client's history in trying to cope with this problem by himself or herself, eliminate those methods that failed and begin with methods that have worked, if any.

Also consider whether there are aspects of the sleeping environment that could be altered to eliminate or reduce the trigger aspects of going to sleep. For example, the client's bedroom or sleeping area may contain noises, smells, or colors reminiscent of the trauma. Walls can be painted a different color or the client might change bedrooms. Earplugs can be used to help drown out certain kinds of noises.

Relocation may also have to be considered. For example, a client who was assaulted near a Chinese restaurant or who is a Korean War or Vietnam combat veteran might find the smell of Asian food a trigger. Thus, living next to an Asian restaurant subjects this client to constant reminders of the past. If such a client has a choice, such as moving to a different area of the apartment building where the smells are not as intrusive or to another place entirely, such a move might be considered. The costs of moving need to be weighed against the costs of lost or interrupted sleep and other trigger reactions. On the other hand, desensitization with guided imagery on this trigger may prove effective, enabling the client to tolerate the smells of Asian cooking without being plunged back into the past. In this case, relocation might be unnecessary.

Similarly, it may be that some of the bedtime habits of individuals who sleep with the client serve as triggers or make sleep difficult for the client. For example, suppose your client is hypervigilant at night due to having been attacked at night while on guard duty during a military tour. Such a client may wake or otherwise react to every noise and movement. His or her chances of sleeping would be enhanced by having a sleeping partner who does not move much, doesn't snore, and otherwise makes minimal disturbances. On the other hand, if such a client has a sleeping partner who also has sleeping problems or is a restive sleeper, problems may arise. Separate beds or bedrooms or some kind of compromise may have to be considered.

You might also want to inquire if there are any present emotional or physical dangers associated with going to sleep. For example, is the client in danger of being victimized by a family member or a criminal? Is the client's bed or bedroom in an unsafe place or are there unsafe aspects of the sleeping area that need to be attended to, such as an old heater the client fears might catch the room on fire or windows that are easily jimmied open?

Habits and Techniques for Improving Sleep

Certain practices improve the chances of good sleep for anyone, whether or not they are trauma survivors. The following are suggestions for improving sleep hygiene:

• Taking some physical exercise during the day, although not immediately before sleeping.

• Listening to relaxing music at bedtime.

- Listening to a relaxation tape or practicing relaxation techniques (if this has proven helpful in the past).

- Praying or meditating (if this has proven helpful in the past).

- Talking to others (if the client finds it soothing). Note that this does not include confrontation or argument.

- Writing about thoughts or feelings or speaking them into a tape.

- Eating something light an hour before sleeping. Foods with carbohydrates and calcium tend to be relaxing, such as milk products, fruit juice, bran muffins, and oatmeal. In contrast, protein and chocolate tend to be stimulants.

- Avoiding stimulants, such as coffee, tea, cola drinks, and cocoa.

- Doing boring tasks or reading a boring book before going to bed.

- Establishing a standard wake-up time. Often clients cannot control when they go to sleep, but can control when they wake up, which assures that they will be tired when they do go to bed. Likewise they should avoid taking naps.

- Sleeping in the same place consistently.

- Keeping the sleeping area at a temperature that is comfortable for the client. Also most people prefer dark and quiet for sleeping, but if your client needs a light or the radio or television on to feel safe or fall asleep, there is no problem with such a practice.

In addition, clients should not read material or watch movies that relate to their trauma or that are otherwise emotionally upsetting to them in the evening. For example, in general, combat veterans should not watch war movies before going to sleep; rape victims should not read feminist analyses of women's oppression as bedtime reading.

Suggestions for helping clients cope with nightmares and intrusive thoughts are offered in the preceding section on reexperiencing phenomena.

Baker and Salston (1992) propose the following technique for helping clients with insomnia. In preparation, clients make a list of the ten things they most hate to do, with the worst task listed first and the rest in descending order. These should be activities that can be completed inside the home and that the client considers safe, physically and psychologically. Clients are also to advise their family members that they may be engaged in these activities in the middle of the night so that they are prepared.

Clients are to stop drinking water two hours before bedtime. If they are thirsty, they are to sip water only. They should also do something that relaxes them before going to bed: relaxation exercises, reading, listening to music, following the guidelines above.

They then have half an hour to fall asleep. If after a half hour, they are still awake, they are to get up and do the first thing on their list. After completing the task they hate the most (for example, cleaning toilets or cleaning out the refrigerator) they are to go back to bed. If after fifteen minutes they are not asleep, they are to arise and complete the task they have identified as the second most hateful. They then return to bed, and if after another fifteen minutes they are not asleep, they are to rise and complete the third most hated task on their list, and so forth. If they complete all ten tasks, they are to start over with the most hated task.

During the initial half hour when they are trying to go to sleep and the fifteen minute intervals between tasks, clients can use relaxation tapes and imagery to help them relax.

Numbing and Dissociation

As with the intrusive symptoms of flashbacks, nightmares, and so on, clients need to be educated about the protective or survival function of numbing and dissociation. Numbing and dissociation (or "tuning out") are less dramatic than reexperiencing phenomena, but just because they do not show does not mean that they do not cause clients considerable emotional pain.

"My father died and I couldn't even cry at the funeral," "I know I love my children, but I hardly ever feel that love," and "I let that man rape me and felt nothing, as if it were happening to someone else," are statements of numbing or dissociation. The statements that immediately follow these are usually along the lines of "What's wrong with me? Why can't I feel? How did I become so weird?"

You can help clients understand and depathologize their numbing and dissociative symptoms by explaining that originally numbing, even to the extent of dissociation, protected them from the intense emotion which might have shattered them during the trauma. Had they experienced their emotions in full during the trauma, it would have been difficult, if not impossible, for them to think or act in a manner that maximized their safety and chances for survival.

It is important that you obtain as complete and concrete a clinical picture as possible of the client's numbing or dissociative symptoms. For example, when clients state that they "go numb," what does this mean? Are they physically unable to move or speak or are they unable to experience an emotional reaction or feel physical pain? Does it mean they doze off or fall asleep? If so, how long do they sleep?

If the symptom is dissociation, where do clients imagine they are? Are they simply not attending to the present, or are they in a corner of the room, on the ceiling, outside the room, or having some other type of out-of-body experience?

If the dissociative or numbing symptoms are extreme or prolonged, hospitalization may be needed. With less severe cases, the nature and extent of the numbing or dissociative symptoms will help you understand the client's present living problems as well as give you a clue as to how difficult or prolonged the therapy will be. If a client tends to go numb or dissociate frequently, ask if she or he is willing to let you know when she or he goes numb or dissociates in your sessions. Let the client know that if you feel she or he is going numb or dissociating, you will check out your hypothesis by asking whether you are correct.

When a client goes numb or dissociates in your sessions, you might decide to stop and ask how the client feels and if she or he is aware of what caused the numbing response. Was it something that was said or that happened in the session or at other sessions? Was it an event that occurred outside the therapy room that triggered memories from the past? Or was it simply anxiety about a present life stressor?

Like intrusive symptoms, numbing symptoms can be expected as reactions to trigger events, anniversaries of the trauma, and current pressures; they will also occur unexpectedly. As the roots of the client's PTSD are explored and understood in therapy, the numbing and other symptoms will diminish in frequency and intensity. However, until such progress is made, clients who are uncomfortable with their numbing or dissociative responses may simply want help in managing their symptoms.

The first step is to have clients identify when they become numb or dissociate and, if possible, make a list or keep a running log of the times during the week where they felt "dead inside" or "in a faraway world." Then discuss with them not only what they feel like when they are numb or dissociating, but also their judgments about having such symptoms. For example, are they full of self-loathing for having times of numbing? Are they simply "bored" while feeling numb? Or have they reached some level of acceptance of their numb states? Also, what feedback, if any, do they receive from others when they are in one of these states? What is the problem: their own discomfort with their symptoms or the discomfort of others, for example, a family member or an employer? Are there ways the symptoms limit their ability to function or pose a threat to their safety or the safety of others?

Some clients, especially those who have been multiply traumatized or abused as children, may try to break out of numbing or dissociative states by self-mutilating or by turning to some sort of substance abuse. In this case, you will want to explore other ways the client can break out of numbing. For example, could the client ground him or herself in physical reality by changing clothes, taking a bath, touching a safe object (such as a stuffed animal), doing some exercises, or completing some mindless chores around the house? Could the client ground him- or herself in emotional reality by writing or talking to someone?

Anxiety and Panic Attacks

Your client may experience anxiety or panic attacks in anticipation or in the presence of a trigger or as the result of a flashback. You need to assess whether your client is experiencing a panic attack as outlined in *DSM-IV*. If so, consultation with a physician for possible medical contributions to or complications stemming from the panic attack is necessary. Similarly, anxiety attacks, which vary in intensity, require medical consultation if they involve physiological problems such as an outbreak of rash, numbness in a limb, blurred vision, or any significant physical problem. Some psychiatrists also prescribe anti-anxiety medication for anxiety attacks.

Many of the interventions already discussed for coping with flashbacks and other reexperiencing symptoms, with trigger situations, and with anger may also prove useful to clients in coping with anxiety or panic attacks. The first step, however is to obtain a history of the symptom from the client, including a history of how the client has tried to handle these attacks in the past. It is also necessary to educate the client about the nature of the symptom and its possible causes in order to normalize it and put it in perspective. For example, having an anxiety attack is not the same as having a stroke, a heart attack, a psychotic break, or dying, even though fear of dying may be present during the attack.

After this preliminary work is completed, and on the basis of the information gathered, possible interventions can be discussed and agreed on with the client. Possible interventions include, but are not limited to, the following:

- Deep breathing exercises
- Physical exercise

- Muscle relaxation exercises

- Positive self-talk

- Writing and other expression of feelings

- Systematic desensitization

- Stress inoculation

- Visualization

- Examining negative self-talk

- Changing mistaken beliefs

- Assertiveness training

- Nutrition counseling

- Medication

Numerous resources are available for use as sources of instruction in these areas.

As with any other intervention presented in this book, the cautions noted in the section of this chapter on triggers need to be ever before you, and the client. The purpose of these interventions is to promote well-being, not to create additional problems. If with any intervention a client should react, or even begin to react, in any of the ways outlined in the Warning Signs handout (in the introduction), stop using that technique (no matter how beneficial it may be with other clients), and assist your client in recovering from problems it has caused.

Self-Mutilation

As with every other aspect of the healing process, the therapeutic interventions presented in this chapter depend entirely on your having a positive therapeutic alliance with the client. They may work in the short run, but will not in the long run, if they are not grounded in a cooperative relationship based on mutual respect and trust. Without such a relationship, even your most brilliant suggestions become virtual gimmicks and will fail to meaningfully replace the client's self-limiting or destructive coping mechanisms.

In order to maintain a viable therapeutic relationship, you need to make a continuing effort to stay in touch with your client's ever-changing needs and emotional states. This degree of connectedness requires considerable sensitivity and effort on your part; clients with PTSD will sometimes come to you in a state of numbing, other times in a state of hyperalertness or with intrusive symptomatology.

Furthermore, PTSD clients, like any other clients but especially clients in recovery from addictions, often go "two steps forward and one step back" in the healing process. Healing is not a linear process. A survivor may make significant progress in several sessions, only then to regress.

Nowhere is this process more evident than in self-mutilating clients, with whom apparent progress is often made in tempering, or even eliminating, the self-mutilating habit, only to be followed by a regression into self-harm. Some of this regression may be caused, in part, by the client's unfamiliarity and discomfort with success or self-love. Intense survivor guilt often prevents combat veterans, prisoners of war, refugees, rescue workers, and others from acting on their own behalf (Langer 1987; Williams 1987b; Lee and Lu 1989; Kinzie 1989). Domestic violence survivors also commonly experience anxiety and discomfort when they begin to practice self-nurturing or self-loving ways of being rather than self-abusive ways (Walker 1979; Herman 1992).

In classic domestic violence cases, the abuser attempts to make his or her victim as emotionally dependent as possible, so that most if not all of the victim's self-esteem is dependent on the abuser's approval. This enables the abuser to wield great power over his or her victim. If your client is still living in the abusive situation, or the abuser maintains contact with the client, the abuser may punish the client's emotional independence from him or her as expressed in the cessation of self-mutilation and growth of self-love.

Even if your client is no longer in fear of the abuser, she or he may have internalized the abuser's punishing attitudes toward the client's self-love or taking positive steps toward goals. Your client may revert to self-mutilation because of such internalized punishing attitudes, or as a way to please the abuser.

Some regression, unfortunately, may be caused by therapist error. If the therapist probes for memories or pushes the client to examine feelings before she or he is ready to do so, the client can become emotionally flooded and may self-mutilate as a sedative or means of containment (Calof 1992). However, even when therapy is conducted at the client's pace (rather than the therapist's), the very progress made in unearthing memories and getting in touch with long-buried emotions may cause the client to reach for the old method of relief if this traumatic material carries with it elements of shame (Nathanson and Turkus 1992).

Some combat veterans (Wong and Cook 1992), prisoners of war, (Langer 1987; Oboler 1987) and domestic violence survivors (Walker 1979; Herman 1992) especially have been found to experience great shame in acknowledging to themselves, not to mention to others (even therapists and members of their support group) how they "allowed" themselves to be abusive or abused. In addition, both domestic violence survivors and prisoners of war often erroneously feel that there was something they could have done to stop or escape the abuse. In reality, POWs are usually held in most severe forms of captivity, and abused women and children, once the full battering syndrome—with its economic, psychological, social, and legal components—is operative, become literally as powerless as if they were locked in a prison.

Unfortunately, many domestic violence survivors' assumptions that they were "too weak" to fight back or escape, or were otherwise deficient or incompetent, are also held by large segments of society and by uninformed members of the mental health and medical professions. Similarly, prisoners of war may have been accused of being traitors, of letting comrades die or participating in torture executions so they could live, and of otherwise "giving in" to the enemy. These attitudes add to the shame of whatever humiliating experiences the survivor has had. Battered women, formerly abused children, and former POWs frequently self-mutilate in response to this shame, creating yet another source of shame: the self-mutilation itself.

In sum, a resurgence of self-harming behaviors among these clients may, strangely enough, be the result of the very progress made in resurrecting memories of the trauma and feelings associated with those memories in your sessions, possibly in combination with other healing efforts on the part of the client. This is especially the case when shame is a part of those memories. If this is the

case, you, the therapist, can help reframe the client's regression so as to minimize the shame involved. For example, you could say this:

> As I explained to you during our initial sessions, it is part of
> the nature of healing process that as you come closer and
> closer to the truth about what happened to you and how you
> felt about it, you begin to experience more pain and, perhaps,
> more symptoms. However, this process of greater
> self-awareness leading to greater pain will not go on endlessly.
> Eventually, you will obtain a more complete picture of what
> happened, and, as you talk about or otherwise process your
> reactions to what happened, your symptoms will gradually
> lessen in frequency and intensity and your sense of inner
> peace, self-acceptance, and even your self-love, will grow.
>
> You and I are working toward these goals, but we haven't
> reached them yet. Therefore, it's only natural that as you start
> feeling more deeply, you will want to go back to the ways
> you comforted yourself in the past, for example, by hurting
> yourself [or binging and vomiting, drinking, drugging].
>
> I know how painful it is for you to be seemingly going
> backward, and you've told me how hard it is to get back on
> track after you slipped into your old self-destructive ways. But
> let me assure you, you haven't obliterated all your progress.
> You can never go back to where you were when you first
> started coming here and working on understanding yourself.
> You simply know too much to go all the way back there.
>
> It really is all right that you went "backwards" a little. In
> fact, as I explained, it isn't really going backward at all, but
> rather a sign that you are going forward and, if you continue
> to go forward, you may sometimes find yourself reverting to
> some of your old coping mechanisms. I'm not saying that you
> *must* go back to hurting yourself, but if you do, beating
> yourself up about it will only increase your desire to hurt
> yourself again, as a form of self-punishment.
>
> It's a vicious cycle. The only way to break it is to practice
> self-acceptance and self-love and—this is very important—to
> process the experiences by writing, drawing, or otherwise
> sharing parts of your story with people who will listen to you
> carefully and respectfully. The more you can get your feelings
> out, in a safe way, especially your feelings about your
> experience of "going backwards" the closer you are to being
> healed.

A question you might ask at this point, or at any point in dealing with a
self-mutilating client is whether she or he is able to imagine what it would feel
like or what she or he might do without the self-mutilating behavior. Some self-
abusive clients will be able to answer these questions. Others will not be so fortunate. To you, a clinician, the language and knowledge of feelings are almost
second nature, the very essence of your profession. But for some self-mutilating
clients, identifying feelings is almost an impossible task. They, like an undeter-
mined number of other survivors, may suffer from a condition called *alexithymia*,
an inability to verbalize feelings.

This condition was first described by Sifneos (1975; Sifneos, Apfel-Savitz, and Frankel 1977) in reference to traumatized clients, especially males, who could not name their feelings. According to recent research, such clients may need antidepressants or other medication before they can respond usefully to psychotherapy (Kosten et al. 1992).

Not just clients who suffer from alexithymia but many of the rest of your self-mutilating clients will lack the language of feelings. You may need to educate them concerning issues such as what is a feeling, how to distinguish a feeling from a thought, the names of different feelings, and so forth. (Discussion and exercises pertaining to these areas can be found in chapter 9, "Feelings Work.")

As is discussed further in chapter 11, perhaps the worst "technique" for reducing self-mutilating behavior is scolding clients and accusing them of hurting themselves only to get attention. If we do this, we become part of a vicious cycle of the client's self-dislike, if not self-hatred. In fact, as Calof (1992) asserts, self-mutilating survivors are "probably seeking shame and rebuke more than true nurturance."

The work before you is intense. Hopefully, you will make use of professional consultation and supports, otherwise you can very easily slip into a blame-the-victim mentality out of sheer frustration, fear, and fatigue. Remember, self-mutilating clients have had years of trauma, and therefore healing may take a long time. Do not beat yourself up, or berate the client, when progress seems slow. Furthermore, if you should somehow "slip" and shame your client by one of your responses, admit your mistake and apologize.

Choosing Methods of Change

This first step in choosing methods of arresting and ultimately eliminating self-mutilating behavior is to try to determine the functions of the behavior. As explained in chapter 4, self-mutilating behavior can serve a variety of functions and a single behavior can serve more than one purpose. Assessing the functions of these behaviors constitutes a major professional challenge, not only because the same behavior can serve more than one function, but because the same behavior at one stage of the therapy may serve a different function than at a later stage of therapy. For example, self-cutting may initially function as an expression of rage at the perpetrator, but then take on the function of testing the therapist as well. If the therapist can accept cutting behavior, the client may reason (unconsciously) that perhaps the therapist will be able to tolerate listening to certain horrific memories.

The following list of methods of coping with self-mutilating behaviors is only a beginning. For maximum effectiveness, explain to clients that self-mutilation can be a way of telling their story or showing their feelings. Then ask them if they would be willing to try a different way of telling their story or showing how they feel, or if they would be willing to examine any events, feelings, or acts about which they experience shame. If clients are hesitant, ask if they would at least be willing to consider some of the ways you are going to suggest. Such concern for the client's autonomy may seem excessive; however, in the case of trauma survivors such as domestic abuse survivors, combat veterans, and rape and crime victims, it is essential.

It would not be unusual for a combat vet, for example, who is struggling with having had to carry out objectionable orders, to simply walk out of your office and never return if he felt you were ordering him about. Similarly, individuals who have been tortured or otherwise abused are often particularly sensitive in being told what to do. Conversely, survivors who go along with suggestions only because you are an authority figure and they feel it necessary to please you will never achieve the deep-rooted healing that is your ultimate goal. In the worst of cases, clients may cooperate with you because they feel they are supposed to, and then, because your suggestion feels forced upon them, they rebel against you, causing your entire plan to backfire.

As Calof (1992) stresses, self-mutilating clients are usually people whose lives have been, for the most part, in the hands of other people, usually people who did not have their best interests at heart. For some, self-mutilation was a means, perhaps the only means, of self-assertion and expression of independence tolerated. Your role is to encourage the independence while helping clients find other ways of expressing it, which is why it is essential you discuss any method you plan to use and secure the client's feedback and agreement. In addition, clients may have excellent suggestions for modifying these strategies so that they will work for them.

Most of the methods listed below are appropriate primarily for the beginning stages of therapy, rather than the middle or later stages. The material on grounding and emotional containment chapter 8 and the anger and grief work in this chapter and chapter 9 may also be of assistance. However, the exercises in the later chapters assume a certain degree of affect recognition and specific remembrance of the trauma—qualities that may still be in the nascent state in clients who are actively harming themselves.

As always, the most basic intervention is to, without pushing, make it clear to your clients that you are willing to listen to every detail of their experience, no matter how sad or gruesome. You can reinforce your interest by asking, "Is there anything else you'd like to tell me about this? I'm willing to listen to whatever you have to say, but remember, you only need to share what you want to share. If you feel you have shared enough with me, that's fine."

Normalizing Client Responses Through Education

Whenever possible, clients need to be educated about the relationship between self-mutilation and shame and the nature of their specific trauma (Nathanson and Turkus 1992; Peterson 1992). Do not assume clients have information that may seem like common knowledge to you. For example, some of your sexual abuse survivors may need basic education on normal psychosexual development. Many feel tremendous shame at having experienced sexual arousal during molestation. Nathanson and Turkus (1992) give the example of abuse survivors who literally carved words such as *dirt*, *ugly*, or *whore* on their bodies as an expression of their shame. They did not know that it was normal for young children to have sexual feelings and to respond to sexual stimulation.

Similarly, rape victims who experienced sexual arousal, along with fear, anger, and grief during the rape, may harbor tremendous shame regarding their arousal. They may need basic education on the physiology of arousal and climax. For example, they need to learn that sexual organs lack cognitive abilities and will therefore generally become aroused when stimulated, regardless of any mental effort to feel no pleasure.

Combat veterans and other war survivors can suffer from a variety of shames: shame at having killed, shame at being unable or unwilling to kill, shame at having enjoyed killing, shame regarding atrocities witnessed or committed. Such individuals need to be educated about the age-old conflict between the "man" and the "warrior" and about phenomena generated by war (rather than individual personalities), for example, blood lust and combat addiction. While such education is not intended to reduce appropriate guilt, it does help to normalize client feelings and behavior.

Reframing Verbal Abuse

For clients who have been verbally abused, either in their homes, on their jobs, in prison, in the military, in prisoner of war camps, or elsewhere, it is important to generate a list of the insults and other forms of abuse they endured. Clients who can't remember and who are returning to the original site of the abuse (for example, abuse survivors who are planning to visit their nuclear family for a holiday), can be given a "homework assignment" of listening for verbally abusive statements. Often the verbal abuse is so ingrained in the family system that it goes unrecognized as abuse. However, it is abuse, and will remain powerful until it is identified as such.

Another way to generate this list is to ask clients if they ever verbally abuse others. If so, what names or epithets do they use to attack others? Are any of these, by chance, similar to epithets which were hurled at them? While survivors are victims, some are also perpetrators of verbal abuse. In a sense, such abusiveness can function as a form of self-abuse, because it ultimately results in social rejection and loneliness. These, in turn only affirm the client's feelings of personal inferiority and social deviancy.

Once some of the original verbal abuse is identified, Nathanson and Turkus (1992) suggest taking a piece of paper and drawing a line down the middle. On one side, the client (or therapist) lists the verbally abusive statements, on the other side, an adult perspective on the abusive statement. For example, an adult countering statement for an incest survivor who was called a whore by her perpetrator needs to be more than simply, "I am not a whore." A rebuttal such as, "I am an adult woman with normal sexual capacities. Under conditions of my choosing, I can engage in sexual activity with appropriate partners," is much more powerful.

Consider the case of Joe X. who was called a "dumb-dumb" by his alcoholic father. His adult countering statements needed to include specific statements of actual intellectual, mechanical, artistic, and other real abilities, as well as areas where skills were lacking. Joe X.'s countering adult statements went as follows:

> I finished high school with a B average. I am skilled in the
> following areas ... and my skill levels have been recognized
> by ... I am extremely adept at ... but not as skilled at ...
> However, the fact that I am not an expert at everything
> doesn't mean I am a dumb-dumb. My father suffered from a
> terrible illness and had self-esteem problems himself. He
> needed to put me down to feel better about himself. His
> statements about me are more a reflection of his despair than
> the reality of my skills or intelligence level.

Identifying Present Behaviors That Cause Shame

Is the client doing anything in the present which he or she feels is shaming? Clients need to be aware of how shame generated by the trauma is perpetuated by their behavior in the present. Furthermore, their present behavior, although shaming in itself, may also, by association, carry with it the weight of the shame from the past.

Substituting a Less Harmful Behavior

For clients who somatize their feelings, you can suggest that they put the pain in one of their little fingers. It is important not to take away the pain entirely because it "needs to be there for it is a way of telling the story and telling about pain without telling the story" (Calof 1992).

Using Symbols

Instead of cutting, burning, or hitting themselves, clients could cut, burn, or hit a picture or some other concrete representation or symbol of themselves, the perpetrator, or some other aspect of the trauma. For example, clients could make a clay or other artistic rendition of some aspect of their traumatic experience or their feelings, especially their aggressive feelings toward themselves or others, and attack this rendition, rather than themselves (Calof 1992).

Reducing Emotional Intensity: Rage Dumps

If self-mutilation serves the function of helping to contain feelings associated with the trauma and, through physical pain, of distracting survivors from their intense emotional pain, then reducing their level of emotional intensity may help reduce the need to self-mutilate. Calof (1992) suggests that "rage dumps" may be helpful for clients who have a great deal of primitive rage. This method, he stresses, should be used in the early (not the later) stages of the therapy. It is addressed to rage so primitive that it must be acted out in some physical manner. Simply talking about this kind of rage will not suffice.

These rage dumps, Calof stresses, are not therapeutic in the sense of functioning to help integrate the meaning of the anger into the client's self-awareness. Neither can they be classified with some of the more sophisticated forms of anger management presented above, but they can serve an important purpose: They reduce levels of rage so that true therapy can begin. Otherwise, the rage interferes with cognition (the client literally can't think because of the anger) which limits the usefulness of the dialogue that occurs in therapy.

Rage dumps include the usual techniques of hitting sofas with plastic bottles or plastic batons, cutting up material or phonebooks, beating up old cars or other objects, and engaging in an aggressive sport such as boxing (if medically permitted). The client needs to contract to engage in these rage dumps for a specific amount of time for a specific purpose in the presence of the therapist. The therapist monitors the client, assuaging any fears the client might have of losing control. The therapist also functions to encourage the client to express his or her rage to the point of satiety. In Calof's experience none of the clients who participated in such managed rage dumps later went on to act in uncontrollable aggressive ways outside the therapeutic setting.

Using Imagery

It can be suggested to clients that they engage in their self-mutilating behaviors in imagery, rather than in actual practice. For example, if they cut themselves because being beaten to the point of bleeding preceded receiving food in their refugee or POW camp or preceded the honeymoon stage of the battering cycle, suggest that they instead imagine the blood.

Imagery can also be used to cope with self-mutilation that represents rage at the perpetrator. The perpetrator can be first visualized by the client as she or he seemed during the trauma: big, strong, wielding a weapon, and so on. Then, in imagery, the perpetrator is imagined as weak and impotent. Calof (1992) suggests the perpetrator be visualized as wearing diapers. Alternatively, the perpetrator could be visualized as sucking her or his thumb, on crutches, or extremely old and frail.

Countering Depersonalization

Some clients cut or otherwise injure themselves in ways that would cause most people acute pain. However, these clients do not experience physical pain because they were so depersonalized and dehumanized during the abuse that they learned to tune out all forms of pain, emotional and physical.

As therapist, you need to teach clients that certain forms of self-injury hurt. For example, you can suggest to clients that when they cut themselves, they will feel pain.

Preventing Revictimization

Self-mutilation also occurs in response to client revictimization (Nathanson and Turkus 1992). Reread the section earlier in the chapter on creating a safe environment for the client, and help your client in identifying dangerous places. For example, for some abuse survivors, danger lies primarily at home. They may abandon their ordinary sense of caution outside their homes because they associate being away from home as being safe.

Revictimization can also be reduced by strengthening the client's sense of pride and dignity. Clients, for example, could be asked to generate a list of the rights of persons. As Nathanson and Turkus point out, we cannot assume that many of our trauma survivors know the basic rights of being a human being, such as the right not to be hit or sexually abused, the right to speak about feelings, the right to make a mistake, the right to have the needs for shelter, food, water, and love met.

Another way of strengthening clients is to make a distinction between spirituality and religion. This is especially important for individuals who were tortured or physically abused in the name of some perversion of religious faith (Nathanson and Turkus 1992). Such clients need to know that not all forms of spirituality are the same as sadistic cults.

Chapter 7

PTSD-Related Problems

In addition to its symptoms and its reexperiencing-numbing cycle, PTSD usually brings with it several additional problems. These include survivor guilt, self-blame, secondary wounding experiences, low self-esteem, and victim thinking. Although these problems are not listed in the *DSM-IV* either as diagnostic criteria or symptoms of PTSD, they are present among a great number of help-seeking trauma survivors (Ochberg 1988; Herman 1992; Courtois 1988; Williams 1987b; van der Kolk 1990a). Some of these PTSD-related problems stem directly from the nature of trauma itself, others result from societal and familial reactions to the trauma survivor.

Survivor Guilt and Self-Blame

Self-blame and survivor guilt are found among survivors of many different kinds of trauma, from concentration camp survivors and combat veterans to abused wives and children (Ochberg 1988; Walker 1979; Courtois 1988). In fact, trauma survivors, including those who harbor a great deal of fury about the trauma, are notorious for blaming themselves for the traumatic event or one or more of its negative outcomes. A part of this self-blame stems from society's blame-the-victim attitudes (discussed later in this chapter); another part comes from the survivors' difficulty accepting their powerlessness.

When clients say, "The trauma was my fault" or "My behavior [or personality] played a major role in creating the trauma," they seem to be assuming that they could have stopped the trauma from occurring or could have exerted a significant influence on it. In reality, however, traumatic experiences are either random events or situations so full of double binds that no matter which alternative is chosen, the victims must risk their health, their values, or their very lives.

Even in instances where survivors did contribute to a traumatic event's occurring or increased the negative impact of the trauma, they often acted in the context of nearly impossible situations. Traumatic circumstances are fraught with forces that make it easy for most people to make mistakes, exercise poor judgment, betray their own moral values and human attachments, or engage in other actions that increase the negative effects of the trauma. Some of these trauma-related forces, such as cognitive shut-down and perceptual distortion, are discussed below. In sum, when survivors blame aspects of the trauma on themselves, they are failing to perceive the bigger picture—the conditions that

existed at the time of the trauma that made their self-assessed undesirable behavior almost inevitable.

Basically, self-blame serves as an escape from feelings of powerlessness and
helplessness. These feelings, inherent to trauma, are two of the worst feelings
any human being can experience. In fact, trauma can be defined as being, and
feeling, powerless or helpless in the face of great danger. Since these feelings are
so devastating, people generally prefer to think that they are able to control their
lives. Thus, they must blame themselves for negative events, rather than acknowledging that sometimes life is unfair or arbitrary and that innocent people
can be victimized for no reason. In order to maintain a sense of being in control,
survivors may view themselves (rather than chance or forces greater than themselves), as responsible for one or more aspects of the trauma—perhaps even for
all of it. In short, self-blame can be a means of regaining the power lost during
the traumatic event.

When clients express survivor guilt, they are expressing something more than
just compassion for those who have suffered more than they have. Survivor guilt
is also a way of saying, "If I had suffered more, you would have suffered less,"
or, in its extreme, "If I had died, you would not have died. I could have died
in your place." Such thinking is not logical, but it makes emotional sense. It can
also be a defense against the pain clients experienced at seeing others hurt.

Survivor guilt also hearkens back to atavistic notions about making sacrifices
to the gods in order to assure a desired outcome. With survivor guilt, the notion
is, "If I punish myself, I can undo the damage, or at least keep bad things from
happening again." But of course safety and security cannot be purchased by
such means.

Survivor guilt also sometimes arises among those survivors who find it difficult to accept being grateful that someone else suffered more than they did or
that somehow they managed to live while others died. Although these clients
may someday come to accept that their gratitude is nothing more than an expression of their natural and vital instinct for self-preservation, this does not
mean they will necessarily be free of survivor guilt.

The first reaction of some therapists is to point out to clients how illogical
survivor guilt is or to otherwise indicate to clients that they shouldn't feel that
way or are foolish to feel so guilty. When a survivor of an earthquake or hurricane or other event that is clearly beyond human control begins to express
survivor guilt, it is difficult not to react with disbelief. But, as always, your task
as a therapist is to respect the client, including her or his self-blame and survivor
guilt. No matter how illogical these feelings may seem, do not disparage them.

For example, you should not say, "That doesn't make sense. You had no
choice but to . . . If you hadn't, you might have been killed." Instead, a more
empathic response would be, "You feel so badly about that, don't you? Can you
tell me how bad it hurts?" or "Are you saying that right now it seems as if what
you did will haunt you until the day you die?" or "I bet you'd give anything
to go back and do it over."

Building a More Accurate Picture

Only after you have shown some empathy and respect for the client's pain
surrounding self-blame and survivor guilt should you begin to help the client
distinguish "justified" from "irrational" guilt. For example, you could ask, "What

were your real choices in that situation—not the choices you *wish* you had, but the choices you really had?"

The client can then enumerate those choices, after which you take each choice in turn and ask, "What would have happened if you had made that choice? Then what would have happened? After that, then what?" until the client reaches a natural conclusion or endpoint to the story.

You can then ask the client to rank the choices in terms of practicality, morality, and any other relevant considerations. If it is therapeutically advisable, you can also ask the client to compare the choices he or she made with the real choices available and ask why he or she made those choices. You might also point out that none of the choices were truly desirable by any standard or measure. This process should help the client cognitively sort out "true" guilt from "false" guilt.

Some therapists use the terms "healthy" versus "unhealthy" guilt rather than "justified" versus "irrational" guilt or "true" versus "false"; however, the concept is basically the same. Justified or healthy guilt refers to instances where the client's carelessness or thoughtlessness actually caused or significantly contributed to the trauma. For example, clients who were raped while walking in what they knew were dangerous locations or who were burglarized when they left the back door unlocked, might feel with some legitimacy that their actions contributed to the trauma's taking place or to its negative outcome. Similarly, combat veterans who were involved in friendly-fire incidents, in which they inadvertently killed their comrades, sometimes report that they had a feeling they were firing on their own men, but obeyed orders anyway. Their remorse over these actions can be enormous. Yet they, like other trauma survivors, need to view their behavior from a trauma perspective and to call their guilt "healthy" would be an insult to their pain and their predicament.

For example, if the combat veteran had paid attention to his intuition and refused to fire on what he felt were friendly troops, he might have been court martialed or shot on the spot for disobeying orders. Unless all the soldiers in his unit mutinied, the attack on friendly troops would have probably continued. Therefore, it is highly unlikely that his refusal to participate would have greatly affected the outcome.

Also, he did not know for a fact that the target was friend, not foe. Suppose he had had the power to stop the military operation because he felt the target was friendly, only to be mistaken? Enemy troops might have advanced and slain even more of his comrades than were killed in the friendly-fire incident.

This combat example illustrates the importance of looking at individual survivor behavior from a wider, more complete perspective. Using the previous example, if a rape victim you are counseling feels she set herself up for sexual assault by walking in a dangerous neighborhood, you need to help her put the rape in its social context. Rape is fundamentally the result of the violence that runs rampant in our society, not the result of individual actions.

You also need to educate your guilt-afflicted clients about two conditions of trauma that sometimes contribute to mistakes, poor judgment, and other acts that can lead to self-blame and survivor guilt. Under conditions of trauma, difficulties in thinking and perceptual distortions are frequent occurrences. Some trauma survivors report that during a crime, vehicular accident, natural or technological disaster, or other traumatic situation, they made a decision that in retrospect was not the wisest. If your clients feel likewise, they may wonder why they "couldn't think." This impairment in their reasoning powers needs to be considered from a trauma perspective.

During the traumatic event, they were probably thinking to the best of their ability—under the circumstances. However, the turbulent emotions and high anxiety level that trauma creates sometimes militate against calm, rational thinking. This varies from one individual to the next. Some people remain remarkably coolheaded during traumatic episodes, but they are not in the majority; they mainly appear on the movie screen, not in real life. During a traumatic episode, most people's judgment is affected, to one degree or another, by the very real dangers involved in the situation and the strong fears such dangers can produce. Thus, for many people, it is difficult, if not impossible, to think clearly under extreme pressure.

There may also be biological bases for this "inability to think" under stress. When the body goes into an emergency alert during trauma, it normally has available to it three responses: fight, flight, and freezing. Thinking and reasoning slowly and carefully is not one of these responses.

Similarly, because trauma is by its nature sudden and overwhelming, people are often not able to adequately assess the situation, no matter how intelligent, brave, or physically fit they are. Indeed, it is often difficult for victims even to realize that the trauma is occurring.

Tom Williams (1987b), a psychologist who has worked with police officers, armed robbery and assault victims, combat veterans, and former prisoners of war, has discovered in his work that sensory data often becomes distorted during traumatic events:

> Some victims report perceptual changes in which time is altered and events seem to be happening in slow motion. Visual perceptions may be modified so that people sometimes have a derealized "out of body" experience, or at least feel that they are simply observing rather than participating in the trauma. Another frequent perceptual alteration is a hysterical-like tunnel vision that focuses on the trauma scene itself to the exclusion of the rest of the environment. For instance, a robbery victim focuses on a weapon directed at him or her and doesn't recollect what the robber was like, what was happening, or who was standing next to the robber.

In this initial denial and shock, it is easy for people to make "mistakes," or to act in a manner that later confuses them and causes them to doubt and criticize themselves.

In addition, you may want to suggest that clients talk to other survivors of the same or a similar trauma to get a broader perspective. They could also read newspaper accounts or other materials to the same end. Then discuss their research with them.

You should point out to the clients the ways the physiology of trauma may have affected their responses. If they experienced a fight-or-flight reaction, for example, that contributed to the detrimental outcome of the trauma, they need to be reminded that they did not choose to react that way.

Clients may also be judging all their behavior during the trauma as bad because they made one or two "mistakes." The rest of what they did may have been neutral, even admirable or resourceful, but this is overlooked in favor of the bad side. Clients need to be helped to remember and give themselves credit for the good they have done. It may help for clients to rate their faulty behavior as a percentage, for example, "About 30 percent of me was scared to death, but 70 percent was still holding on and coping," or "About 10 percent of the time I was selfish, but 90 percent of the time I did my best to help the other survivors" (McKay, Davis, and Fanning 1981).

Recognizing the Problem

Self-blame and survivor guilt are major issues for trauma survivors. Making progress in lessening self-blame and survivor guilt helps to lessen the frequency and intensity of any self-punishing behaviors that began or were exacerbated by the trauma. However, reducing self-blame may also lead to survivors' experiencing greater anger and grief over the events that occurred, as well as their own loss of innocence.

Although therapy can help diminish self-blame and survivor guilt, the degree to which "irrational" or "unhealthy" survivor guilt can be mitigated varies from one survivor to another. Nevertheless, even if the irrational guilt persists, it helps clients to put their guilt in a trauma perspective.

The Self-Blame and Survivor Guilt handout is designed to help clients identify their survivor guilt, self-blame, and other negative feelings about themselves stemming from the trauma. This exercise can be done as homework and then discussed in a therapy session, or you can work on it together with the client in a session. Also, you can revise this exercise to fit the needs of your client in any manner you deem therapeutically helpful.

Effects of Self-Blame on Present Life

Your clients may or may not be able to rid themselves of self-blame to the degree you would like. Much to your disappointment, they may leave therapy still burdened with an exaggerated sense of guilt over what they did or did not do during the traumatic event. Despite your educational efforts on the impact of trauma on human beings, unjustified self-blame may persist.

However, regardless of the degree to which your clients are able to divest themselves of unjustified self-blame, they can be made aware of the impact of self-blame on their present life. The following questions can be used as a follow-up to the preceding exercise to strengthen clients' awareness of the costs of self-blame.

How did it feel to look at the ways you blame yourself and any other negative feelings you have about yourself? Did you feel angry, sad, confused, afraid?

Did the exercise require considerable effort or thought on your part, or was it easy to complete?

Can you identify any of the feelings you had while completing the exercise or did you have no feelings at all? Did completing the exercise put you in a numb state or at any time make you feel hyper, agitated, or even hostile?

Were you surprised by the number of ways you took responsibility for the traumatic event or saw yourself in a negative light? Or were you already all too well aware of all these thoughts and feelings?

Were the feelings and other reactions you had in response to completing the exercise at all similar to the feelings and reactions you have when

Self-Blame and Survivor Guilt

As a trauma survivor, it is critical that you identify any feelings of self-blame and survivor guilt you may have. For each traumatic event you experienced do some writing on the following questions. As always, if you begin to feel over-whelmed or experience another of the warning signs your counselor has mentioned, stop doing the exercise. You can always come back to it.

1. In what ways, large or small (if any) do you blame yourself for the event's occurrence?

2. Do you blame yourself for the way you acted or didn't act during the trauma? If so, why?

3. Do you feel responsible for the extent of the injuries or damage or other negative results of the trauma? In what ways?

The following list identifies some common sources of guilt and shame among trauma survivors. You can use this list as a starting point in completing the exercise.

I believe that the traumatic event and/or its negative consequences were due, in whole or in part, to:

- An innocent mistake I made

- My general inability to make good decisions

- A one-time act of incompetence

- My general lack of intelligence

- A one-time thoughtless act on my part

- My general carelessness and failure to take adequate precautions

- An impulsive or immature act on my part

- My general lack of emotional maturity

- My lack of skill in a particular area

- My general inability to learn

- A specific act or feeling that I feel is immoral or not right

- My generally sinful or bad nature

You may still not remember the event completely. However, based on what you do remember, make as complete a list as possible of the ways you feel responsible. Be as specific and detailed as possible. Closely examining these self-blame statements is fundamental to your healing.

Include both rational and irrational thoughts on your list—the "crazy" thoughts may be the most important ones. For example, someone who had been abused as a child might write the following:

> I blame myself for my father's beating me because I spilt the milk on his newspaper when I was five years old. I don't know if I spilt it by accident or on purpose because I was mad at him for not buying me a bike for my birthday and I knew that he loved to read his morning paper without any interruptions. I think I spilt the milk by accident, but I may have been just trying to get back at him. I don't know, but I do know that if I wasn't such a sloppy kid, the beatings would have never happened.

Other examples include these:

> The earthquake happened because I was leading a sinful life and God was trying to punish me.

> When I had to leave my foxhole because of my injured arm, my buddy took my place. A few minutes later he was blown up. I had been ordered to get medical treatment, but I still feel guilty because if I had stayed in my place, he would be alive today.

Remember to also write about the aftereffects of the event. Remember that this is not a writing contest. Your sentences and thoughts can be long, complicated, and garbled.

For example, a battered woman might write this:

> I blame myself for my son's depression and emotional problems while I was married to John because I blame myself for the beatings because I should have been more mature when I was 19 and seen that John was capable of violence and never married him at all. I blame myself because I didn't measure up to John's expectations and that's why I was beaten. If I had been a better wife, I wouldn't have gotten beaten and my son would not have been affected. The beatings were also my fault because after a few beatings I hated my husband. It's a sin to hate and the rest of the beatings were partly my punishment for hating him and for causing my son emotional damage.

someone or something reminds you of the traumatic event, especially of those aspects of the event that tend to make you feel guilty or ashamed?

If the answer to the last question is yes, ask clients to identify three or four situations in which they reacted in such a manner during the past week or month. Also find out how they reacted.

Following are three examples of typical reactions to such situations:

> I saw a newspaper article saying that divorce was bad for children, and it touched off my guilt about divorcing my husband. But underneath that guilt was guilt about not having been able to stop the violence. Despite all the therapy I've had, I still feel that if I had been a better wife—prettier, more pleasing, more something—he would have stopped abusing me and we would have had a good marriage. After reading the article, I felt enraged, like I wanted to kill the person who wrote it.

> The grocery store clerk mentioned that one of her relatives had been in an earthquake in California. She was only trying to be friendly, but it reminded me of the fire I was in. I didn't get hurt, but two of my neighbors and my dog died. I shut down entirely. I couldn't smile or cry. For hours I felt dead inside, and I didn't go to that store anymore.

> I don't know why, but something made me remember how I hit some little children who were begging for food after a firefight. It seemed okay then. Everybody was doing it, but now I can't stand thinking about it. If therapy is going to make me think about these things, I think I'll quit because after thinking about those kids I went around for days as if I was in a black cloud.

The goal here is for clients to begin to see some relationships between the trauma and some of their problems in coping with daily life. Remind them that part of healing involves becoming aware, little by little, of the ways in which the trauma continues to affect their feelings about themselves and their reactions to people and situations in the present.

Working on Self-Forgiveness

The Self-Forgiveness handout is designed to help clients begin to consider forgiving themselves for aspects of their behavior about which they experience considerable shame or guilt. Clients are often helped in achieving self-forgiveness, as well as awareness of their emotions and their conflicts, if they are led to distance themselves from the trauma and see it from the viewpoint of an objective or third-party observer, as if it had happened to someone else.

Secondary Wounding

In some mental health circles, PTSD is currently used to explain every aspect of a survivor's concerns, so that pretrauma differences between clients are overlooked or ignored. In my view, however, pretrauma, trauma, and post-trauma

Self-Forgiveness

Forgiving yourself for some of the choices, behaviors, and feelings you had during the traumatic incident is crucial to your healing. You may find this a long and difficult—even a life-long—process. But whatever progress you make toward forgiving yourself will be invaluable. To begin, consider the following questions. You can also write about them, if you wish:

1. What would it take for you to forgive yourself for some of the behaviors, attitudes, and feelings for which you still blame yourself?

2. Is it possible for you to do whatever you need to do so that you can forgive yourself? If so, what is keeping you from pursuing whatever you need to make peace with this part of your past?

3. Do you need to know something to forgive yourself that you will never be able to find out? If so, your options are to try to forgive yourself anyway or to continue to punish yourself. Who are you helping and what good are you doing in the world by punishing yourself? Who would you harm if you forgave yourself?

4. Think of family members and friends, people you dearly love. If you can't think of anyone you truly love, imagine a child of about ten or eleven. Now rerun the story of your trauma or an imaginary movie of the trauma, but make the "star" one of the people you love or the young child. Have the person do, think, and say exactly what you did during the trauma.

5. Now, make notes about the actions (or inactions) you condemn or blame the person for. Are you being kinder to that person than you are to yourself? Would you be able to forgive him or her for some of the things you blame yourself for? If you can forgive that person, why can't you forgive yourself for the very same behaviors, attitudes, and feelings?

factors all need to be taken into account to form a complete picture of the issues facing the survivor in need of help. It is a great disservice to our traumatized clients to lump them all together, ignore their backgrounds, and hence lose the opportunity to make any connections between their pretrauma and post-traumatic histories, when such connections exist. The making of such connections is not intended to blame the victim for the trauma, but rather to help clients understand the meaning of the trauma for them.

Likewise, special attention needs to be given to the client's post-trauma experiences, particularly any personal losses that followed the trauma, such as a divorce, the death of a parent or child, and the loss of a job. Secondary wounding experiences must also be explored and factored into the equation. Secondary wounding occurs when the people, institutions, caregivers, and others to whom the trauma survivor turns for emotional, legal, financial, medical, or other assistance respond in a way that is damaging to the survivor, emotionally, psychologically, financially, or otherwise. The most common forms of secondary wounding are discussed below.

Forms, Effects, and Causes

People commonly deny or disbelieve the trauma survivor's account of the trauma. Or they minimize or discount the magnitude of the event, its meaning to the victim, its impact on the victim's life.

For example, after a hurricane, Sandra, a concert violinist, was taken to a makeshift hospital, along with others who were injured. When she was told that three of her fingers would have to be amputated, she began to cry. "Hush now, you big crybaby," the nurse said. "Look around you. Bed number one lost his arm, and bed two has to have both legs removed. Count your blessings and don't upset the others."

It is also common for people to, on some level, blame survivors for the traumatic event. This, of course, only increases survivors' sense of self-blame and low self-esteem. Similarly, stigmatization occurs when others judge survivors negatively for normal reactions to the traumatic event or for any long-term symptoms suffered. These judgments can take the following forms:

- Ridicule of, or condescension toward, the survivor

- Misinterpretation of the survivor's psychological distress as a sign of deep psychological problems or moral or mental deficiency, or otherwise giving the survivor's PTSD symptoms negative or pejorative labels

- An implication or outright statement that the survivor's symptoms reflect his or her desire for financial gain, attention, or unwarranted sympathy

- Punishment of the victim (rather than the offender) or in other ways depriving the victim of justice

Trauma survivors are also sometimes denied promised or expected services on the basis that they do not need or are not entitled to such services. An example of this is Alvin, a railroad worker who lost his left leg in a train accident. When he sought compensation from the railroad, he was told to wait and see if his leg would "get better." After presenting medical documentation showing that it would not, Alvin's request was again denied because, despite his disability, he had found gainful employment.

Four years later, with the help of an attorney whose fees Alvin had to pay himself, Alvin was granted compensation. However, he was awarded neither attorney fees nor payment for the four years he had to struggle to obtain the benefits he was entitled to.

Ignorance and insensitivity can take many forms in addition to those listed above. It is their effects, however, that are often most devastating. Claudia H., for example, was trapped in an abusive marriage. Back in her small town, in the early sixties, there was little awareness of wife abuse and only minimal legal protection for battered wives. Whenever Claudia could, she would call the police when her husband threatened her. Their responses were less than helpful:

"Lady, he's your husband, not mine."

"You're both animals."

"There's nothing we can do about it until he does something. Call us after he actually starts beating or cutting you."

After repeated threats on her life, Claudia took her children and fled.

During the divorce proceedings, mental health experts testified that Claudia was a masochist who also suffered from other "severe psychiatric disturbances" (unspecified), as evidenced by the fact that she had stayed in an abusive marriage as long as she did. On the other hand, they also faulted her for "breaking up a happy home" and subjecting her children to the "horrors of divorce."

And, whether out of sheet incompetence or for some darker reason, Claudia's attorney failed to bring up the husband's own personality problems.

The judge awarded the divorce to Claudia's husband. According to the law in that place and time, Claudia had not been "battered enough"—seven years of hospital reports and other documentation of the abuse were necessary for a battered woman to win the divorce. And because Claudia was labeled a deserter who left her marriage for insufficient cause, the judge allotted the lion's share of the property, including the house, to Claudia's husband, leaving Claudia homeless and almost penniless. He then told Claudia that if she could not adequately support her children, custody would be given to their father.

Claudia's case is a rather extreme example—one that we all hope could not happen today. But such things do happen, more frequently than most people would believe. Although some progress has been made in providing legal help for abused wives since Claudia went to court, the laws vary from state to state and county to county. Some areas offer strong protection for abused wives, others do not. Even where good laws exist, however, they are not always enforced.

For example, in a recent study, the American Psychological Association found secondary wounding experiences rampant among victims of crime and violence. Some victims reported that their secondary wounding experiences were more painful and devastating than the original traumatic event. Police officers, lawyers, and court officials, were cited in the report. However, medical personnel, mental health professionals, and a myriad of others not usually associated with causing psychological injury to the people they serve were also found guilty of secondary wounding (American Psychological Association 1984).

In essence, secondary wounding occurs because people who have never been hurt sometimes have difficulty understanding and being patient with people who have been hurt. Secondary wounding also occurs because people who have never confronted human tragedy are sometimes unable to comprehend the lives of those in occupations that involve dealing with human suffering or mass casualties on a daily basis.

In addition, as discussed earlier some people, even some therapists, simply are not strong enough to accept the negatives in life. They prefer to ignore the fact that sadness, injustice, and loss are just as much a part of life as joy and goodness. When such individuals confront a trauma survivor, they may reject or disparage the survivor because that individual represents the parts of life they have chosen to deny.

It also happens that trauma survivors are rejected or disparaged by other survivors—those who have chosen to deny or repress their own trauma and have not yet dealt with their losses and anger. When trauma survivors who have not dealt with their own traumatic pasts see someone who is obviously suffering emotionally or physically, they may need to block out that person in order to leave their own denial system intact.

The following paragraphs give a brief rundown of some other common causes of secondary wounding.

Some secondary wounding stems from sheer ignorance. Especially in the past, there were few if any courses on victimization, domestic violence, or child abuse available to medical, legal, and mental health professionals. Today, such courses are available in many locations; however, they are not a required part of the training in any of those fields.

Increasing numbers of police departments are sensitizing their staff to the problems of victims. And where the training is sufficient, the police have been shown to be more responsive to victims. Yet not all police departments are able to devote adequate training hours to this subject.

Another major cause of secondary wounding is that many helping professionals (police, rescue workers, doctors, and other emergency room staff), are themselves suffering from burnout (or even some form of PTSD). As a result of having worked for years with trauma survivors, like those survivors, they are emotionally depleted. They may also, like many trauma survivors, feel unappreciated and unrecognized by the general public and by those in their workplace.

Nurses, for example, are notoriously underpaid and undervalued, and paramedics and police officers often feel betrayed by the criminal justice system, which they feel fails to adequately deal with the criminals they have risked their lives to apprehend. In some places, police officers are ostracized in their own communities.

In the mental health field, social workers and other mental health workers assigned to child abuse and family violence cases, or who work in public mental health agencies, often stagger under enormous caseloads and are hampered in helping victims by the massive amounts of paperwork and red tape and lack of support services.

Another hurdle victims face is the prevalence and persistence of what can be called the "just-world fallacy." According to this philosophy, people "get what they deserve and deserve what they get." The basic assumption of the just-world fallacy is that if you are sufficiently careful, intelligent, moral, or competent, you can avoid misfortune. Thus, people who suffer trauma are somehow to blame for their misfortune. Even if the victims aren't directly blamed, they are seen as causing their victimization by being inherently weak or ineffectual.

American society is particularly prone to this sort of thinking. The United States was founded by individuals who overcame massive political, economic, and social obstacles by means of hard work, self-sacrifice, and physical and emotional endurance. As a nation today, as in the past, we pride ourselves on our can-do spirit and our American ingenuity—we are certain we can overcome almost any hardship. The American dream tells us that our country is so bountiful and so full of opportunities that anyone who wants the good life can have it; all they have to do is pull themselves up by their own bootstraps.

Abraham Lincoln is quoted as saying "People can be as happy as they make up their minds to be"—implying that in the personal realm, as well as in the economic realm, man can be master of his own fate. If only that were true.

Treatment Implications

Secondary wounding experiences can be as painful and powerful as the original traumatic event. Just as clients need to heal from trauma, they will need healing from any secondary wounding experiences they have had as well.

Healing from secondary wounding experiences requires first that clients be able to identify what hit them—what secondary wounding experiences they experienced—and then that they be able to distance themselves from the negative responses involved in these experiences.

The distancing needs to be achieved on both emotional and mental levels. On the emotional level, the goal of distancing is for clients not to be devastated by the experience. In all likelihood, they will still be troubled by others' insensitivity, but they can learn not to allow it to destroy them emotionally. On the mental level, the goal of distancing is that they become less likely to believe the negative judgments of their worth that secondary wounding experiences can so easily generate.

Clients need to learn that, generally, the rejection, humiliation, or attack says more about the ignorance, insensitivity, fears, or prejudices of the other person than anything about themselves, and that it reflects larger societal problems, including the prevalence of blame-the-victim attitudes and lack of adequate funding for victim-compensation services. Once they learn the technique of viewing their secondary wounding experiences from this perspective, they will have some armor against the pain involved in many interactions.

It may also help your traumatized clients to know, and keep in mind, that in addition to the emotional vulnerability that results from trauma, biological changes can occur that make them exceptionally sensitive to and observant of others' responses. Thus, very subtle cues in the behavior of others will affect them much more than they would a nontraumatized person.

A second technique you can teach your clients is that of countering the negative messages of those who lack understanding and compassion with affirming "self-talk" of their own. Together, these two approaches will enable them to gain a measure of objectivity. This objectivity in turn gives them increased control of their lives by acting as a brake on two destructive but legitimate reactions many trauma survivors have to secondary wounding experiences: sinking into helpless-hopeless thoughts and feelings, and being overwhelmed by the urge to strike back, verbally or physically.

Even when the desire to retaliate is entirely justified (as it often is), an aggressive response only confirms the other person's belief that the client is "a nut case" or otherwise undeserving of assistance—which can lead to that person withholding something that the client does in fact deserve and need.

Countering the powerful negative messages of secondary wounding experiences is not done effortlessly or quickly. Such experiences will probably always trouble your clients to some extent. But they can make progress in affirming their worth as a person and their strengths as a trauma survivor, in addition to increasing their objectivity and control.

Naming the Demon

The first step toward helping clients overcome secondary wounding is to educate them on the subject. You can explain what secondary wounding is and identify its forms and causes either orally or using a handout. The exercises provided below, or exercises you evolve on your own, can help clients identify their secondary wounding experiences and their emotional and other reactions to these experiences. You can then help them "name the demon" involved in their particular secondary wounding experiences.

This analogy may actually be helpful to your clients: In certain societies, psychological distress and its symptoms are conceptualized as attacks by supernatural beings. Typically these demons or spirits are given specific names—jealousy, revenge, bad memories, depression—and a healing ritual is performed to rid the suffering person of the particular spirit or demon that is causing the problem.

The efficacy of the healing ritual aside, it is probably helpful to suffering individuals simply to know that their affliction has a name, since for human beings, words are a way of making the unknown knowable, and therefore controllable, just as it is helpful for clients to put the name PTSD to their trauma-related symptoms. For example, because they are aware of what PTSD is, when they experience a PTSD symptom, they can tell themselves, "I don't have to panic. I am only having a PTSD attack. What I'm experiencing now is predictable and limited. It will not last forever and it cannot cause me to lose my mind."

Likewise, for your clients to achieve some distance from the secondary wounding experiences they have had in the past and will probably have in the future, they need to learn to name the demons of those experiences. For example, instead of acting on their feelings or allowing themselves to become increasingly hopeless, they can tell themselves, "It's not my fault this person is treating me with so little respect and appreciation of my difficulty. But, if I lose control of myself, or sink deeper and deeper into depression, I will only be lessening my chances of getting what I need from this person. Maybe if I can figure out this demon's name I will know what I'm dealing with. Just what kind of secondary wounding is this anyway?"

Secondary wounding responses can be divided into six categories:

- Those showing denial or disbelief

- Those that involve discounting

- Those in which the victim is blamed for his or her problems

- Those that exhibit ignorance

- Those involving generalization or labeling

- Those stemming from sheer cruelty

Once clients are able to identify the responses of others along these lines, they will be better able to view these reactions for what they truly are. Giving them a name will increase clients' ability to cope with secondary wounding experiences in a constructive manner, and will lessen, though not eliminate, the pain and humiliation.

Denial and Disbelief

When people respond to clients with statements such as "You're exaggerating," "That could never happen," or simply, "I don't believe it," they are denying the reality of your client's trauma.

Abusers and criminals are often the first to deny their victims the reality of their experience. "Please don't take my purse," says the victim. "I'm not taking your purse. It's your imagination," replies the thief. Or, "Stop hitting me," says the victim. "I'm not hitting you. You're hitting yourself," the abuser says. Unfortunately, they aren't the only ones who practice denial. For example:

- Sally B.'s three-month-old daughter was raped by Sally's boyfriend. When she told the admitting clerk at the emergency room, he replied, "That's impossible. Nobody would rape a baby. Come on now, tell us the real truth."

- Friends and family members also sometimes practice denial, as in Dan K.'s case. When Dan told his mother that his father was verbally and physically abusing him, his mother replied, "Your father is a good man. You've been watching too much TV."

Discounting

In denial, people do not believe the client's story. When clients are being discounted, people do not deny that the traumatic event occurred. They simply minimize its effect on the client or the magnitude of the event, as in the following examples:

- Jane S. explained to her boyfriend that she sometimes has trouble responding to him sexually because of having been raped three years before. "How could one little rape have affected you that much? I know some women who have been raped three or four times, but they still like sex," the boyfriend replied.

- Bill T., a policeman, confided to a colleague that he had been suffering from headaches and nausea since a shoot-out where three people were killed. The colleague replied, "They were a bunch of crooks. They are where they should be—six feet under. You should be in ecstasy, not having headaches."

- Carl J., a flood survivor, went to his doctor for the "shakes." "I've been shaking for two years," he said, "ever since that flood washed away my . . ."
  "Come on, now, Mr. Jones," the doctor broke in, "that flood wasn't that bad. Only a few people died and about a hundred homes were destroyed. When I was a boy, I was in a flood that wiped out over half the town. Now *that's* a real flood."

Blaming the Victim

Victim blaming responses may be more frequently delivered by strangers, but friends and family members are also sometimes guilty of them:

- After Howard L.'s house was burglarized and vandalized, he took a second job to pay for the repairs and replace his stolen camera gear. When he complained about how tired and upset he was to a friend one day, she replied, "I told you, you should never have moved into that neighborhood. The least you could have done was buy more insurance."

- Ross N., a former serviceman who had been discharged after losing an arm in a training accident, met a cousin at a family gathering. The cousin said, "So you're a lefty now, eh? I guess that's what you get for enlisting."

Ignorance

Ignorance of trauma and its effects plays a major role in secondary wounding experiences. If people have not experienced trauma themselves, or have not learned about it in other ways, they often do not know what to say or do. Also, as mentioned before, often the fact that a person has been victimized threatens other people's defenses against the idea that they too could be victimized.

People are often also ignorant about the possible economic, social, and psychological consequences of trauma. Ignorance can even result in inappropriate medical or psychological treatment methods being applied. These methods may be perfectly appropriate for nontraumatized people, but can be unhelpful, even harmful, to trauma survivors. Consider these examples:

- "Jen, I'm sorry, I can't make it to your party. Ever since my accident I try to avoid Route 97 as much as possible. And I can't get to your house any other way," Betty C. said.

    "That's crazy," her friend replied, "you're acting like a superstitious nut. And selfish too. You're just thinking of yourself."

- "No more vacations at the beach! After seven months in Saudi Arabia, I don't want to see another grain of sand as long as I live!" said Hank R., a veteran of the Persian Gulf war.

    "You are going to deny your family a trip to the beach just because you had to sit on the sand for seven months?" his father replied. "And don't go claiming you have that TSP or PSSD or whatever that Vietnam thing is called. You didn't fire a shot."

Generalization

One of the social consequences of being victimized is being labeled a victim. Once a person is so labeled, there is a tendency for others to interpret most, if not all, of that person's emotions and behavior in light of that label. For example, the deaf are often assumed to also be blind or mentally retarded. Furthermore, once one is labeled, it is very difficult to escape from that label (Taylor, Wood, and Lichtman 1983).

For instance, it may be assumed that because your client has been through a trauma he or she is now "emotionally scarred"—forever. For example:

- Roger S. lost an eye in a chemical explosion at work. Otherwise, he was not injured. But when he returned to his job, he was offered a wheelchair and told that his company did not employ "cripples."

- Juanita P., a dental hygienist, confided to her employer that she was seeking counseling for having been robbed and beaten.

    "That's fine," he replied, "you can take the receptionist's job; she's leaving us anyway," implying that somehow being a victim of crime had impaired Juanita's ability to work.

Cruelty

Most secondary wounding experiences *feel* cruel. Therefore it is often difficult to assess whether the secondary wounding arises from a desire the other person has to cause pain or whether it is caused by ignorance, generalization, or some other secondary wounding process. In many cases, a mixture of cruelty and some other process or processes is at work, as some of the preceding examples demonstrate.

Sometimes the fact of the client's traumatization and PTSD may be used by people the client knows. In the absence of the trauma they would have found something else to use as a weapon against the client. However, perfect strangers are also capable of gratuitous cruelty. A feature of our culture that helps lay the groundwork for these behaviors is an increasing emotional detachment among people, even in families.

According to some observers, contemporary American culture in general is experiencing an "increase in psychic numbing, alienation, isolation and difficulties with intimacy" (Young and Erickson 1988). This generalized numbing throughout the population can be attributed at least in part to economic and social changes that make it difficult for people to empathize with each other's pain, even within their own families, much less with that of strangers.

Client Exercises

The Secondary Wounding handouts can be completed by the client as a form of homework to be shared with you in a later session, or you can complete them with the client in session.

Low Self-Esteem

Low self-esteem is the hallmark of PTSD-afflicted trauma survivors in this and many other countries. The numerous origins of this low self-esteem include the internalization of blame-the-victim attitudes, the self-blame and survivor guilt almost inherent to traumatization, and the pain of experiencing helplessness and great fear, anger, grief. Low self-esteem results from the latter cause when the survivor lives in a society or in social group that places a high value on self-sufficiency and emotional moderation and looks down on individuals who need help or are in emotional pain or feel other forms of emotional torment.

There is nothing inherently humiliating about being a victim of trauma. Historically, in countries that have been repeatedly besieged by internal strife, military invasion, or frequent natural catastrophe, the powerlessness and feelings associated with being a victim of trauma affect so many people that they are considered part of the normal range of the human experience. However, in countries that have been relatively more fortunate, and among social groups that hold to the just-world fallacy and highly value self-reliance and self-confidence (rather than family, tribal, or community dependence and cohesiveness) many trauma survivors experience their intensified need for protection, assurance, and other kinds of support from others as a form of humiliation or personal defeat.

Yet clinical experience has shown that when the trauma is fresh, the need for help, is especially intense. If that help is provided, the need for support may diminish, provided the trauma was of minimal duration and severity. However, if initial help is not provided, or if the trauma was either severe or of long duration or both, the survivor's dependency needs may be stronger than those he or she

Identifying Your Secondary Wounding Experiences

1. Write down as many secondary wounding experiences that you have had as you can remember, including any current ones, one experience to a page. (You need to leave space for analyzing and commenting on each experience.)

2. When you have finished, review your list and categorize each experience as denial or disbelief, discounting, generalization, victim-blaming, ignorance, or cruelty. Include as many labels as apply; for example, a single experience can contain elements of ignorance, cruelty, and blaming the victim.

3. After you have completed the labeling for each experience, identify your emotional response. Did you have no feeling at all? Did you experience irritation, anger, rage, hurt, disappointment, disgust, a desire to retaliate, or any other feeling? List as many feelings as apply.

4. Now take some time to reflect on the process you have just been through. Were you surprised at how many secondary wounding experiences you have endured? Did labeling the experiences help ease the pain or did it make you more furious or sad?

5. Finally, consider whether any of the secondary wounding experiences ignited your anger or rage, lowered your self-esteem, or made you feel hopeless or helpless. In your journal, write more about those particular experiences.

Once the feelings stemming from your secondary wounding experiences are faced, their intensity may be lessened. You will likely never feel completely neutral in the midst of a secondary wounding experience—or when you are remembering one. If you are aware enough to feel your feelings, you are going to feel angry, sad, powerless, betrayed, and a host of other emotions. But this does not mean that you are hopelessly bound to the past and will never feel joy again.

Secondary Wounding and Your Attitudes Today

Do some writing about how your secondary wounding experiences affect your life. More specifically, for each secondary wounding experience, consider whether that experience had the following effects:

1. Did it alter your views of your social, vocational, and other abilities?

2. Did it change your attitudes toward certain types or groups of people or certain government or social institutions?

3. Were your religious or spiritual views affected?

4. Did it affect your family life, friendships, or other close relationships?

5. Did it alter your ability to participate in groups or belong to associations or your attitudes towards the general public?

6. Now look at what you've written, and ask yourself, "Which of these attitudes do I wish to retain? Which of them are in my best interest to reconsider? Which ones would I like to discard because they hamper my life in the present?"

Secondary Wounding and Your Activities

Suppose that one of your worst secondary wounding experiences was being treated like the criminal, rather than the victim, in court. Because of this, you have concluded that all judges and jurors are insensitive at best and corrupt and heartless at worst. Yet now someone owes you several thousand dollars, and in order to get it you need to take that person to court.

If you hadn't had the experience you did in court, you would probably already have begun the groundwork for the lawsuit. However, because of your hatred of courts and fear of being, once again, denied justice, you procrastinate about pursuing the litigation.

At this point, what do you think is in your best interest—avoiding the courtroom, with all its secondary wounding memories and the risk of repeated victimization, or pursuing the thousands of dollars you are due?

The decision is yours. It may be that if you receive some healing assistance for your courtroom-related secondary wounding experiences you will be able to tolerate the aversiveness of being in court.

Counseling can assist you in differentiating your past courtroom experience from the present situation. And, with support, you might be able to manage any PTSD symptoms that emerge as a result of placing yourself back in that setting. For example, you could take some friends along, rather than facing the situation alone.

On the other hand, you might decide that you simply can't handle it. You'd rather do without the money than subject yourself to another courtroom experience. This is not cowardice. Rather it is a respectable life-preserving decision. At all times, it is vital that you know and respect your limits and not be pushed into activities that are emotionally overwhelming or otherwise destructive for you.

Your emotional health comes first, not conforming to some inner voice that says you "should" be able to handle anything. (The same voice that has probably been telling you, "You should have been able to go through the trauma, and everything that's happened since, without its getting to you. You just aren't strong enough.")

By the time you finish therapy, you will know beyond a doubt that this "should" has no basis in emotional reality. But even after you have let go of this unrealistic expectation of yourself, others may still believe in it. They may encourage you to do things you know are not in your best interests emotionally, or denigrate you for letting your "fears and neuroses" or "skeletons from the past" control your life.

Close your ears to these voices and listen to your own inner voice—the one that knows what you have been through and what you can tolerate without arousing excessive anxiety, pain, rage, or other symptoms. In all probability, you will be able to stretch the limits of what you consider tolerable, but you can only do so one small step at a time. Great leaps forward can send you spiraling downward into a depression or flying off into a hyper state.

With that caution in mind, first list the activities your secondary wounding experiences have taught you to curtail or avoid. Then, for each of them, do the following:

1. Ask yourself whether at this particular time, in your view (not someone else's) you can tolerate the activity. What will be the emotional cost? Is it worth it to you?

   Once again, the main point is to realize that you have a *choice*. During the original trauma and during the subsequent secondary wounding experiences, you had either no choices or very few choices or all the options available were so aversive they were not really choices.

2. For the activities you have decided you cannot currently tolerate (or feel it's not in your best interests to attempt), consider whether counseling or some other form of assistance might make them tolerable. Do you want to make the attempt? If you don't feel you can or want to at present, might you want to in the future, at some point further along in the healing process?

had prior to the trauma or than those of others in his or her family or peer group. For this need, the survivor may be punished or looked down upon by others.

Alternatively, the survivor's vulnerability may prove attractive to others. Some of these others may genuinely wish to be supportive of the survivor, whereas others may exploit or manipulate the survivor for their own ends. Regardless of how the survivor is treated, however, in general the individual in the relationship who is "hurting" tends to be seen as less strong and holds less power.

Accepting Dependency Needs

At some point in your counseling sessions, you need to tell your clients that their heightened dependency needs and their increased needs for protection, assurance, and emotional support from others are entirely normal and appropriate following a traumatic incident. It is only cultural values that make this emotional state shameful or degrading. Clients who do not seem to understand this, and who need help in accepting their temporary dip in self-reliance, may be helped by a discussion of what usually occurs when animals or children are wounded.

The following sample dialogue uses the example of an injured dog; however, you could use the example of any other kind of injured animal or the example of an injured child. Be sure to pick an animal or human being toward which your client has a natural sympathy or liking. For example, if your client can't stand certain kinds of animals or dislikes children, do not use these as examples.

Therapist: Now suppose you had a dog that was hit by a car. Its leg was badly injured, and you weren't there to take it to the vet right away. What would the dog do?

Client: Go into a corner, lick its wounds, whimper and sleep a lot.

Therapist: That's what most animals do. They find a safe spot and lick their wounds. Do you have any idea why animals do that?

Client: Well, in licking they are trying to heal the wounds, and they go into a corner because it's quieter there.

Therapist: Any other reason?

Client: For protection. If an animal is injured, it can't protect itself very well from attack, so it kind of hides in a corner or in another place with some natural protection.

Therapist: And what did you do after the trauma?

Client: I wanted to stay home. I didn't feel I could face people because I was so shaky that I was afraid they might ask me to do something I couldn't handle. I was certain that the fact that I couldn't handle it would show and I'd be humiliated.

Therapist: Do you see an analogy between how you acted and what a wounded animal does almost instinctively? It's almost as if what happens to an animal on a physical level happened to you on a psychological level.

Now let's carry this analogy further. If your dog was injured, would you bring its water and food bowl near its resting spot, or would you expect the dog to go down to the basement or wherever you usually kept its food and water?

Client: Of course I'd bring the food and water near.

Therapist: And if the dog whimpered a lot, would you pet the dog and say loving things, or would you tell it it was acting like a sickeningly dependent child who should shut up or that it was only feeling sorry for itself and should toughen up and not whimper.

Client: Come on, who do you think I am, Simon Legree?

Therapist: I'm trying to make a point here. How did you feel about yourself when you stayed home after the trauma and so desperately wanted your wife to stroke you and baby you a little bit?

Client: Like a whining fool. Like a crybaby. Certainly not like a man.

Therapist: If your best male friend had his leg smashed in a car accident, would you think he was a whining fool and crybaby if his wife brought him his food in trays and gave him a little extra loving attention while he was recuperating?

Client: Of course not. I'd say he deserved it.

Therapist: Then why didn't you deserve it?

Client: I don't know.

Therapist: It's something to think about, isn't it: why you wouldn't think twice about treating a dog better than you let others treat you and why a male friend of yours could receive attention and care and still be a man, while if you receive those things then somehow you are emasculated?

Client: I don't know.

Therapist: I hope someday you can think of the trauma as something that ran over your life the same way a car might run over a dog. Instead of a broken leg, you have a broken spirit or a broken view of life.

Now consider this question: What if there was no one to help the dog after his leg was hurt? What might have happened?

Client: Well, if he could get to food and water, he might live. But the strain of walking on an injured leg might injure it more. And if his leg was hurt too bad and he couldn't make it to food and water, he would eventually die.

Therapist: So do you see the analogy? It's appropriate for you right now to take a rest from the usual pace, lick your wounds and otherwise take care of them, and not stress yourself so much that there is no chance for healing or the healing is so prolonged that you want to give up the entire effort.

What do you think might happen to people who are denied emotional "food and water" and the concrete kinds of help they need when they are run over by life? Does it help them or hurt them to get help? Does trying to do everything on their own, just like before the trauma, speed up or delay the healing process? And what if they are so injured they just can't take care of themselves? Couldn't they die, psychologically if not physically as well?

If you really want to return to your pretrauma state of functioning and your previous level of self-sufficiency, then the smartest thing to do is look for and accept the help you need to heal whatever is broken in you. If you had been physically injured in an accident, but acted as though nothing that bad had happened and started walking on a leg that still needed a rest and bandaging for support, the leg might never heal and you'd be crippled for life. Then you really would be dependent.

It sounds like a contradiction, but it isn't. The only way to get back to however independent you were is to allow yourself to be dependent when you need to be.

You can then point out that just as the dog will begin to leave his corner and start taking care of himself as he used to once his leg is better, so will your client leave her or his social isolation or other form of "safe place" as soon as she or he is healed enough. Like the dog, the client will soon resume normal activities, maybe with a scar or two or a limp, but she or he will be up and about and will no longer need as much special attention as right after the trauma.

Your therapeutic task then, is first to help clients accept their post-traumatic emotional state and their need for help, even if this clashes with the high value the culture places on self-confidence and social outgoingness. Basically, the message you wish to impart is this:

> It's okay if right now you are somewhat introspective and full of self-doubt and remorse. In fact, true mental health requires a balance between self-confidence and self-doubt. Self-confidence is necessary for normal functioning, but perpetually self-confident people are usually arrogant and shallow. Those that never question themselves cannot grow.
>
> Also, no one can be "together" all the time. Eventually everyone, no matter how fortunate, encounters a situation that baffles or breaks them. Some people seem unaffected by a major loss or crisis, but their apparent solidity is built on shaky ground. Externally, it may seem as if they are handling the situation, but in reality they are either denying it or hiding it under a calm facade.
>
> You, on the other hand, are in the process of acquiring the skills with which to handle life's inevitable blows—a process that requires considerable self-examination. The work you have done so far in therapy is part of that process, including the realizations you may have come to where you see yourself as blameworthy or deficient in some areas.
>
> Those negative feelings toward yourself can be very painful, in and of themselves. So it may be comforting for you to know that the low self-esteem and other bad feelings you may have about yourself are not immutable parts of your personality. It may also help to know that low self-esteem is, for a variety of reasons, common among trauma survivors.

Self-Esteem and Self-Blame

No doubt some of your clients already will have had areas of low self-esteem prior to the trauma. For clients who entered the traumatic situation with existing problems in that area, the trauma may have increased their negative feelings about themselves.

Alternatively, if clients entered the traumatic situation with relatively high self-esteem or with a mixed view of themselves, the trauma may have created serious self-doubts. However, the good news is that since much of this self-blame stems from the traumatic event and secondary wounding experiences, there is considerable hope that once clients better understand the trauma and how it affected them, they can be delivered from some of the negative feelings they have about themselves.

You can assist your clients in overcoming some of the low self-esteem attached to being a trauma survivor by helping them identify the specific ways in which their self-esteem has suffered as the result of the trauma. The Self-Blame and Your Self-Esteem handout is designed to assist in this process. After you have explained the purpose of the exercise, the client can complete it as a homework assignment, to be discussed with you in session later, or together with you as part of counseling session.

Victim Thinking

The lives of PTSD-afflicted clients are limited not only by survivor guilt, self-blame, low self-esteem, and the psychological and other burdens imposed upon them by secondary wounding, but by what can be called victim thinking. "Victim thinking" refers to a negative, fearful worldview born of being in a trauma. In the midst of trauma, victim thinking, like emotional numbing, is entirely appropriate, if not life-preserving. However, in safer circumstances, victim thinking diminishes the survivor's creativity, energy level, and ability to trust in and communicate with others.

The Three Levels of Victimization

As briefly discussed in chapter 1, victimization can potentially occur on three levels (McCarthy 1986): the traumatic event itself, secondary wounding experiences, and the acceptance of the victim label.

During the traumatic event (level 1), three basic assumptions about life are shattered: the belief in personal invulnerability, the belief in an orderly world, and a positive view of one's self. Once a client has been traumatized, he or she can no longer think, "It can't happen to me," because it did happen. Even if the client is assured that it can't happen again (which you should never do because people can be revictimized repeatedly), the client will fear that the trauma will repeat itself. This feeling of vulnerability can develop into the sense of doom or foreshortened future, which is one of the classic symptoms of PTSD.

The loss of a sense of invulnerability shatters the survivor's sense of safety. The loss of a sense of an orderly world shatters the survivor's sense of life as meaningful and comprehensible. If your trauma survivor clients were like most people, they probably believed that if they tried to be careful, honest, and good people, they could avoid disaster. Trauma taught them differently.

In order to make sense of the trauma's occurrence, some survivors blame themselves. Others begin to question their previous views of human and social justice and some find that their religious or spiritual views fail to provide them with adequate answers to questions about why the trauma happened and why it happened to them or their loved ones. The result is that the survivor is left in a state of turmoil and confusion.

Trauma also shatters assumptions about the self, in ways discussed elsewhere in this book (see, for example, the section in chapter 2 on depersonalization and entrapment). In the course of trauma, people often involuntarily behave in a manner that violates their beliefs, morals, and self-image. These actions, though understandable in the context of the trauma as attempts to survive, can be difficult for the victim to reconcile afterwards.

Self-Blame and Your Self-Esteem

You may want to use the following list as a guide to identifying the ways in which the trauma has affected your self-esteem. Keeping in mind the work you have done on identifying your areas of self-blame, write about how that self-blame has contributed to lowering your self-esteem.

As a result of the trauma, I now see myself as:

- Lacking in intelligence
- Less intelligent than I thought I was
- Evil or bad
- Less sexually desirable
- Unworthy of love or affection
- Ugly, disgusting, or deficient in some way
- Emotionally abnormal
- A very angry, hostile person
- Not as good and honorable as I used to be
- Inadequate in many ways
- Difficult to talk to
- Difficult to live with
- Unlovable
- Too emotional
- Fearful
- A big baby
- A weakling

Secondary wounding experiences (level 2), previously discussed in this chapter, serve to reinforce the shattering of assumptions and the low self-esteem of many trauma survivors.

The third level of victimization occurs when clients internalize the victim status. Even though they are no longer in the original traumatic situation, they think and act as if they are still being victimized. This third level is not a sign of pathology, but one of the unfortunate, but natural, outcomes of the first two levels.

The statements on the Victim Thinking handout reflect this type of thinking. Either in a session or as a homework assignment, ask clients to identify the statements that characterize their view of life. You can discuss in detail those thoughts with which your client agrees, or you can have the client write more about how such thinking may be affecting his or her life.

Countering Victim Thinking

You can then assist your clients in countering victim thinking—and, hopefully, slowly reducing it and eventually cutting it off—by speaking to them (at an appropriate time) as follows:

> Once you have decided that some of your victim thinking is hurting rather than helping you, you need to fight back aggressively. It is natural for the feelings and thinking patterns corresponding to being a double victim (of trauma and secondary wounding) to reappear in many life situations, especially in those that are stressful. However, if you would like to approach situations in your life today from a different perspective, devoid of a victim mentality, you can help yourself by doing the following:
>
> Remind yourself of the original traumatic event or secondary wounding experiences that created your need for the victim thinking. For this you have to determine how and why you acquired the victim thinking in the first place, as we have discussed before.
>
> Also remind yourself of the main reasons a victim mentality doesn't fit the current situation or doesn't serve you now. Consider that the best revenge, and perhaps the only revenge available to you, is first to survive and second to live well. You might also remind yourself that the negative consequences of following your victim thinking usually outweigh the positive.

Preventing Revictimization

Clients may be involved in situations in the present in which they feel misused or maltreated and in which they are, consciously or unconsciously, acting as powerless as they did during the original trauma. Once they identify these situations, they may or may not choose to take action in order to rectify matters. However, they need to be aware of as many instances as possible in their present life, large or small, in which they are assuming the role of the victim.

When you give the Avoiding Revictimization handout to your clients, or have any other kind of session devoted to their identifying ways they feel they are being taken advantage of, stress that their adoption of a victim or passive role

Victim Thinking

To begin, check the boxes beside those statements that sound like something you find yourself thinking or feeling.

☐ I have to accept bad situations because they are part of life and I can do nothing to make them better.

☐ I don't expect much good to happen in my life.

☐ Nobody could ever love me.

☐ I am always going to feel sad, angry, depressed, and confused.

☐ There are situations at work and at home that I could do something about, but I don't have the motivation to do so.

☐ Life overwhelms me, so I prefer to be alone whenever possible.

☐ You can't trust anyone except a very few people.

☐ I feel I have to be extra good, competent, and attractive in order to compensate for my many defects.

☐ I feel guilty for many things, even things that I know are not my fault.

☐ I feel I have to explain myself to people so that they will understand me. But sometimes I get tired of explaining, conclude it's not worth the effort, and stay alone.

☐ I'm often afraid to do something new for fear I will make a mistake.

☐ I can't afford to be wrong.

☐ I feel that when people look at me, they know right away that I'm different.

☐ Sometimes I think that those who died during the traumatic event I experienced were better off than me. At least they don't have to live with the memories.

☐ I am afraid of the future.

☐ Most times I think things will never get better. There is not much I can do to make my life better.

☐ I can be either a perfectionist or a total slob depending on my mood.

☐ I tend to see people as either for me or against me.

☐ I feel pressure to go along with others, even when I don't want to. To avoid such pressures, I avoid people.

☐ I am never going to get over what happened to me.

☐ I find myself apologizing for myself to others.

☐ I have very few choices in life.

If you checked ten or more of these statements, then you probably suffer from victim thinking. Such thinking may have been appropriate during the traumatic event. It may even have helped you to cope with your secondary wounding experiences. For example, if you were suspicious of certain officials, you may have been correct in requiring written documentation of their interactions with you. However, in your present life, victim thinking may be seriously hampering your opportunities for personal growth, vocational development, and the satisfaction of loving human relationships. For example, if you continue to require extensive or inappropriate documentation of interactions with your current coworkers, you could be seen as creating unnecessary work and perhaps as being hostile to them as well.

Can you identify any areas in your life that are currently being adversely affected by your victim thinking, including but not limited to the personal, professional, family, or creative parts of your life? Write about the effects of victim thinking on these areas of your life or discuss them with your counselor.

Avoiding Revictimization

Take some time to consider and write about the following questions.

1. In what ways have you internalized the blame-the-victim attitudes of certain people and institutions in society?

2. To what extent, if any, did the victim-blaming attitudes of others reinforce any low self-esteem or self-doubts you had prior to the trauma and your secondary wounding experiences?

3. Did your trauma or secondary wounding experiences subject you to the learned helplessness syndrome? If so, in what ways are you manifesting the learned helplessness syndrome in the present?

4. To what extent has the healing process helped you to overcome the low self-esteem and negative thinking that being victimized created or reinforced in your life?

5. In what ways are you being victimized or misused in your present life? List all the situations in which you feel mistreated or ignored, if not outright victimized.

6. Which of those situations can be changed?

7. Of the situations that can be changed, which situations do you want to work on changing?

8. For each situation you choose to work on, list at least three constructive steps you can take towards rectifying matters.

For example, you might want to lighten your load at work, but until recently you felt you had to accept whatever tasks were given to you. You now realize you may be being revictimized at work, and you want to change the situation. To do so you could begin by rereading your job description to ascertain whether or not the tasks you are being given fall into your job category. If the tasks are not part of your job description, you can choose to discuss the matter with your supervisor, delegate work whenever possible, and/or ask for help with difficult assignments.

in the situation is not a sign that they are "sick" or masochistic. Rather, ask if they may be doing so because such a position was taught to them as a child, because it was a survival mode during the trauma, or because they were psychologically beaten down by secondary wounding experiences after the trauma.

Emphasize to your clients that, as they consider the questions in the exercise, no situation is too minor to consider, even one as seemingly petty as loaning a coworker five dollars that was never returned. A lot of small victimizations and abuses can result in one big depression.

Chapter 8

Uncovering the Trauma

Although memory retrieval, cognitive restructuring, and working with the feelings, are presented separately in this book, the processes are not inherently separate. Memories can return with or without affect or with varying degrees of affect. For example, whereas some clients have little or no emotion at all as they recall the events of the past, others may become so emotionally flooded that you must stop the memory retrieval process and focus instead on helping clients contain their feelings.

Ideally, returning memories will come with or will eventually generate sufficient emotion so that they can be reprocessed both cognitively and emotionally. This reprocessing allows clients to grow in self-understanding so that they need not waste significant portions of their lives stymied by, reenacting, or destructively reacting to the trauma or trauma-related stimuli. According to van der Kolk (1989), the sole purpose of uncovering the trauma is to "gain conscious control over the unbidden reexperiences or reenactments" of the trauma so that ultimately clients become increasingly able to control their present life.)

The Purposes of Memory Retrieval

Clients may ask you why they should engage in memory retrieval. If you are facilitating a therapy group for survivors, you can call upon senior members of the group to help answer this question. Usually those who have made strides in their healing will make statements such as, "I never knew why I was doing certain things until I remembered what happened during the trauma," or "I always blamed myself for . . . until in therapy I remembered that that's what I was taught by my abuser," or "Only after remembering the trauma did I realize how I was setting myself up for failure in order to punish myself for . . . ."

If you do not have the advantage of such group feedback, you can explain to your questioning clients that memory retrieval is important because until the trauma is uncovered, it may continue to influence their lives in unknown ways. For example, some physical and medical problems may have their origins in or be exacerbated by unprocessed memories. Such memories may also be contributing to clients' present problems with addiction, relationships, vocational or other achievements, and self-esteem. In my experience with adult survivors of childhood physical and sexual abuse, I have found very few who were initially able to link their addiction to the abuse. Instead of seeing the obvious relationship between the abuse and their addiction, clients tended to see the substance abuse as yet another indication that they were "no good" and therefore deserved the abuse. One reason for their difficulty in making the connection between the abuse and their alcohol, drug, or food addiction was this inability to piece together their personal story.

At the same time, however, you need to stress that your prime goal is client safety, that you will never push beyond what you feel the client can handle, that in fact you will not push at all. You will simply facilitate memory retrieval when the client expresses the desire and need to delve into his or her untapped reservoir of self-knowledge. You also need to stress that, in the words of a Vietnam veteran, "It wasn't necessary to remember every mosquito and relive every firefight to make my peace with Vietnam." However, this man did need to remember enough of what occurred to identify and own his feelings about his trauma and, eventually to be able to articulate the existential crisis the war represented to him before he could stop making his war experiences the center of his psychic life.

The Order of Memory, Feelings, and Cognitive Work

As stated before, the healing process does not necessarily follow a prescribed sequence. For some clients, memories do not generate emotions but vice versa: emotions generate the memories. A client may come to a session feeling emotionally out of control and from that starting point will work backward to the memory that gave birth to the emotion.

For example, Allan D. arrived for his session both suicidal and homicidal. His presenting issue was his fury with his employer for having failed to dispose of poisonous materials as promised. During the course of the session, it was revealed that Allan had a double anger: anger at his present employer but also anger at his commanding officer during his military tour of duty. This commanding officer had failed to place certain ammunition in a safe place. When the ammunition exploded, several of Allan's buddies were killed.

However, Allan's issues ran even deeper than anger. The incident with the commanding officer presented Allan with an existential crisis regarding his manhood and his value system. Both before and, even more so, after the ammunition blew up, Allan felt like fragging (killing) his commanding officer, but refrained out of respect for authority, as well as fear of punishment. Apparently others in his unit had the same hatred toward the commanding officer, who soon after was "accidentally" killed by two of his own men. Allan felt guilty: first, for being so "animalistic" as to want to kill the commanding officer; second, for not being "man enough" to kill him before the explosion; and third, for leaving it to others by not killing the officer after the explosion. He felt torn, as many soldiers do, between his training and belief in the necessity of obeying commanding officers and the obvious need to take action against a potentially dangerous situation.

The situation at work was so similar to the military incident that many times Allan considered reminding his employer of the necessity of removing the hazardous materials from the work site. Indeed, Allan had reminded his employer several times, only to incur the man's annoyance. Allan needed his job and did not want to risk the well-being of his family by continually pressing the point with his boss. On the other hand, Allan felt responsible for the safety of his coworkers, not to mention his concern for his own safety. Once again, as in the military, Allan felt trapped. The only way out, he felt, was suicide or homicide.

Ideally, memories are retrieved with an eye not only toward identifying emotions, but toward weeding out cognitive distortions. As discussed in chapter 5, cognitive distortions are beliefs or attitudes that helped the client survive the trauma but do not accurately fit present-day realities and do not help the client function well in present life. For example, a common cognitive distortion is all-or-nothing thinking regarding trusting other people: some survivors either trust someone entirely or not at all.

In many kinds of trauma, a person is either a friend or an enemy, with few in-between categories. However, in nontraumatic situations shades of gray exist. All individuals cannot be classified as a friend, to whom one could entrust one's life, or an enemy, whom one can trust with nothing. In everyday life, some individuals can be trusted with some information and for some activities, whereas other individuals can be trusted with other matters. The more free survivors can become from all-or-nothing thinking in regard to trusting others (as well as in regard to their self-esteem and other issues), the more functional they will be in their present-day family and vocational roles.

Memory retrieval is also important in this respect, because the more coherent and detailed a picture survivors can generate of their trauma, the more progress they can potentially make in eliminating cognitive distortions. There is then a greater probability that the experience of feeling the feelings associated with the trauma will be an emotionally corrective experience rather than a retraumatizing one.

In some cases, the same memory will have to be processed many times: to obtain a more complete picture of the trauma; to examine the various emotions involved, such as terror, anger, sadness; and to uncover and correct cognitive distortions.

It cannot be overemphasized that the memory retrieval process, along with other aspects of recovery, is a highly individual matter. Clients will go through these stages of the healing process in their own unique manner and at their own pace. Likewise, the specific application of any of the interventions suggested in this chapter or elsewhere will vary from one client to the next. Methods that work with one client may not work with another. In addition, methods that work at one stage of therapy may not work well at another stage.

When Clients Never Remember

You will not need the material in this chapter for all your clients, because some trauma survivors never reach the stage of remembering the trauma. Nor do these clients ever significantly experience the feelings associated with the trauma or embark on the process of reconsidering the trauma on a cognitive, emotional, or existential level.

This does not mean you have failed. If your work with a client results in an improvement in the client's outer or inner (psychic) safety, you can consider your counseling endeavor a major success. For example, if as a result of therapy a client leaves an abusive relationship or an environment where she or he was vulnerable to repeated exploitation, or takes increased measures to protect against crime or other forms of danger, then you have accomplished a great deal, especially since such changes may have taken years to achieve.

You can also congratulate yourself (more than once), if as a result of therapy a client makes strides in controlling his or her anger, self-destructiveness, responses to trigger events, and other trauma-related reactions which had previously seriously disrupted and limited his or her social and vocational lives and sense of self-control.

Even if some of your clients never recall a single detail of the trauma, other than that it happened (and sometimes they aren't so sure about that either), if therapy has contributed to their ability to become increasingly engaged in their lives today, rather than in the past, and to be able to love, work, and play despite their PTSD symptoms, then your input to their lives can be considered invaluable.

Memory Problems

Some clients desire or need to delve further into their traumatic histories than they are currently able, but have problems in doing so. Memory distortions of various types, for example, amnesia (either partial or total) and inaccurate sequencing are possible.

In a series of studies of sexual abuse survivors (Briere and Courtois 1992), it was found that approximately 50 percent entered therapy with memories of the abuse and 50 percent came with amnesia. These studies also found certain consistent differences between survivors who were originally amnesic and those who were not. Those who suffered from amnesia tended to suffer more violence in association with the abuse and were abused beginning at a younger age. In one study, the violence suffered by amnesic survivors was so severe that 35 percent had required medical treatment.

In general, those who were amnesic were abused two years earlier than those who had recall. According to available data on sexual abuse in the family, the average victim's age is between six and seven. It can then be assumed that those with amnesia suffered abuse at the age of four or five. In addition, those who were amnesic reported more fear of death, abuse of a longer duration, and a greater number of perpetrators than those who could remember.

Richard Kluft (1992b), a leading psychiatrist in the field of dissociation, points out another disorder of memory: pathological doubting. The client remembers the trauma—for example, the client knows he or she was abused—but cannot remember the identity of the abuser or other aspects of the experience and may resequence the events. As Kluft points out, when one is being abused, one may have to turn reality upside-down in order to survive. One of the frequent ways family abuse survivors do this is by rearranging the events so that they can blame themselves for the abuse.

Memory problems seem to plague survivors of long-term or repeated trauma more than one-time trauma survivors. For example, typically the former survivors are more likely to have trouble recalling what occurred than the latter. However even one-time trauma survivors can suffer from partial or total amnesia, depending on the nature of the incident—the kinds of physical and psychological injuries and losses sustained.

Another important aspect of remembering the trauma is uncovering the core trauma. When certain symptoms persist, despite numerous sessions discussing the traumatic experiences in an honest, open manner, the problem may be that the client has yet to uncover the core trauma. The core trauma may be the trauma which was the most violent, the one which the client experienced as the most shaming or humiliating, or the one fraught with the most emotional or spiritual conflict.

The core trauma may, in fact, not emerge during the course of your work with a given client. In the case of survivors of long-term or severe trauma, it is not uncommon for clients to stop counseling after a certain measure of recovery is achieved. They may simply need a break or may not be ready to face the core trauma or other events that are more horrible or shaming than the ones discussed to date.

In cases where the core trauma is revealed during the course of therapy with you, you may be surprised to find that it is unrelated in theme to material discussed at length in previous sessions. For example, a combat veteran may spend months discussing feeling the horrors of seeing scores of dead bodies, but the core trauma may be that he believes he made a mistake that caused the death of a buddy.

Conflict, Shame, and Pain Avoidance

It has been postulated that people "forget" traumatic episodes or portions of their traumatic experiences because these incidents created moral or emotional conflicts for them. In the case of family violence, sexual assault, and other such traumas, the trauma may also be repressed because of the humiliation and shame involved. However, the fundamental cause of memory loss is probably more simple then either conflict or shame: People just don't like to hurt.

Once a certain threshold of psychological or physical pain is reached, and the pain becomes intolerable, people find ways of not feeling it. Numbing is one defense against such pain, as are dissociation and various forms of substance abuse. Simply "forgetting" the abuse, or certain parts of it, and rearranging the memories so that they are more tolerable are also ways of reducing the pain to a manageable level or eradicating it entirely.

Physiological Overload

According to van der Kolk (1990a), dissociation can occur when the state of physical hyperarousal experienced in traumatic situations is so intense that people's ability to reason and remember decreases. Some traumatic experiences are so frightening that the brain cannot comprehend or make sense of them. Consequently, these memories become split off from the conscious mind and exist as fragments on the semiconscious or unconscious level.

Later on, the memories return. However, when they emerge into consciousness, they may not return as coherent stories but rather in bits and pieces, as fragmentary memories of the event. Alternatively, the memories can return as "terrifying perceptions, obsessional preoccupations, somatic complaints," or as a number of other symptoms (van der Kolk 1990a).

When the memories are fragmented and unconnected with one another, survivors sometimes find it nearly impossible to make sense out of their inner life. Until these memories can be pulled together into (at least) a semicoherent story, they may have difficulty understanding themselves. Carol Y., was sexually abused by her father. Years after the incest, her father unexpectedly came for a brief visit. He behaved appropriately and acted as if he had never molested her, but after he left, Carol developed serious leg cramps. Since there were no injuries, the doctor concluded she was suffering from psychosomatic spasms. He suggested aspirin, tranquilizers, and bed rest. The word *psychosomatic* put Carol into a panic; she was more convinced than ever that she had a screw loose.

Years later, in therapy, Carol discovered the origin of her leg cramps. In order to make her submit to the incest, her father had told her that if she wasn't a "nice girl" who would do what he wanted, he would break her legs. Her mind had forgotten the threat, but her body remembered.

Not just incest survivors, but other trauma survivors who have totally or partially repressed their trauma, can suffer from symptoms they do not understand. Joanne, a 30-year-old secretary, could not understand why she would hyperventilate and sweat anytime she was near an elevator. Although she had been raped in an elevator when she was thirteen, her mind had blocked out the event. Consequently, she could make no sense out of the fact that she would rather walk up several flights of stairs than go near an elevator. She also could not explain why she became furious whenever her boyfriend wore a blue shirt. Had she remembered that her rapist wore a blue shirt, she might have been better able to cope with the situation.

The Issue of Coding

Some memories are coded (stored) at very high or otherwise unique levels of arousal. Some specialists even argue that there are situations where the individual is so anxious or aroused that the memory is not stored at all. Others argue that all memories are coded, but that some simply cannot be retrieved unless the individual is subjected to the same degree of traumatization as existed at the time of the event in question, which is clearly not a therapeutic option. In terms of psychotherapy, the issue of whether everything human beings experience is coded in memory is academic. The functional reality is that some memories may simply not be available to the client or the therapist.

For example, Briere (Briere and Courtois 1992) cites the example of a woman client who was taken captive, then raped and mutilated by a number of perpetrators over many hours. After several counseling sessions, she was able to recall what occurred during some of the hours, but other hours remained totally blank for her. Despite her therapy with a world-renowned trauma expert, some of this woman's memories of her torture may remain total blanks forever, unless she is once again traumatized (and consequently physiologically aroused), to the same degree that she was during the kidnapping and gang-rape for which she sought treatment. Obviously, it would be unethical and counterproductive to retraumatize this woman in such a manner simply for purposes of memory retrieval.

The State-Dependent Nature of Some Memories

The forgetting of certain incidents may also be caused by the fact that some memories may be state-dependent (Briere and Courtois 1992). For example, experiences that occurred when someone was drunk or high on a certain kind of drug may not be recalled until that person is drunk or on that same drug again. In a parallel manner, experiences that occurred when an individual was sober or clean may return when that individual gives up addiction and is once again alcohol or drug free.

This aspect of remembering contributes to the high rate of recidivism among substance abusers who have been traumatized. Those survivors who used a substance as a form of self-medication for the symptoms of PTSD or to dull or obliterate memories of the trauma, may find that once they become clean or sober they are confronted with memories and feelings related to the trauma. Without help, they can easily revert back to the addiction they used as a coping mechanism in the past.

Preverbal Memories

Other memories are not available because the trauma occurred preverbally, or prior to the time the client's mind was able to code with language. Preverbal memories, however, can emerge through dance, art, and other expressive therapies or in the form of physical or psychosomatic pain.

Since children vary developmentally, the ages at which they learn to speak and relate on a verbal level also vary. Therefore the ages that can be classified as preverbal will differ from survivor to survivor.

The Nature of Memory Retrieval

According to Courtois, an expert in the field of memory retrieval, the memory retrieval process is characterized by "approach-avoidance." Those survivors who remember, want to forget, and those who can't remember, or remember only partially, often desperately want to remember. However, once they begin to remember, like those who are fully cognizant of their traumatic histories, they also want to forget what they worked so hard to remember. Consequently, as Courtois states, the memory retrieval process is one of "two steps forward, one step backward" (Briere and Courtois 1992).

Re-repression

Re-repression, or the forgetting of memories that have been remembered, is a "normal" part of memory retrieval. As explained by Briere and Courtois (1992), every day all people, whether or not they have survived trauma, sort their memories between those that will and will not be repressed. The human brain does this so that it does not enter a state of cognitive or information overload.

When we are on role overload, or processing a larger volume of information than we can comfortably handle, our minds tend to suppress certain relatively nonessential information so that we can tend to the more important matters. For example, have you ever had so much to do for an important project, a sick relative, a wedding, or some other matter of great significance that you forgot relatively minor matters such as picking up clothes from the cleaners or answering a letter? Although necessary, the forgotten tasks, at the time were not priority and hence were repressed or forgotten.

This same process of forgetting or repression occurs when the information is emotionally overwhelming in a negative manner. Consequently, a survivor who remembers the trauma may re-repress it or parts of it if other life events make dealing with the trauma a matter of emotional overload or if the traumatic material is more than can be safely handled. In some cases, re-repression is a life-preserving act: Certain traumatic material could make some survivors homicidal, suicidal, or otherwise self-destructive if they are not equipped to handle it or do not have adequate supports for handling it. Consequently, it is in the survivor's best interest that the material be re-repressed.

The process of "re-repression" fits in with the approach-avoidance tendencies many survivors exhibit toward their experiences, and it should be expected when doing memory retrieval work. Just as you need to inform clients of the possibility that they will both want to know and not know what happened to them, you need to prepare them for the possibility that they will re-repress incidents they have worked hard to remember.

Varying Modalities of Memory Retrieval

Just as memories may come and go, they may also return in whole or in fragments. They may "make sense," or they may be fraught with cognitive and other distortions. According to Courtois, "cognitive distortions are an acceptable part of memory retrieval" (Briere and Courtois 1992).

It is also possible that a client will recall a memory in one fashion during one session and then present a revised version at a later session. This does not usually mean the client is lying or fantasizing, but rather that the memory emerged initially in a confused manner because the client had to "mix it up" for self-protective reasons. Clearly, memories will not necessarily return in the form of a complete coherent story or narrative. A client may remember one aspect of the trauma, then another, and only after time has elapsed be able to weave the memories into a sequenced, meaningful story.

If you do have serious doubts about a client's truthfulness, or there are legal or disability issues you must address, it may be possible to corroborate parts of the client's story. For example, you could take a history of the client, talk to others who know the client, and compare their accounts with the client's story. (See the section on assessing PTSD for nonclinical purposes in chapter 11.) However, your primary role is not that of detective. In cases of extreme trauma, your client may have a multiple personality disorder or some other severe disorder that makes his or her story seem unreasonable or fabricated, when in actuality it may be true. In the end, there is no real way of knowing whether a client's story is true or not or what portions are "true" and which portions are "false." There may or may not be proof, and different people see things in different ways and will inevitably disagree about what occurred.

The issue of truth or falsity is complicated by the fact that memories may not return as memories as we customarily think of them. For example, memories return not only in the form of pictures or stories but in clients' reexperiencing phenomena: nightmares, night terrors, age regression, fight-flight-freeze reactions, smells, and bodily sensations, both comfortable and uncomfortable.

Sharon L. came to therapy at double her ideal weight. She had problems with assertiveness and self-esteem, as well as depression. Neither she nor her therapist suspected that Sharon was an incest survivor until after Sharon lost about seventy pounds. She then discovered that she became sexually aroused whenever she was with someone who talked a lot in a boisterous manner. However, she was uncomfortable with her arousal and did not experience it as pleasurable.

In the past, Sharon had used food to cover up her discomfort. But now that she was committed to not eating to her emotions, she had to face her reaction and try to understand it. Much to her chagrin, she found that she was simultaneously attracted and repelled by men who were exuberant and verbose. Within months, she began having memories of being sexually abused by her brother, an extremely articulate, boisterous man.

In Sharon's case, the memory returned first in the form of a sensual experience. In a case cited by Courtois (Briere and Courtois 1992), memory retrieval in a sexual abuse survivor was first signaled by extreme body-temperature changes during the therapy session. Apparently, this client had learned that if she didn't move, the abuse hurt less. Her inactivity, however, lowered her body temperature.

Memories can also return somatically, in the form of nausea, back pain, rashes, tremors, breathing problems (such as sleep apnea and asthma), and other such symptoms.

The Therapist's Role

All of the basic therapeutic principles presented in this chapter apply to memory retrieval work perhaps even more than they do with other types of interventions. In particular, clients need to be educated about the following topics (described in preceding sections of this chapter):

- The causes of amnesia and dissociation

- The idiosyncratic nature of memory retrieval

- The approach-avoidance tendency toward memory retrieval exhibited by many trauma survivors in therapy

- The possibility of re-repression

- The various ways memories can return

- The purposes of memory retrieval

In addition, clients need to be advised of the necessity of going slow, the need for emotional containment, and that your role is to serve as facilitator, not judge.

Keeping Clients to a Slow Pace

Many clients are in a great rush to remember the trauma, deal with it, and "get it over with." Their urgency and motivation can be commended and respected; however, such clients also need to be warned of the danger of retraumatization occurring if the memory retrieval process is rushed. They also need to be reminded that remembering what occurred is only the beginning. The purpose of memory retrieval is not simply to remember the traumatic event, but to process the emotions and cognitive distortions associated with what occurred during the event, and such work takes time.

For example, Larry S. wanted to read every book available on his particular form of trauma in order to quickly overcome his addiction to sugar and alcohol and "be normal." He knew that in order to be sober he needed to attend both AA and OA meetings, as well as PTSD counseling sessions, and he did so faithfully. But he was exasperated when, after a year of counseling, he was still overeating, still having nightmares, and still having interpersonal problems related to his PTSD.

Larry was continually reminded of the necessity of going slow, but he did not believe it until after uncovering a particularly painful memory, he went on a five-day eating binge and then failed to show up for the next three sessions. At the next session, we discussed the role of food in sedating the emotions aroused by the memory and the necessity of his coming to therapy with the intense emotions generated by the memory, rather than staying away from therapy at these times.

There are several ways to assist clients in slowing down and giving them some control over the pace of memory retrieval. First, you can ask them whether or not they feel they can handle a particular memory before they begin a detailed description. For example, you could ask, "Have you ever talked about this incident before? What was it like for you? How did it feel afterward? Did you find yourself feeling freer for having shared it or more burdened? What about your PTSD symptoms [or problems with addiction, depression, or some other disorder]? Did these problems increase or decrease after talking about the incident?"

Second, you can suggest to clients that they need not tell the entire story in one session; that is, they can stop at any time. They can also simply give the "headlines" or an overview of the story, if they desire, without going into detail. They can save the details for another time or to express in some other way, in a poem or piece of art, dance, or some other form of expressive therapy.

Third, when clients state that they would like to share the entire story, or as much as they remember, you can remind them to try to be aware of their emotional and physical reactions to telling the story. Give them permission to stop the storytelling at any point, to talk instead about how they are feeling physically or emotionally.

Fourth, tell your clients that if you notice they are hyperventilating or having other physical symptoms or are beginning to dissociate, you will call a halt to the memory retrieval process, help them identify how they are feeling, and help them center themselves.

If the client is especially distressed or is dissociated, you might want to try some of the grounding techniques described below.

Facilitating, Not Digging

Therapists frequently ask, "How far should we dig into the client's past?" Experts in the field, such as Judith Peterson (1992), answer "Not at all." In fact, Peterson says, therapists should not even "own a shovel." Memories will surface at their own pace, when the client's inner self feels safe enough to let the memory emerge. (See "The Issue of False Memories," in chapter 11.)

Your role is not to dig for memories, but to gently nudge the client toward greater truth, when the client is at a place where such nudging would be useful, not traumatizing. The stance of the therapist should be this:

> I am here to help you remember. I am not here to push you,
> but since you want to know, while at the same time you don't
> want to know, I am here to carry along the part that wants to
> know just a little further each time. But we are going to stop
> the minute it becomes too much for you to handle.

When the client is in a state of relative peace or comfortable numbing, you might nudge the client by introducing a memory trigger, such as suggesting that the client begin one of the memory retrieval techniques listed below. Being in group therapy with survivors of similar traumas can also serve as a memory trigger. However, if the client is in the reexperiencing phase, you will need to help the client contain the affect. Such methods for containing affect are presented below in the section on grounding techniques.

As some clients go through the memory retrieval process, they may question whether or not you believe their accounts. From the very beginning, you need to divest yourself of the role of judge and clarify that your role is to facilitate and listen. What matters is whether they believe their own memories and how they feel about their pasts, not what you believe or feel. If a client repeatedly asks for your opinion about the truth or falsity of their stories, you might ask why your opinion is so important. Your question may give rise to transference issues, which, if appropriate, could be discussed.

Clients who are confused about their memories, who one week remember certain incidents and other weeks "forget" or deny that such incidents occurred, may also want to know if you believe them. In such cases, you might want to reiterate your didactic material on the nature of memory problems, as discussed above.

Grounding and Emotional-Containment Techniques

Grounding the client means helping to bring the client away from the trauma and back to the here and now. The following are some suggestions (Courtois and Briere 1992):

- Ask the client to focus on the room and describe the color of the walls or carpet or touch the chair he or she is sitting in (this works better if the chair is upholstered).

- Ask the client to focus on you, say your name, and look you in the eye.

- Ask the client about his or her evening or weekend plans.

- Ask about non–emotionally charged interests or activities, for example, a pet, a sports team, recreational activities, or any other matter that is not trauma related or conflict ridden.

- Ask the client if he or she would like to walk around the room, write, or draw. Have some writing or drawing materials available; often these activities soothe clients.

Minimizing Retraumatization

PTSD therapy cannot help but retraumatize clients to some degree, because the trauma is resurrected from the past. However, you can minimize retraumatization by planning memory retrieval sessions, by keeping recall to a minimum when you feel the client is ill-prepared to be engaged in remembering the past, by monitoring the client during the retrieval process, by assuring that there is support for the client after the session, and by giving structure (especially closure) to your sessions.

Planning for Remembering

Since in PTSD therapy there should be no "secrets" on the part of the therapist, if you are planning to nudge the client toward remembering, you need to plainly state what you are doing. For example, you could say, "I think it's time I encourage you to talk more about . . . ." Then spell out as specifically and concretely as possible why you feel the client might be ready for reconstructing the trauma by recounting the progress she or he has made since the inception of therapy. You also need to provide the clients with solid reasons why you think the process might be important. For example, you could say this:

> You began coming here two years ago, because of your fear of striking out at police, employers, and other male authority figures. Since that time, you have learned to identify those situations where you feel you might lose control and avoid them as much as possible. However, since such situations are unavoidable, when you find yourself in them, you now know to reach for the telephone and call me or a friend or use anger management techniques such as time-outs.
>
> In two years, you have essentially stopped drinking and fighting, learned to respect your limits, and learned to turn to people instead of alcohol for help when you become afraid of yourself. In my view, the fact that you have come this far might mean you are ready to think about the events that contributed to your having so much anger.
>
> You have only talked about your trauma now and then, which is fine. But now, if you want, we can go back, or start to go back, to understand better what happened and how it might be influencing you today.

You need to receive the client's feedback and consent before you engage in memory retrieval (or feelings work). "What do you think about this?" you could ask. The client's response will determine your next move. If the client agrees to proceed with memory retrieval, you can then outline the various safeguards that you plan to use to assure the client that he or she will not lose control emotionally or mentally during this process.

Uncovering the trauma, like the feelings work described in the next chapter, is often more effective when it is planned in advance. First, planning gives clients a role in the therapy, which enhances their sense of mastery. For example, clients can be involved in generating safeguards for themselves. Prior to the session, you can ask the client whether she or he has any suggestions for making memory retrieval less traumatic. Clients are often adept and creative at suggesting therapeutic interventions. You do not want to lean on them or make them feel as if you are at a loss as to what to do; however there is no harm in telling the client that you are trying to minimize the retraumatization inherent in PTSD therapy and are therefore open to suggestions.

Second, planning ahead permits clients to voice both their fears and their hopes, which you can correct as appropriate. For example, in planning sessions you can address a common fear such as that talking about the trauma will make it recur. Rationally, most clients know that talking about it won't cause it to happen again. However, the ever-present fear that the trauma will repeat itself, and the sense of doom, which is a symptom of PTSD, may be triggered by talking about the trauma.

A common false expectation you might need to address is that telling the story will deliver the client once and for all from the trauma and its effects. The truth is that, ultimately, telling the truth about what occurred is extremely healing. However, uncovering the events is only part of a process that involves working with emotions and existential crises as well as more fully remembering the narrative involved in the traumatic episode. Uncovering the trauma involves grieving not only what occurred but the loss of the client's fantasies and illusions and the loss of the defenses that served to protect those fantasies.

Dealing with Spontaneous Recall

Remembering the trauma, like the therapeutic process itself, cannot always be planned—nor should it always be. Consequently, there will be times when you are confronted with clients who begin to talk about the trauma spontaneously. At such times, you should listen attentively. Also listen to whatever else they are saying, such as complaints about symptoms, concerns about current stresses, and fears about anticipated stressful events. You also need to look at the clients' gestures and appearance, which may reflect their emotional state, current level of self-esteem, and so on.

Putting together all the information you have about the client from the current session, as well as past sessions, you may have to quickly assess whether the client has sufficient ego strength and external supports to delve deeper into the traumatic memories. If you decide the client can work well with the memories and most of the preconditions for successful memory retrieval have been met (see "The Memory Retrieval Process," below), then you can proceed to support the client's internal momentum.

However, if in your professional opinion the client would become emotionally overloaded or would otherwise be unable to constructively handle or process the sharing of memories, then simply continue to listen attentively, without asking the client any probing questions or otherwise encouraging this sharing. You can also steer the client away from the past toward present concerns (without appearing to be disinterested, disgusted, or afraid of the description of the trauma), by asking questions that link the past to the present.

For example, you could say one of the following things:

> Do you think what you have just described relates to your present crisis?

> You've never mentioned (or rarely talk about) these incredible events which you managed to survive. I'm wondering if something happened lately that reminded you of the past?

> I can see that the trauma is still bothering you, which is perfectly appropriate given the horrible time you had. I'm wondering, though, if you want to talk about it more now, or if you'd rather wait until some other time when you aren't so stressed. Just now, when your marriage is falling apart [or you are losing your job, you just found out your mother has cancer, you are coping with your son's drug problem], you might want to put the subject of the trauma on the back burner for a while and deal with the present, instead. Unless, of course, you really need to talk about it.

Monitoring the Client

At all times during both the remembering process feelings work, you need to monitor your clients, both psychologically and physiologically. Psychologically you can ask clients not only what they are feeling but if they are feeling safe within themselves. Also, continually give them the choice of either continuing the process or stopping it. Physiologically, you need to observe your client carefully for signs of sleepiness, shaking, hairpulling, or other signs of anxiety or withdrawal.

Processing the Session

In all sessions, keep in mind the rule of thirds. In the first part of the session, identify what is going on or the agreed-upon purpose of the session such as recalling the memories. In the second part, the client is engaged in the activity: remembering, identifying feelings, and so on. In the third portion, you process whatever occurred. For example, you can ask, "How was it for you to remember?" or "How was it for you to try to remember but not be able to?"

Remember, if the client reports, and you can see, that the remembering sessions are becoming too stressful, you can plan vacations from remembering. Also, if necessary, you can help the client arrange for a leave from work or other stress reduction measures during this time.

Providing for Supports

You may want to review the cautions listed in the Warning Signs handout in the introduction and remind clients of the sources of assistance available (in addition to yourself) should they have an extremely negative reaction following the session. Ask clients to whom they would turn or what they would do should they find themselves having any of the symptoms listed as cautions or other symptoms that frighten them.

Then ask your client to make a commitment to you to try to find help should there be a need. Also make a notation in your records of the support plan. This is necessary for your own protection, as well as for future reference. For example, if your client becomes extremely troubled and symptomatic, and then does not use the supports you have discussed together in session, you could refer back to your notes when the two of you discuss why the client deprived himself or herself of needed assistance.

Retraumatization can also be minimized by avoiding memory retrieval work under the conditions listed in the section "When Remembering Is Not Advisable," below.

The Memory Retrieval Process

In both the process of remembering the trauma and in feeling the feelings associated with the trauma certain prerequisite conditions need to be met. Ideally, you and the client should have established a strong therapeutic alliance, or at least a trusting relationship. In the words of van der Kolk (1989):

> The trauma can only be worked through after a secure bond is established with another person: the presence of an attachment figure provides people with the security necessary to explore their life experiences and to interrupt the inner or social isolation that keeps people stuck in repetitive patterns. Both the etiology and the cure of trauma-related psychological disturbance depend fundamentally on the security of interpersonal attachments.

Furthermore, clients should have at their disposal some skills in containing their feelings, so that they have some defenses against feeling emotionally overwhelmed. Clients should also have achieved a fair degree of mastery of any secondary elaborations:

> Prior to unearthing the traumatic roots of current behavior, people need to gain reasonable control over long-standing secondary defenses that were originally elaborated to defend against being overwhelmed by traumatic material, such as alcohol and drug abuse and violence against self or others."
> (van der Kolk 1989)

Note: If you are working with a severely traumatized person, it is wise not to do memory retrieval, or any of the subsequent work on emotions, alone in a building or office suite. For example, if you work in private practice, you might want to have a fellow therapist on call. If you work in an office with others, do not do this kind of work late at night or at times when you are the only therapist there.

Some therapists ask another therapist to sit in with them (with the client's permission of course) is they anticipate the possibility that memory retrieval might generate an unmanageable or even psychotic reaction. However, if you suspect that the memory recall will produce such a negative effect, you will probably want to discourage the client from memory recall until he or she is more prepared. Yet if the client insists on sharing, you may have little choice but to listen, in which case you will want to have professional support readily available.

When Remembering Is Not Advisable

There are no hard and fast rules about when to encourage or nudge the client to remember the trauma. In general, however, nudging the client towards remembering is *not* advisable under the following conditions:

- If you have not established a strong therapeutic alliance or trusting relationship with the client. For example, the client does not keep appointments regularly and is consistently distrustful or degrading of you, or you do not like or believe the client or feel morally or otherwise repelled by the client.

- If the client is not familiar with PTSD therapy and you have not had the opportunity to explain the nature of memory retrieval and other aspects of PTSD counseling or to provide for adequate supports for the client.

- If the client is still engaging in out-of-control addictive behavior, self-mutilation, or is in danger of committing suicide or homicide, or the client has a history of decompensating or become self-injurious or other-injurious when the subject of the trauma is discussed.

- If the client is under current severe or multiple life stresses.

- If the client does not have a support system other than yourself.

- If the client is currently in the intrusive/hyperalert phase of the PTSD cycle; that is, the client is currently having nightmares, flashbacks, irritability, rage reactions, and so on.

- If the client has stated she or he does not wish to remember the trauma.

- If the client is suffering a psychotic episode or is manifesting psychotic symptoms.

- If the client begins to talk about the trauma during the last few minutes of your session, leaving little time to finish the story or for you to provide whatever necessary assistance might be necessary.

- If you have completed some memory retrieval work in a session, but the client has forgotten the retrieved memories by the end of the session or by the beginning of the next session. Such re-repression usually signifies that the material is, for the time being, more than the client can handle.

Assume a Mr. X. comes to you for assistance because he finds himself having crying jags almost every other day. He has been in an earthquake and two fires within four years and his wife had recently left him. He was able to "handle" and start over again after the first two catastrophes. However, after the last one destroyed his home, he became numb for several years.

When he came out of numbing, he began drinking, which led to the loss of his job, as well as the departure of his wife. Now he is sober through AA, but sobriety has resulted in his losing motivation to seek employment, in sleeping problems, in thoughts of death, and in a cycle of, "feeling so bad all the time all I can do is cry. But if I'm not crying, I feel nothing at all." These are symptoms of depression and PTSD; however, a more thorough evaluation is needed to be firm about these diagnoses.

At this initial interview, an inexperienced therapist might probe for details about the earthquake and the fire or about the specifics of the marital breakup. However, there has not yet been time to build up a therapeutic relationship, nor an opportunity to explain to the client the nature of counseling in general or PTSD therapy in particular. There has been no "contract" established, in which the client agrees to allow the therapist to nudge toward uncovering the trauma while at the same time taking measures to protect the client from unnecessary retraumatization.

At this juncture, or even by the fifth or sixth session, the therapist may not be in a position to ascertain the client's preparedness for memory retrieval. Without being relatively certain that the client can survive the emotional upheavals that usually follow the resurrection of memories, a therapist could be taking risks asking questions such as, "Can you tell me more about the earthquake and fires?" However, the therapist could say this:

> It must have taken a lot of courage for you to come here and
> talk to a total stranger about how bad you feel. Your
> description of your life tells me you have been in many
> life-or-death situations, and that makes you a trauma survivor.
> If, in the future, you would want to talk at length about the
> traumas you have been through, I would be more than willing
> to listen. But, for now, let's look at what's going on in your
> life in the present. Is there something about your life today
> that's making you suffer so?

If Mr. X. cannot identify the reason for the tears or sadness, the therapist could help out the client (who is probably overwhelmed and confused) by suggesting possibilities, for example:

> You must be hurting a great deal to be crying so hard. People
> who I've seen before have cried this hard over losing someone
> they loved, over a medical problem, over some regrets they

have, or over some part of their life or self they feel they have lost. Do any of these reasons apply to you?

On the basis of the client's responses, the therapist can then try to have the client focus on the one or two areas of his life that are causing the greatest stress.

Reconstructing the Traumatic Event

One of the principal tools of the healing process is the reconstruction of what happened. As the healing process progresses, the client's memories of the trauma may expand and his or her perceptions of the trauma will change. However, uncovering the trauma must start somewhere. The two handouts provided here, Recording the Traumatic Event and Visualizing the Trauma, are offered as possibilities for helping clients record their traumatic experiences.

As with the other handouts in this book, these exercises can be completed by the client as homework assignments, to be reviewed by you in session, or you can work through the handout with the client in a session.

Before beginning or giving clients these exercises, be sure to review with them the cautions listed in the introduction, and give them a copy of the Warning Signs handout if they will be doing an exercise on their own. Whether clients complete these exercises through writing, by making an audiotape, or by drawing pictures or creating some other artistic expression, stress that they need to be as detailed as possible in their descriptions. Details may not be traumatic in and of themselves, but are still important in understanding and anticipating trigger reactions, as discussed in chapter 6.

In her work with rape victims, S. L. Williams (1990) found that many of her clients tended to give detailed descriptions of what they did before the rape, but failed to truly describe the rape itself. They would write, "I had toast and coffee for breakfast. I wore a blue dress. I walked to the bus stop. Then I was raped." Williams had her clients rewrite their accounts to include as many graphic and sensual details as they could remember, including what the rapist looked like, what he smelled like, and the particulars of the room or environment in which the rape occurred.

Note: If your client has difficulty completing the first exercise, you might suggest that she or he write or speak about the trauma as if it had happened to someone else. Recording the trauma in the third person may provide the client with sufficient emotional distance so that the task can be completed. The visualization exercise also uses the third-person technique.

Using Visualization

Another way of helping clients who have trouble recording or speaking about the trauma is to have them visualize the trauma as occurring on a videotape whose speed they can control. If they need to "fast forward" or rewind some sections, or skip over certain parts, they may do so. Alternatively, you can have them talk about trauma as if they were watching a movie, only they are in the projectionist's booth, somewhat far from the screen, and they can turn the movie on or off at will, as well as skipping over or replaying sections as needed.

Advise clients that completing this exercise may take anywhere from thirty minutes to an hour or longer. Their response to this exercise can be as long as needed, and they should feel free to add on to their description as often as necessary. Out of this exercise, for example, an entire book could be written. Indeed,

Recording the Traumatic Event

Before you begin this exercise, you might want to center yourself by taking a few deep breaths, stretching, taking a walk or some other form of exercise, or by some other method which works for you.

As you begin this exercise, keep in mind the warning signs discussed in therapy and listed on your handout. If you start to develop any of the problems on the handout, stop the exercise immediately.

List in writing what happened immediately before, during, and after your trauma. If you have endured more than one traumatic event, you will need to describe each one. If you prefer to speak into an audiotape or draw pictures of the trauma, these are also acceptable alternatives. What you need, however, is a concrete description of the trauma to which you can refer as you progress through the healing process. You will also need to add to it and revise it as your understanding of the trauma grows and changes.

As you describe your traumatic incident, make it come alive with as much sensory detail as possible. For example, if you are a combat veteran describing a traumatic battle, mention the temperature and terrain, the weapons or other objects you were carrying, your medical and physical condition, the noises and sounds you heard, and any other details you can remember.

As you list the events, also describe your thoughts and feelings as the traumatic event progressed. Also describe what others thought or felt about what was happening or about you. You may only know what you thought they were thinking or feeling, but write that down.

Take as much time with this as you need, and don't try to do it all at once. If you start feeling overwhelmed, stop. Then come back to it later. If you can't remember everything now, don't worry about it, you will be returning to it later. You can add details then or at any point between now and then.

Don't be self-conscious about your writing, speaking, or drawing. The idea is to remember and have a record of events, thoughts, and feelings—not to win a contest. No one ever needs to see your description of the trauma, but yourself, unless you choose otherwise. You don't even have to show it to me.

When you've written, spoken, or drawn as much as you can remember, do one more thing: Congratulate yourself for being willing to look at and deal with these events. It takes a lot of courage.

Visualizing the Trauma

To begin this exercise you need to center yourself. Take a few calming breaths, do a relaxation exercise, pray, or go for a long walk—do whatever lets you feel calm, relaxed, and at peace. As you begin this exercise, keep in mind the warning signs you've discussed with your counselor. If you start to develop any of those problems, stop the exercise immediately.

Now imagine that you are watching a television show or movie about your trauma, or that you are seeing your story being acted out in the next room, a room from which you are separated by a one-way mirror. You can stop the film anytime you wish, fast-forward through some parts, replay others. You are the projectionist and the only member of the audience. As best you can, pretend the star of this show is not even you (even though it is).

When you have watched the whole movie, or as much of it as you want to right now, take some time to write about what you saw. (You may also make a recording on a tape or draw or paint scenes from the movie.) Try to record as much detail as you can for now. Later you can watch the movie again (when you feel ready) and get further details of what occurred.

many first-person accounts of dramatic traumatic incidents have begun with such descriptions.

Aids to Remembering

To stimulate the process of remembering, you can ask clients to follow any of the suggestions below that might prove helpful.

Using Prompts

Objects can help trigger memory, especially photographs. Clients can be asked to find photographs of themselves before, after, or even during the traumatic event or photographs of significant others from that time. If clients bring these photographs to sessions, you can ask them to explore these questions: What was I like then? What did I feel like? What was I interested in? How did I change? (They can also explore these questions on their own, outside of therapy.) If the photographs are of significant others, clients may want to explore how that person changed in attitude or behavior toward them after the traumatic event.

Questions arise about using photographs involving painful memories, for example: Should a combat vet bring pictures of the dead? A family abuse survivor, a photo of the abuser? A natural catastrophe survivor, a photo of the disaster?

There are no hard and fast rules. Clients need to trust their gut reactions. If they want to look at such pictures, they should do so. If they don't want to view such reminders of the past, then they need not. There is no point in clients forcing themselves to look at the "raw truth" when doing so might be self-punitive and destructive to their inner serenity and the healing process.

Assure clients that if they don't want to view some photos or reminders, this is not a sign that they aren't "ready" or "strong enough." It may just be that viewing certain photos is not needed or helpful. They can make good progress in their healing without ever looking at pictures of the persons or places involved in their trauma.

If clients are concerned about their reactions to certain photos, you might ask them to have someone be with them as they gather these photos or other prompts and to look at them only in session with you or in another supportive context.

Other potentially useful prompts include pieces of clothing or other personal artifacts and movies, newspapers, magazines, music from or about the era during which they were traumatized.

Revisiting the Scene

Clients can also stimulate memories by returning to the original site of the trauma. Under no circumstances should you consider suggesting this idea, however, unless you are certain that the client can manage the encounter. There have been numerous cases of individuals completely falling apart when they returned to the scene of the trauma without adequate preparation or support. In a few cases of severe and repeated trauma, survivors lost their ability to function on the job and suffered long-term impairment in their ability to relate to others.

Thus, if the client wishes to return to the original site of the trauma, and you think he or she can undergo the experience without severe negative effects, you need to spend time in your sessions preparing for the visit and discussing and preparing for the range of possible reactions the client might have.

Researching the Trauma

Similarly, if the client plans to find and talk with people who knew him or her, or who were present during the trauma or otherwise have information about it, you need to discuss this plan and lay out how the client might expect to feel before, during, and after such a venture. For example, clients may hope to find the "missing link" or "the answer" in their search, only to be disappointed. Furthermore, even if they do discover valuable information, they may find that the increased knowledge does not take away the pain. In fact, as a result of the new information the client's symptoms may increase.

Consequently, you need to consider whether the client can deal with additional anger, grief, and possible disappointment at this point in his or her life. If the client has many current stresses or is feeling vulnerable or overwhelmed for other reasons, it may be wise to defer the plan of returning or contacting people from the past to a later time.

If clients, with your approval, decide to talk to individuals who have knowledge of them or the trauma, they need to remember their goals. They should not expect these people to provide them with unconditional love or emotional support. Clients need to be warned that even if these people love the client, it does not mean that they will be able to supply the empathic listening the client would expect from a trained therapist or knowledgeable survivor. In fact, there are no guarantees that sharing with others about the trauma will receive any kind of supportive response.

Thus, it is better for clients to ask neutral questions, such as, "I've been thinking lately about my past. I've forgotten so much that I'd like to remember. I wonder if you can help me remember what I was like when I used to live next door to you?" They may also want to inquire specifically about the incident. For example, they could ask, "What is your memory of that hurricane we had in 1965?" or "Do you remember my Uncle Joe? I remember him as tall, with blue eyes and a lot of charm. Is that how you remember him?"

Also make sure clients understand that seeking out information from others is not the same as confronting those who abused or otherwise victimized them. Such confrontations are highly complex matters that are well beyond the scope of this book. They require far more thinking, preplanning, and preparation than does simple information gathering.

The preceding cautions are not meant to suggest that clients should not take an active part in their healing. They are included merely to minimize possible negative effects. Some trauma survivors, in their initial enthusiasm for healing, charge ahead with such plans, only to suffer as a result because they were unprepared for their possible emotional reactions, disappointment, and the potentially negative reactions of others they sought out.

On the other hand, it takes much courage and a dedication to one's healing to take the time, effort, and risk involved in returning to people and places from the past to find out what happened. Many survivors have found great peace in finally uncovering some of the missing pieces of their story. "It was worth the pain to find out the truth," is the feeling of many who were finally able to use the facts they gathered to make peace with the past. And if they did not find out everything they had hoped to discover about themselves and the trauma, they still felt pride in having done all they could to heal themselves.

Traumatic memories can also be stimulated by talking to other trauma survivors—in a support group or at the client's school, community, or workplace.

Also, today there is a wealth of reading material about certain kinds of trauma, especially physical and sexual abuse, rape, and combat. Less is available on the subjects of natural catastrophe, technological accidents, and crime.

Clients can go to libraries to obtain books and articles on the type of trauma they endured. Not only news articles, but literature can deal with their experience. For example, the mythologies of various cultures have numerous accounts of the struggles of incest and rape survivors and those of warriors. These topics are also central to much modern fiction, drama, and poetry.

Autobiographical Writing

Clients can be asked to write an autobiography. Clients who are illiterate or otherwise cannot write can record their life histories on audiotape. If you think this task would be helpful to some of your clients, when you discuss the idea with them, ask if they would like to set a page or time limit on the autobiography or if they would rather leave it open-ended.

Once again, stress to clients that they are not entering a writing contest and that no one will see what they have written unless they choose to share it (this includes yourself and other therapists). If you suspect your client is a perfectionist, the fact that the autobiography need not be perfect cannot be emphasized enough.

If the task of writing an autobiography seems overwhelming to clients, break it down into smaller pieces. For example, they could write about a certain period of their life (early childhood, late adolescence, early adulthood) or trace a certain relationship or theme throughout their life (relationships with parents or friends or their interest in music or machinery).

Note: If and when you review clients' autobiographies, take special notice of any periods of time when their memory is hazy, confused, or absent entirely, because this may indicate that significant events that were difficult for the client to cope with occurred. These events may have been traumatic, or they may have simply been tumultuous or life changing. If they were traumatic events, they may need to be dealt with in therapy. Even if these events were not of traumatic or life-threatening proportions, they may have made the client more vulnerable to the impact of the trauma or created conflicts that later trauma exacerbated. On the other hand, hazy or absent memories about particular periods of time may simply indicate that nothing of significance took place.

Clients who are addicted often benefit from writing a history of their addiction. The Writing Your Addiction History handout gives directions for how the client could proceed.

Hypnosis and Flooding

In hypnosis, clients are put into a trance state during which partially or totally repressed memories can emerge. During flooding or implosive therapy, clients are barraged with stimuli reminiscent of the original trauma to desensitize them to such stimuli. For example, combat veteran clients are exposed to vivid war movies or tapes of war sounds. Another technique is to have veterans listen to their own most horrible experiences repeated back to them by the therapist. In the presence of memories, sounds, pictures, and so on, of the original traumatic event, using relaxation techniques, survivors learn to not be anxious or afraid, thus remembering is facilitated.

Writing Your Addiction History

If you are addicted to alcohol, food, drugs, gambling, or compulsive spending or sexual behavior, most likely your addiction patterns reflect the traumatic event you endured. One way to help resurrect your memories of the trauma is by writing, recording, or telling another person your addiction history, as follows:

1. Write at least three pages on how your addiction has adversely affected your life. Go back to the first time you ever used your substance (whether food, alcohol, or drugs) or engaged in a compulsive behavior, and tell how you felt about it. Then go through the rest of your life, noting the times you were practicing your addiction, and remembering how you felt about it. You can write less than three pages if that is all you want to do. But the more you write, the more you will learn about yourself.

2. Make a list of all the people in your family who suffer from some form of substance abuse or addictive behavior and/or are trauma survivors themselves.

3. Think back over your life. Which events in it seem to be related to your practice of your addiction?

4. How did people around you react to your addiction?

5. What was the role of the trauma in creating, perpetuating, or increasing your addictive behavior?

6. Make a list of everything in your life that prevents you from giving up your addiction.

7. To what extent do you think healing from the trauma affects your recovery from substance abuse or compulsive activity?

Both hypnosis and flooding are highly controversial techniques. In a few cases, they have been used with select samples of trauma survivors with considerable success. However, our knowledge of the effects of these techniques is limited. For example, so far flooding techniques have been primarily used with PTSD-afflicted veterans and little with other populations. Furthermore, both of these techniques take away control from the client, which is not the best method of working with trauma survivors as has been noted previously.

Courtois (1988), a leading authority on trauma therapy, asserts that flooding may be countertherapeutic and should only be used as a last resort. Similarly, Judith Peterson (1992), an expert in working with traumatized family abuse survivors, stresses that hypnosis should only be used for specific purposes and observes that, unfortunately, this valuable technique has been misused by many therapists. Her suggestion is to use hypnosis in a subtle fashion: the therapist sends the message to clients that they can be successful, can create as safe an environment as possible for themselves, and can learn to contain their feelings and behavior: success, safety, containment.

Even when hypnosis or flooding is used properly, it does not assure a "magic cure." Such techniques may bring back memories, but memories not only have to be remembered, they have to be processed. Once clients recall a specific memory, they still have to go on to understand its meaning to them and their feelings about it.

These techniques should only be used very carefully and only if you are very skilled in this area. A weekend course, or even a two-week training course, is not adequate training. Skill in the area of hypnosis involves more than the ability to put a client in the trance state; it includes awareness of the pros and cons of the procedure, consideration of the ethical questions, and rigorous training and supervision. Although hypnosis can be an excellent tool in helping some trauma survivors, it can spell disaster if the therapist is superficially trained and makes exaggerated claims about the procedure.

Chapter 9

Feelings Work

Working on feelings is as essential to the healing process as working on the mental aspects of the trauma (see chapter 8, "Uncovering the Trauma); it is also similar in many ways. Many of the suggested modes of therapeutic intervention discussed previously, such as stimulating memory retrieval, reframing the trauma in terms of the dynamics of traumatic situations, and correcting cognitive distortions, also apply to helping clients work on their feelings.

Once again, it is important to adhere to the following preconditions and guidelines:

- To have developed a trusting relationship with the client

- To have the client's substance abuse, self-mutilating, or other problems under some control

- To have educated the client on the basics of PTSD and PTSD therapy and of any other conditions from which the client may suffer such as depression

- To continue to educate the client regarding the nature of PTSD, trauma, and other specific problems as appropriate topics arise in counseling

- To respect the client's timetable (while keeping to a slow pace, as much as possible)

- To respect the client's defenses and *ask* the client for more information, *ask* judicious questions, and *make suggestions* (which the client can accept or reject), rather than handing the client definitive or authoritative comments or pejorative-sounding interpretations

- To continually assess the client's ability to handle certain feelings, for example, by periodically asking the client if he or she remembers what was discussed during the previous session or earlier in the same session and by remembering the rule of thirds and processing the session at the end by asking the client to reflect on your session together

- To stop any trauma work if you notice or the client reports any of the warning signs listed in the introduction to this book, and to slow down trauma-related work if the client has trouble remembering traumatic incidents or emotions dealt with in a previous session or earlier in the session

- To reinforce a message of hope for healing and renewed possibilities, while at the same time acknowledging irreparable losses

It is also important to plant safeguards in the sessions against clients becoming overstimulated or emotionally overwhelmed. Remind them that feelings, or abreactive, work will not cause a rerun of the trauma. Such work is not a reliving experience, but can be perhaps a "first living" experience, in that it may be the client's first experience with feeling the feelings associated with the trauma. That is, during traumatic events, many feelings are suppressed either through the natural anesthesia of psychic numbing or through artificial numbing agents such as alcohol, drugs, and food. Therefore, it may be that encountering those feelings in therapy is the first time the powerful feelings associated with trauma emerge and are released, at least in part.

You need to prepare clients for this fact and urge them not to be unduly alarmed by the intensity of emotion they might feel. For example, you might say this:

> You are supposed to feel strong feelings when you go through this. After all, being in a hurricane isn't like losing a bingo game. It's okay if you feel angry enough to want to hurt something or someone, if you feel so sad you think you'll never stop crying, or if you feel so scared that you want to hide in an armored vault and never come out as long as you live. Not only is it okay if you feel this way, but the books say you are supposed to feel this way. If the feelings involved with trauma weren't so strong, you wouldn't have had to bother using denial to suppress them.

Planning Feelings Work

In chapter 8, the possibility of planning memory retrieval sessions with the client was discussed. During such planning sessions, the goals and purposes of memory retrieval and the fears and hopes of the client would be discussed. Planned memory retrieval sessions, as opposed to spontaneous recall of the trauma, can be doubly therapeutic: First, memory retrieval sessions are more likely to be productive if clients' expectations and concerns are discussed beforehand, so that they know generally what to expect. The therapist also provides assurance that he or she will safeguard the client against becoming overstimulated, overwhelmed emotionally, getting out of touch with reality, and so on. Second, planning memory retrieval sessions enhances the client's sense of mastery and control and sense of being an active agent rather than a passive recipient in the healing process. For example, in the planning sessions, clients could decide in advance with the therapist how far to go in retrieving memories, such as dealing with only certain incidents. Practice in setting limits this way also enhances the client's sense of self-control.

The same principles apply to working with feelings. You can deal with spontaneous emotionality regarding the trauma; however, you can also plan sessions with the client specifically to work on trauma-related feelings. Once again, you would review with clients the goals and purposes of knowing their feelings and help them with their fears and concerns.

A common fear in abreactive work, as with memory retrieval, is the fear of going "too far" and "losing control." Once again, you can suggest to the clients that you will be there to closely observe signs of loss of control and to help them stop the abreactive process if there are signs that he or she may become overwhelmed. You will be there to ask them how they are feeling at different points. And, in addition, they can simply say "Stop!"

Furthermore, in planning, you and the client can anticipate where the hard parts might be. For example, after the client decides which traumatic incidents (or incident or portion of an incident) will be worked on in the session, you can briefly review those incidents and ask the client where in the sequence of events he or she might like to plan "rest stops," or points at which he or she can decide whether to proceed or halt the process. These rest stops will be safe havens. You will make note of them so that you can remind the client when they have been reached (Peterson 1992).

In the abreactive session itself, before beginning feelings work, you need to carefully go over the sequence of events involved in the trauma. If the client has written down his or her story, you can use the written account. If the client has not, the events need to be reviewed orally. According to Peterson, it is important to ask the following questions before planned abreactive work:

What did you do to prepare for this session?

Do you remember the whole story? Are you sure?

Do you expect any unexpected incidents to arise as you tell the story?

Is there any possibility you might have an explosive or out-of-control physical reaction to this session?

Is any part of you afraid you will lose control?

I can touch your hand or arm if that will help you to feel safe. But I need to ask you if you want to be touched. If so, of the two alternatives, which do you prefer?

Is there anything else I can do to help you feel safe other than what we talked about in the planning sessions?

Emotional Awareness

Your work in helping clients with their feelings will be heavily influenced by the clients' degree of sophistication about their feelings. Some clients are unable to label their feelings, to distinguish one feeling from another, or to distinguish different degrees of intensity of the same feeling. For such clients, for example, all feelings ranging from mild irritation to murderous rage may be given the anger label.

Some clients do not even know what a feeling is. When asked what they are feeling, they lack the words with which to communicate their inner experience. Other clients cannot distinguish their feelings from their thoughts or from physical sensations such as bodily pain. Under such circumstances, you will necessarily have to provide some basic education on feelings before you begin to tackle the feelings associated with the trauma.

On the other hand, if a client has already had years of therapy or experience in a psychiatric hospital unit or a twelve-step program, she or he will most likely be familiar with the language of feelings. In that case, your work may involve helping the client sort out feelings or decide what to do with feelings once they are identified, especially with so-called unacceptable feelings such as rage and desire for revenge.

A client's sophistication about feelings is not related to his or her age, race, sex, intelligence, educational background, or emotional maturity. For example, I have worked with physicians who could not distinguish anxiety from sadness and expressed most of their feelings psychosomatically. On the other hand, some of my semiliterate clients have been able to talk with great clarity about their emotional state, often because of prior participation in a twelve-step program.

Clients' degree of awareness of feelings and their ability to talk about feelings usually reflects how emotions were handled in their family of origin and childhood peer groups and in subsequent family, peer, and work groups. In some environments feelings are never talked about or are considered "bad," a "sign of weakness," or "unnecessary." In some families showing emotions is associated with violence, out-of-control screaming and crying, or other frightening behavior.

You can assess clients' degree of familiarity with feelings simply by listening to them. When they describe an event, do they talk about their emotions or the emotions of others, or do their descriptions sound more like police reports or narratives without any emotional commentary? If they talk about emotions, do they distinguish between various emotions, or do they lump all their emotions together?

When clients are obviously emotionally upset during a session, as evidenced by a sign—such as sweating, hand wringing, crying, eyes darting around the room, tearing paper, biting their fingernails—do they deny having any feelings? Do they have trouble articulating what they are feeling? Can they only make statements such as "I don't know," "I'm confused," or "What do you mean?" Can they only state what they are thinking, rather than feeling? When the answer to any of these questions is yes, your client likely needs some basic education on feelings.

Exercises in the following sections are designed to educate clients about feelings; to help clients distinguish feelings, thoughts, and actions; and to help clients overcome obstacles to feeling awareness and expression.

Distinguishing Feelings from Thoughts and Actions

If you suspect your client has trouble distinguishing feelings from thoughts and actions, you might help clarify these differences by dissecting some of the client's responses into these categories. For example, suppose a client were to say, "I was so angry at my boss that I wanted to kill him; I even plotted his murder." You could respond in the following manner:

> Your feeling was anger, but anger is not an action. Even plotting the murder is not an action, but a thought, provided all you did was think about how you would do it and didn't make phone calls to arrange a killing and didn't buy a gun or make any other physical moves. The thought of wanting to kill is different from actually killing. Wanting to kill your boss is a feeling—a feeling that reflects other feelings, for example, being angry and feeling betrayed.

You could also give the client a short lecture on the differences between feelings and thoughts and on the characteristics of feelings. For example, you could say:

A feeling is neither a thought nor an action. Thinking "I should have ... " is not a feeling; it's a thought. Thinking "My friend forgot to pick me up for the party because I'm not smart enough" is also a thought. It's different from feeling inferior, rejected, angry, depressed, or disappointed because you were forgotten. Similarly, feeling angry at a friend or thinking about hitting, cursing, or stealing from that person in revenge is not the same as actually acting on those thoughts.

Feelings and thoughts are not the same, but they are often intimately related. Some feelings arise out of the way you perceive things and the thoughts you have as a result. For example, suppose you were being interviewed for a job and the interviewer had a blank look on her face the entire time. You might leave the interview *thinking*, "I did poorly. I'll never get the job," and consequently *feeling* incompetent, inferior, and rejected.

But suppose you then learned than an hour before your appointment, the interviewer had been told of the death of a friend. How might that information change your thinking about your performance in the interview and your subsequent feelings about yourself?

Or suppose you knew that your friend failed to pick you up because she had car trouble or fell asleep after a hard day. Your thoughts and feelings would probably be entirely different than if you assumed it had something to do with you personally.

Unlike thoughts, feelings involve a physical reaction. Excitement can cause perspiration and an increased respiration rate, for example. Sadness can result in tears or at least a weepy feeling. Joy can make you laugh or smile. Physical pain can be caused by other emotions. Feelings, unlike thoughts, are not just in your head.

Feelings also often appear in combination—they are more often complicated than simple. For instance, a parent whose child is a little late coming home from a date might be both worried and irritated. The fact that people talk about "sorting out" their feelings reflects this complexity.

Fostering Feeling Recognition

When it is said that therapy is work, it means that time, effort, and concentration are required for healing to occur. To work on feelings means setting aside time and making an effort to learn how one feels. The first two handouts presented here—Tuning In to Your Feelings and Separating Your Feelings from Your Thoughts—are designed to assist clients in becoming aware of their emotions and identifying them. You can try any or all of these exercises in session or give one or more to the client as a homework assignment, with the results of the exercise to be shared with you at the next session.

When you review the results of the clients' attempts to recognize and name their feelings, ask your clients which techniques seemed more helpful. Also ask if they have discovered or have used other means of tuning into themselves that they can share with you.

A third handout, Sad, Glad, Mad, or Scared?—A Feelings List (adapted from Bourne 1990), identifies the kinds of feelings associated with the four basic emotions: sadness, joy, anger, and fear. This list will be unnecessary for some clients, but may prove a godsend for others who were never taught the language of emotion and consequently need help in distinguishing one emotion from another.

In addition to giving the list to clients for their personal reference, you could ask clients to refer to the list during therapy sessions when they are struggling with articulating their emotions.

Using Creative Arts for Feelings Work

The creative arts, ranging from art, dance and poetry, to music and writing, offer invaluable outlets for the expression of emotion. Some clients, especially family abuse survivors, can benefit more from art, music, or dance therapy than from talking therapy because as children they were punished for expressing their feelings or were warned "not to tell." Also, some of the feelings that trauma generates are beyond words. They can only be expressed in music, art, or dance.

The purposes of expressive therapies are similar to the purposes of talking therapy: to make previously unbearable feelings (and memories) more bearable and to help clients own previously disowned feelings, especially problem feelings such as anger and grief (discussed below).

Suggesting to clients that they keep a journal of their feelings and thoughts and letting clients know that you would be willing to read or listen to their poetry or other writing or view their art work are all usually extremely helpful activities. However, unless you are a trained expressive therapist, do not attempt to conduct art, dance, poetry, or any other form of creative arts therapy on your own. Without training, you can do clients more damage than good by handing them a box of crayons and telling them to draw whatever comes to mind. For example, such seemingly simple and benign instructions could encourage regression in a client already struggling to maintain control of regressive tendencies.

If you feel a client could benefit from working with an expressive therapist, refer that client to an experienced and accredited art, dance, drama, music, or poetry therapist who has received specialized training both in the creative art and in the psychotherapeutic process. Names of such licensed accredited professionals can be obtained through local mental health organizations, as well as through local hospitals that offer treatment or programs for trauma survivors. In some areas today, there is a proliferation of individuals with various degrees of training, or perhaps no training at all, who claim to work therapeutically with people using one or more of the creative arts. These individuals may be highly skilled and sensitive; however, unless they are accredited, do not refer your clients to them.

Fears About Feelings

Healing requires that clients eventually experience some of the major emotions that were suppressed during the trauma. However, they cannot force themselves into an emotional experience, no matter how desperate they might be for healing to begin (and to be finished). Yet they can prepare themselves for the emotional aspects of healing by identifying and critically examining any fears or obstacles

Tuning In to Your Feelings

At any given time, you are feeling something, even when it seems otherwise. When you feel at peace with yourself, for example, you may not think you are feeling anything. But you are in fact experiencing that wonderful feeling of serenity.

Some of your feelings may be at the surface of your awareness and thus easy to identify. Others you may have to dig for. Some signs of suppressed feelings are muscle tension, physical pain with no medical cause, depression, ennui, or boredom, agitation or anxiety, dizziness, and involuntary urges to overeat, overspend, abuse alcohol or drugs, or hurt yourself.

Try the following techniques to help you tune in to exactly what you are feeling at this moment:

1. Quiet your body—or move it. The most commonly prescribed methods for getting in touch with your feelings involve getting inside yourself—by sitting still for a few minutes, meditating, or practicing muscle relaxation. However, if you suffer from bouts of extreme physical tension and anxiety, sitting still or meditating can be agitating, rather than soothing. Therefore, you may choose to "quiet" your body by moving through exercise, dance, or physical labor.

2. Ask yourself, "What am I feeling?" Don't expect to know right away; give yourself some time to discover your feelings. Also recognize, and indeed expect, that you may be feeling more than one emotion.

   Alternatively, if you are in a numb state, you may not be able to identify any feelings at all. If you are, don't be overly concerned about it. The numbing may serve an important purpose: protection against feelings that are too distressing or too overwhelming for you to handle.

Bear in mind as you practice these techniques that is very common and normal for trauma survivors to have "stuck points" in identifying their feelings. When this happens, don't berate yourself for not being able to come up with an answer. Instead congratulate yourself for trying. To help yourself get unstuck, you may also want to refer to the Feelings List your counselor may have given you.

During the course of therapy, you will often be asked to identify your feelings. As you do so it's important to keep the following in mind:

- Feelings are neither good nor bad, right nor wrong; feelings just are, they exist. You need not, and should not, judge yourself negatively just because you have or don't have a particular feeling.

- Feelings don't last forever. No matter what you are feeling, eventually it will lift and another emotion will take its place.

- When a strong feeling comes, you do not have to act on it. All you have to do is recognize it and feel it.

- The process of getting at your feelings is important. Try not to block it with excessive self-judgment; save that for your behavior, not your feelings and thoughts. Your actions affect other people. How you feel and what you think is no one's business but your own.

Separating Your Feelings from Your Thoughts

If you're like most people, you probably need some practice in distinguishing your feelings from your thoughts. This exercise is designed to do just that.

For one week, carry a small notebook with you, and every two or three hours jot down the time and the thoughts and feelings you're having on the left side of the paper. Also make a notation anytime you have a particularly strong or troublesome thought or feeling. An example is shown here:

Saturday

Time	Thoughts and Feelings	Thought or Feeling?
10:00	I'm angry at myself for staying up too late last night.	Feeling
12:00	He's probably angry at me for what I said last night.	Thought
3:00	I should do better at school.	Thought
3:15	I hate myself for not doing better at school.	Feeling

On the right side, indicate whether what you are experiencing is a thought or a feeling. If you have trouble deciding, try discussing it with someone you trust: your therapist, a friend, or a family member. The distinction should also become more clear as you progress in therapy.

If you have identified your experience as a feeling, try to identify what feeling (or feelings) you experienced. Talk to others and refer to the Feelings List for help.

Sad, Glad, Mad, or Scared?—A Feelings List

There are four basic emotions: sadness, joy anger, and fear. But there are many degrees and shadings of each one; the list that follows gives names to some of them. You may find it helpful to refer back to this list whenever you are trying to articulate or describe your emotions.

Words Associated With Sadness

Defeated	Ignored	Pessimistic	Unappreciated
Dejected	Inadequate	Preoccupied	Unattractive
Depressed	Incompetent	Pressured	Uncertain
Despairing	Inferior	Regretful	Uncomfortable
Desperate	Inhibited	Rejected	Unfulfilled
Devastated	Insecure	Remorseful	Useless
Disappointed	Isolated	Self-conscious	Victimized
Discouraged	Lonely	Shy	Violated
Embarrassed	Melancholy	Sorry	Vulnerable
Guilty	Miserable	Stupid	Weary
Helpless	Misunderstood	Tired	Worn-out
Hopeless	Muddled	Trapped	Worried
Hurt	Needy	Troubled	

Words Associated With Joy

Affectionate	Curious	Lovable	Tender
Alive	Delighted	Loved	Thankful
Amused	Desirable	Loving	Thrilled
Beautiful	Eager	Loyal	Trusted
Brave	Excited	Passionate	Understanding
Calm	Forgiving	Peaceful	Understood
Capable	Friendly	Playful	Unique
Caring	Fulfilled	Pleased	Valuable
Cheerful	Generous	Proud	Warm
Cherished	Giving	Quiet	Witty
Comfortable	Good	Relaxed	Wonderful
Competent	Grateful	Relieved	Worthwhile
Concerned	Happy	Respected	Youthful
Confident	Hopeful	Safe	
Content	Humorous	Supportive	
Courageous	Joyful	Sympathetic	

Words Associated With Anger

Annoyed	Furious	Irked	Stubborn
Bitter	Hateful	Irritated	Touchy
Contemptuous	Hostile	Outraged	Unappreciated
Distrustful	Humiliated	Overwhelmed	Uneasy
Enraged	Hurt	Provoked	
Exasperated	Impatient	Resentful	

Words Associated With Fear

Afraid	Indecisive	Scared	Uncertain
Apprehensive	Helpless	Self-destructive	Uncomfortable
Ashamed	Hopeless	Self-hating	Victimized
Desperate	Horrified	Terrified	Violated
Devastated	Insecure	Threatened	Vulnerable
Fearful	Panicked	Timid	
Frantic	Pressured	Trapped	

they might have about emotions, emotional expression, and the emotional side of their own personalities in particular.

The following two handouts—Identifying Your Fears About Feelings and Examining Your Fears About Feelings—are designed to help free the clients from unnecessary fears about their emotionality. These exercises can be completed in session or as a homework assignment, to be shared with you upon completion, or you may want to do the first one in session and have the client complete the second as homework (or vice versa).

Anger

There can be no PTSD without anger and grief, profound anger, bordering on murderous rage at times, and intense grief, even lifelong mourning for some, stemming from personal losses, social injustice, and human brutalities.

Some clients come to you with a nameless rage which they fear might explode at any moment. Others present with anger over present-day circumstances, anger which is legitimate, but which they themselves somehow sense is not appropriate in its intensity to the present. PTSD clients often have great concerns about their anger, partly because, until the healing process commences, their anger is being fueled by fires unknown and therefore mysterious and frightening. Anger as a symptom of PTSD and an obstacle to clients' leading a full and varied life is discussed in chapter 6. This section's focus is on helping clients, one step at a time, to trace some of the momentum of their anger to trauma-related or secondary wounding events.

Other clients will come to you weeping, but unable to identify why they find themselves crying. Others are unable to cry, but experience a deep sadness, a psychologically based inertia and loss of interest in activities and people that used to interest them and bring them some satisfaction.

Those who cry without knowing why, like those who feel stuck or stalemated (combined with feeling fatigued yet also restless), may be exhibiting signs of clinical depression. However, their emotional state may also signal unresolved grief; they have yet to encounter, understand, experience, and begin to work through their grief and sadness pertaining to the trauma and its aftermath. As with anger, your task will be to help make clients aware of their grief and help them identify the concrete losses which form the basis of their mourning. (This is the subject of the last section of this chapter.)

For PTSD sufferers, anger and grief are intimately related. Some experts feel that the fundamental issue is the grief. Others argue that it is the anger. In my view, the relative importance of grief and anger is not really an issue—it simply varies from one client to the next. Some clients may be volcanic in their rage, but have yet to shed a single tear over their losses. Other clients may have grieved profoundly, but have yet to confront their rage. Some may be stifling either or both of these emotions in substance abuse, overwork, or compulsive behavior. Or, as discussed above, clients may be out of touch with most of their feelings, grief and anger included. For such clients, therapy is more of an intellectual exercise than an emotional experience.

You can help lay the groundwork for "breaking" clients from their numbing, intellectualizing, or entrapment in unwanted anger or grief, first by "normalizing" either the feelings of anger and grief or the suppression of anger and grief (or both). This involves informing clients that trauma generates profound feelings of both anger and grief and that healing from trauma will mean confronting their anger and grief and ultimately reaching some kind of resolution of both feelings.

Causes of Anger

You should explain to clients that during traumatic and secondary wounding experiences, anger and grief, like other emotions, often go "underground" or are repressed for purposes of survival. (Emphasize the emotions with which the client seems to be having the most trouble.) You can also explain that anger and grief are inexorably linked, due to the nature of trauma, so when trauma survivors experience anger, grief may follow (and vice versa).

The losses endured as a result of the trauma inevitably generate a lot of anger, especially if the trauma involved some form of social injustice. Hence, on one level, the anger is pure rage at whatever force caused the damage or death. On another level, however, anger reflects grief for personal losses, as well as sorrow and disappointment over the societal or institutional failure that contributed to or caused the trauma.

For example, a decade ago, drunk drivers who were responsible for the deaths of pedestrians or other motorists were tried in civil courts and sometimes received ridiculously light penalties by today's standards. Relatives of the victims were consequently enraged not only at the drunk driver, but at the court system. Even more infuriating was that sometimes the courts did not even order the guilty drivers to receive treatment for their drinking problem. Many drunk drivers would leave the court free to drink and drive again, perhaps to kill more innocents, not to mention themselves.

As with relatives of victims of drunk drivers in the past, some of your clients' anger may be a legitimate response to victimization and secondary wounding experiences. Some of clients' anger may also be a defense against grief. When people are angry, they feel powerful and full of energy. In contrast, when they grieve, they feel weak and helpless, for grieving involves mourning not only losses, but helplessness in having been unable to prevent those losses. Grieving also involves acknowledging not only the past but present helplessness, in that nothing survivors can do can undo their losses.

For clients who use anger as a defense against grieving, healing may begin when they realize that their anger, no matter how intense, is impotent. Not even their powerful rage can resurrect the dead, restore their sense of innocence, mend scars or crippled limbs, recreate a community forever changed by war or natural catastrophe, or give them back the time they spent enduring the trauma and secondary wounding experiences and recovering from these events.

Clients need to be told, or reminded, of the biochemical changes that can be caused by trauma and of the ways certain situations can trigger angry (or sad) reactions that have more to do with the trauma than with present circumstances. (See chapter 3, on physiology, and in chapter 6, the section on anger and anger management.)

You may also need to present or review information on self-blame and survivor guilt. Self-blame and survivor guilt often result in clients being angry with themselves, instead of or in addition to external forces or other people. Thus, these problems may arise when clients begin to uncover the sources of their anger. In that case, they need to be dealt with somewhat differently from other sources, as discussed in chapter 7.

Identifying Your Fears About Feelings

Although you cannot force yourself to feel, you can prepare the way by beginning to identify some of the fears you have about feelings. In your present life, both at home, at work, and in social situations, you at times need to interact with others on an emotional as well as an intellectual basis. Therefore, both awareness of your fears about emotionality and overcoming some of those fears are critical to the entire quality of your life, as well as your emotional healing from the trauma and its aftermath.

Begin by reviewing your Feelings List and any work you and your counselor have already done around feelings. Remember that feelings are rarely pure. At any given moment, you are probably experiencing not just one, but several feelings.

Now, take time to write about some of the fears you have come to associate with being emotional or showing your emotions. As you write, consider the following questions:

1. Were you ever told by someone important to you that being emotional or showing your emotions was wrong, shameful, weak, sinful, slothful, unpatriotic, or a sign of mental or emotional instability or a lack of faith in God?

    You could have been given this message as a young child, teenager, young adult, or at any other time in your life. The important persons could have been either authority figures or nurturing ones, for example, a parent, teacher, caregiver, friend, lover, or a religious, military, police, or court authority.

2. Are emotional reactions for you associated with a loved one or caretaker doing one or more of the following?

    - Hurting you or someone close to you

    - Hurting themselves

    - Damaging or destroying property or pets

    - Making threats

    - Entering a mental ward or seeking psychiatric medication

    - Committing suicide

    - Committing homicide

    If so, what emotions did this individual display? Was he or she angry, sad, afraid, or was some other emotion dominant? Did you as a result come to fear certain emotions?

    If the answer is yes, which emotions have you come to associate with the negative events surrounding this individual's emotional expression or display?

3. Were you ever verbally abused, physically punished, abandoned, rejected, or otherwise shamed for being emotional or showing your emotions?

    If so, did the verbal or physical humiliation follow your expression of any emotion at all, or certain specific emotions? For example, were you punished for being angry, but not for crying, or punished for crying, but not for being angry? Or were you punished for showing any feeling whatsoever, even joy?

List the ways you were punished. Be specific. What names were you called? What type of physical punishments were used? Did you come to believe the names you were called? If you were physically abused as well, did you eventually come to believe that you deserved physical abuse because you committed the "sin" or displayed the "weakness" of showing emotion?

4. Are you afraid of losing control? In the past have you actually lost control, or is this a possibility that so far has not materialized? (Just because this fear has not materialized, does not mean your fear is unfounded.) Have you ever come close to losing control? Can you specify which emotions, or mix of emotions, you feel would contribute to or cause you to lose control?

Examine your fear of losing control closely. What are your fantasies or thoughts about what you would do or how you would feel if you did indeed lose control? How dangerous or costly would it be if you lost control that way? Consider the emotional, social, vocational, and financial costs not only to you, but to your family or others you care about.

If you have actually lost control of yourself when you allowed yourself to be emotional, what forms did the loss of control take? For example:

- Did you suffer memory loss, inability to concentrate, fainting, dizziness, paralysis, or unexplained, unexpected, or intense pain in some part of your body?

- Did you cut, burn, bruise, or otherwise injure yourself?

- Did you hurt yourself by abusing alcohol, drugs, food, or some other addictive substance?

- Did you attempt to or succeed in damaging property or in hurting animals or people?

- Did you make rash decisions, forget to show up for an important appointment, or act in ways that betrayed your moral values or resulted in lowered self-esteem?

Under what circumstances did you lose control? Were you alone or with others? Were you practicing an addiction? Were there other stresses in your life besides the trauma or a secondary wounding experience? Do you think you would have lost control if you had not been in these particular circumstances? More specifically, do you think you would have lost control if you had been with supportive individuals, if you were addiction-free, or if you had not been burdened by multiple stresses?

Can you identify what feelings, or mixture of feelings, seemed to trigger the loss of control? (Refer to the Feelings List, if necessary.)

5. Do some of your fears of feeling stem from the trauma? From your perspective, did something negative or terrible happen during the traumatic incident because you became emotional or showed your feelings?

   Consider also your secondary wounding experiences. Do you believe that you were in any way unfavorably treated or otherwise the object of blame-the-victim attitudes because of your emotional state? What evidence do you have that your emotional state or actions caused or contributed to any negative outcome during the traumatic event or a secondary wounding experience?

Examining Your Fears About Feelings

Respect all your fears, both those you think are rational and those you believe are not. The distinction between rational and irrational is almost irrelevant when it comes to fear. Fears grounded in emotional threats, such as rejection and shame, may seem trivial compared to fears grounded in threats to life and limb. However, those grounded in emotional issues can be just as controlling and destructive as threats to physical survival. For example, emotional fears can lead to addictions or other self-destructive behaviors that can eventually cause physical disease and even death. According to twelve-step programs' philosophy, fear is one of the major roots of addiction.

Your task in this exercise is to critically examine the fears about feeling that you have identified for the purpose of determining which of them are realistic psychological or physical threats, and which are dinosaurs from the past. With some assistance, you may choose to discard some of these "dinosaurs."

For each fear you have identified, consider the following questions:

1. To what extent does this fear reflect your fear of rejection, abandonment, disapproval, or some sort of punishment by others, as opposed to a genuine fear of emotionality or of a specific emotion?

    Imagine, for example, being in a situation in which the people around you accepted or even applauded, rather than rejected or disapproved of, your emotional state. Would you still be afraid of your feelings?

    If your fear of feeling seems primarily based on the negative responses of others, rather than in some internal fear of emotionality itself, your task is to find people who will be supportive of your emotional life.

2. If you showed your emotions today, would you be punished physically, emotionally, or financially? Are you still living with an abusive person who verbally or physically hurts you when you show certain feelings? Do you have an employer who is intolerant of emotional expression?

    If so, then you need to adjust your behavior accordingly. For example, you need to find a safe place to get in touch with your emotional self. However, if you are still being abused by a family member or caretaker, it may be difficult for you to find the necessary privacy.

    If you are in an abusive relationship, there are no easy routes to obtaining privacy, just as there are no simple means of eliminating the abuse, without also terminating the relationship. If the abuser is rigid and not amenable to discussion and compromise, sometimes a seemingly simple matter, such as obtaining the minimum of privacy and dignity within the relationship, may involve much larger and more serious issues, such as considering the option of leaving the relationship temporarily, if not permanently.

3. If you were taught that being emotional or having certain emotions is shameful, wrong, weak, sinful, or a sign of mental or emotional instability, make a list of all the persons who taught you these views. As best you can, write about why these individuals held such attitudes. Did their attitudes stem from

their personal fears and difficulties with emotions, from certain religious or cultural traditions, from some other outside force or necessity, or from some combination of these factors?

In some cases, fear of showing emotions arises for reasons of survival. For example, according to psychologist Erwin Parsons (1985), historically, slaves learned to keep their thoughts and feelings to themselves to minimize the extent they could be manipulated by their masters. Also, in many instances, the inner life of a slave was the only possession that could not be taken away. This historical necessity for "wearing the mask," as Parsons calls it, can persist into the present among formerly enslaved groups such as African Americans.

You may or may not have a clear idea why the individuals on your list held such negative views towards emotionality. However, the goal in trying to understand their reasons is not so that you can judge these people or become an amateur psychologist. Rather, the goal is to help you distance yourself from their attitudes. Once you realize that their attitudes may stem from their own personal considerations or outside pressures, not from some inherent truth about the negativity of emotions, you can give yourself the freedom to make your own decisions. In the present, unless these individuals can still harm you, you can work toward choosing which of their values about emotionality you would like to keep and which you would like to modify, or even discard.

4. Is your fear grounded in an expectation based on a sex role? We live in an age of women's and men's liberation, yet traditional sex role stereotypes die hard. Some men and boys still feel they need to always be strong and never cry. Some girls and women feel they must always be "sweet" and never get angry. Yet the male survivor needs to grieve his losses and the female survivor, to experience her anger and rage.

   If you are a man, do you fear that others will see you (or that you will see yourself) as a "weakling" or a "sissy" for expressing emotions? Do you have special problems acknowledging and coping with sadness, tenderness, or self-doubt? If you are a woman, do you fear that someone will label you (or that you will label yourself) as "unfeminine," "aggressive," or "masculine," if you experience the power of your anger?

5. If you indeed lost control when you became emotional or had specific emotions, can you identify the source of the loss of control? Did it stem directly from the emotional experience itself, or did it instead come from your fears about how others might react to you if they knew (or saw) how you felt?

   When you lost control, did you experience physical symptoms: hyperventilation, dizziness, or any of the warning signs your counselor has discussed with you? For example, if the last time you truly felt your pain you lost consciousness; became delusional, homicidal, or suicidal; sat immobilized in your bed for days, unable to eat; or found yourself incoherent, stop doing this exercise *immediately*.

Did you become disoriented, out of touch with reality, destructive toward yourself or others, or otherwise undergo significant psychological or physical distress during your last emotional experience?

If so, you need to discuss this situation with your counselor at your next session, if not earlier.

However, if your loss of control stems from anticipated rejection, shame, or punishment from others, or from internalized prohibitions against being emotional, then you may continue.

Keeping in mind your answers to the above questions, review your list of fears and decide which of them are so unfounded that you can discard them. Be sure to discuss those that still seem realistic or strong with your counselor or a supportive, knowledgeable friend.

Obstacles to Anger

Substance abuse, depression, and self-mutilation (including neglect of medical problems) are complex, multilevel, multipurpose behaviors. They can express anger at the self or they can indirectly express anger at others (including inanimate others) by taking out that anger on the self. When societal or familial norms make the direct and open expression of anger toward others a taboo, people are left with two choices: either they express their anger directly, and risk societal and familial rejection, or they take out that anger on themselves and suffer from depression, substance abuse problems, self-mutilation, and psychosomatic disorders. They may even do both.

Some clients may have been taught by their family of origin, caretakers, or religious instructors that all anger, in any form, is a sin and that anger at parents and authority figures is especially sinful, bad, wrong. Trauma survivors with such an upbringing experience exceptionally difficult internal struggles when they are mistreated or otherwise traumatized by someone in an authority position, such as a parent, priest, military officer, teacher, policemen, or an older sibling or relative, or by an institution that represents authority. Their emotions react normally with anger, to the wrongs they experience. But the voice of their upbringing tells them not only that it is wrong for them to be angry, but that they have no reason to be angry because the actions of authority figures are above reproach. This voice is especially strong for clients from social or familial groups where to question the authority figure is to ask to be banished from the family or social group.

Being reprimanded by or even excluded from one's family or from an important reference group is for some people a high price to pay. Therefore they suppress their anger, and for this they may pay another price: a high potential for developing a clinical depression, psychosomatic disorder, substance abuse problem, or problems with self-mutilation.

Prohibitions against anger may arise in families for nonreligious or nonideological reasons as well. For example, rigid rules against the expression of anger may exist in homes where one parent is a trauma survivor with untreated PTSD. This parent may so fear his or her anger that he or she prohibits the expression of anger in other family members. Indeed, research has shown that such sanctions against the expression of anger have been found in the homes of survivors of the Holocaust, in certain refugee families, and among families of veterans with untreated PTSD (Rosenheck 1986; Barocas and Barocas 1973; Trossman 1968; Sigal and Weinfeld 1985; Sigal and Rakoff 1971; Sigal 1976; Matsakis 1988).

In such families, children are often hesitant to express anger at a parent because their parent is already suffering greatly and they do not want to add to that parent's burden. For example, in families in which the mother is overwrought or dysfunctional as the result of being a trauma survivor herself or having a husband who is a trauma survivor, it is not uncommon for one of the daughters to become a "little adult," or to take emotional care of the mother or father. The daughter hides her anger, as she does her other emotions and needs in deference to the needs and emotions of one or both of the parents. As a result, such daughters have been found to suffer from clinical depressions (Sigal 1976; Matsakis 1988). Having learned to check their anger at home, both sons and daughters from such homes may be predisposed to suppressing anger regarding any traumas they themselves might have in their own lives.

Clients may also fear expressing their anger if in their family of origin they were punished for doing so or if the only expression of anger they ever experienced was out-of-control, destructive, or violent anger. For individuals who were never taught the distinction between anger as a feeling and angry acts, or whose parents or caretakers were unaware of the distinction, "getting angry" may mean throwing things, hitting people, shouting hurtful words, making horrible threats, or other negative events. Quite understandably, clients from such backgrounds might tend to suppress their anger—not only because they have learned to fear anger, but because they do not know how to express anger nondestructively.

In fact, any client who has experienced only negative manifestations of anger, who has never seen anger expressed nondestructively or acted out physically in a safe way, will have trouble coping with trauma-related anger and tend towards suppressing it. When the pressure of keeping a lid on the anger becomes too great, however, such a client may "explode" in some harmful or inappropriate way. If the client is a "relatively pure" PTSD case, and does not suffer from a character disorder, tremendous guilt and shame will follow such an outburst of anger. This leads in turn to further suppression of the anger. Thus, helping these clients to understand and manage their anger (as discussed in chapter 6) is a prerequisite to feelings work.

Prohibitions against anger may also stem from cultural group norms, such as those prevalent in some Eastern spiritual faiths, such as Zen Buddhism and others, which have as a goal rising above the cares of the world. Among people of such a cultural or religious bent, becoming angry and expressing it may be seen as a sign of spiritual deficiency. According to such value systems, spirituality includes rising not only above worldly concerns but above worldly emotions, such as anger, and attaining a state that is minimally reactive emotionally to surrounding forces and external events.

In trying to help clients with their anger, you need to be aware of the client's attitudes toward anger and the client's learning about anger gained from family, culture, religion, and other social agents. Some of the client's specific fears about anger may be tapped in the exercises presented earlier in this chapter: Identifying Fears About Feelings and Examining Fears About Feelings. These exercises could be reworded to help the client identify fears about anger.

Another reason clients sometimes have difficulty identifying or experiencing their anger is that the true targets of their anger may be unavailable to them or are so amorphous and diffuse that clients cannot focus their anger on any specific person.

For example, it is harder for abuse survivors to feel anger at their abuser when the abuser is dead (or sick or elderly) than when the abuser is alive, healthy, and still abusing. It is difficult to get angry at an earthquake, a tornado, or fire. Rape victims who are angry at institutionalized sexism in many areas of our society likewise have no person or group to direct their anger toward. Similarly, war survivors who are angry at governments for supporting the institution of war have no readily identifiable, tangible target.

In many cases, trauma survivors suppress their anger or are otherwise "stuck" with it because it is difficult to direct anger toward impersonal institutions, where to some degree, everyone is to blame, yet no one is to blame, than at a specific person.

Identifying Proper Sources of Anger

"You've got the wrong enemy," a wife shrieks to her PTSD-afflicted husband as he slams her against a wall.

One of the major goals of PTSD therapy is to help clients identify the "right enemy." Then they will not waste their energies attacking, defending themselves against, or being otherwise preoccupied with people or organizations onto which they have displaced anger properly belonging to the original offender.

As angry as some PTSD clients may be, do not assume they know what they are angry at. Some may know; others will have no idea or only have a vague idea. Alternatively, they may know intellectually that they are angry but have yet to experience the anger on an emotional or "gut" level.

Whatever the situation, healing involves identifying the people and institutions clients feel contributed to their pain or to the pain of others. Once they identify the "real enemies" associated with their traumatic and secondary wounding experiences, they are less likely to create problems for themselves in the present by confusing their right enemies with wrong enemies such as current problem people or situations. Their insights into some of the traumatic roots of their anger will also help them begin to take control over how they respond to both their right enemies and other people in future interactions.

The exercise that follows asks clients to answer the question, "Who or what are you angry at?" and list all the various sources of their anger for each trauma, secondary wounding experience, PTSD symptom, and other aftereffects experienced. However, bear in mind that such a task can be overwhelming if the client has endured many traumas or has backlogs of repressed anger. You need to use your judgment about how much of the exercise to use with each client.

As with memory retrieval, it is best to deal with anger in doses, in small manageable quantities. As you introduce the idea of dealing with anger and discuss the possibility of completing the exercise, be sure to ask your clients if they feel they can handle the experience or if they feel it will be helpful to them. If your client is afraid to experience even a flicker of anger, for fear that it might suddenly turn into a raging fire that will destroy his or her life or the lives of others, stress to the client that you will only deal with a small piece of the anger at a time, not all of it. If the client agrees, then use only portions of the exercise. If they do not, do not pursue the subject.

You might want to ask those who do not want to talk about their anger why they find this area so difficult to discuss, but your inquiry should not be in the form of a challenge or a confrontation. In other words, your tone of voice or expression should not imply that they are "failing therapy" or are somehow deficient because they do not wish to talk about this subject. Also, do not treat them as if they are abdicating their responsibility to probe deeper into themselves in quest of the "truth." Some truths, for some survivors, are best left unspoken, uncovered, and unanalyzed.

You can help matters by giving the client an "out," for example, by saying something like this:

> You've just told me you do not want to talk about your anger about . . . in our session today or in the near future. That is fine, but I wonder if you are willing to tell me why the subject is so difficult for you, if you know. I am not asking you this question in order to pressure you into talking about anger, but rather to find out more about you.
>
> Many people have difficulty with anger. That's only natural, because anger is one of the most difficult of human emotions to deal with. Some of my clients think I won't

approve of them or like them if they tell me how angry they are. But that's not the case. I don't judge people on that basis, because it is not my judgment that matters, but yours. Other people don't want to talk about their anger because they are afraid of becoming overwhelmed with pain, fear, grief, or agitation, or they're afraid they might do something they wish they hadn't if they start talking about how mad they are. Do any of these reasons apply to you?

If clients reply by telling you that if they discuss a certain area of anger with you, they will be tempted to hurt something, someone, or even themselves, do not press for more information. For example, don't say, "Could you tell me more about that?" Leave the topic alone. Respect clients' inner knowledge. After all, they have lived with their PTSD longer than you have known them in therapy, and they may know their limits better than you do. In your eyes, as a therapist, some of the ways clients have found of controlling their anger may seem somewhat self-destructive, or they may seem to limit clients' activities or potential. But these ways have served the client—and others—well, in that the client is not behaving violently. In such situations, it is not for you to challenge or try to change the client's coping skills, no matter how dysfunctional they may seem. When clients state that they might "go berserk" or hurt someone or something if they talk about certain anger-provoking experiences, believe them—especially if they have training in shooting or killing, as do combat veterans, police officers, and certain others.

If you and the client do agree to begin on the task, first present the full scope of the work ahead and its purpose: that it is helpful to look at the sources of anger in the past so that the past slowly becomes less confused with the present, and so that when anger left over from the trauma and secondary wounding experiences reappears in the present, it will do so with less frequency and intensity.

You should then ask clients to estimate how much of the anger they want to deal with in the session and with which angers they wish to begin. As with all such work, assure clients that should they become extremely uncomfortable or exhibit any of the warning signs listed in the introduction, you can stop the trauma work and help them become centered and calm.

Keeping in mind the above considerations, you can present the following exercise, Identifying the Sources of Your Anger, to your clients in written or oral form. For those clients you feel can handle the task, you can ask that they complete the exercise (or parts of it) as a homework assignment, to be shared with you at the next session. Otherwise, you can simply ask the questions in the exercise in your session. At the end of the session, be sure to process the experience by asking the client what it felt like to try to identify the sources of his or her anger and talk about them.

Grieving

Most trauma survivors have much to mourn, and until this grieving begins, therapeutic progress is difficult, if not impossible. Thus, a critical aspect of the therapist's role is to help clients identify their losses and support them through the mourning process. Identification of losses involves the lifting of denial regarding losses and overcoming obstacles of grieving.

Identifying the Sources of Your Anger

To begin to clarify the sources of your anger, consider all the traumas you have endured. If you have made a list of these traumas, review that list.

1. For each trauma, list the people or thing (besides yourself) you blame for the event. For example, you may blame a person, a specific group of people, or a certain religious, governmental, societal, financial, or other institution. Even if you aren't sure whether certain individuals or groups are actually responsible, if you feel anger toward them, put them on your list.

2. Now go back over the list of traumas and add to your anger list any additional entities you think you might be angry at, even if you can't feel that anger. If you can't think of any additional instances, mentally walk through the traumatic events and secondary wounding experiences as if they had happened to someone else. Write about who or what might have made that person angry.

3. Review your list of angers, and add to it any additional sources of anger you are able and willing to acknowledge. Also consider these possible sources of anger:

   • Are you angry at your PTSD symptoms? Consider how those symptoms have affected or hindered your career, your social life, your spiritual life, and your sexual relations.

   • Are you angry at any physical disability you suffered as a result of the trauma?

   • Are you angry that you became addicted or developed a compulsion as a way of dealing with the trauma? How do you feel when you look back on all the time, money, and effort you spent on your self-defeating behavior?

   • Are you angry that you have not been adequately compensated for having been victimized or traumatized? Do you feel you suffered so much as a result of the trauma that you are entitled to recognition, comfort, financial compensation, or justice? Are you angry because these compensations have been inadequate or completely lacking?

   • Are you angry at society or at life because, in addition to having been victimized, you still must suffer normal life stresses and perhaps even subsequent victimization or traumatization? Did you feel or hope that having been traumatized once would immunize you against future pain and loss?

   • Often trauma survivors blame themselves for things that happened during the trauma, for example, being confused, making a mistake, becoming "frozen" and unable to act. Do you see any relationship between being angry at yourself over such matters and your anger at others? Consider any areas where you blame yourself for what happened during the trauma and afterwards, and then see if you can make a connection between some of your self-blame and your anger toward other people, institutions, or forces. Make note of these instances and share them with your counselor.

Of all the aspects of PTSD therapy, dealing with grief tends to be one of the most difficult. Both client and therapist must overcome cultural prohibitions against intense grief, and the client must be willing to bear any stigma attached to those who are in emotional pain. In addition, grieving itself is excruciatingly painful—emotionally and in some cases spiritually. But despite the suffering grieving entails, it must be done. Otherwise the individual runs a high risk of developing other problems. The saying so-and-so "died of a broken heart," is not far from reality; sorrow that is not expressed and grieving that is not completed through its various stages can lead to behavioral or medical problems that are potentially life threatening.

For example, unresolved grief has been found to be a factor in the genesis or perpetuation of a wide range of psychological problems, including anger, outbursts of rage, restlessness, depression, addiction, compulsion, anxiety, and panic disorders. Unexpressed grief has also been implicated in the development or worsening of medical problems such as diabetes, heart disease, hypertension, cancer, asthma, and a variety of allergies, rashes, and aches and pains.

Clients who cannot grieve or who are afraid to even attempt the process also run the risk of staying psychologically stuck in the loss. When the anger, depression, and sorrow associated with a specific loss are repressed (either partially or totally), the individual escapes having to suffer these emotions directly or in full. However, this does not mean these emotions have been washed away and no longer exist. Indeed, in semiconscious or unconscious states, the emotions associated with unresolved grief can exert considerable control over people's lives. Thinking patterns and major decisions, behavior patterns, visions of the future, and relationships can all be affected by unwept tears and the anger and pain behind those tears.

Those clients who do have the courage to yield to the pain and suffering will, for an unpredictable length of time, be immersed in the grieving process. In fact, for a while, they may be intensely preoccupied with their losses and perhaps even incapacitated by the grieving process. However, in time, they will emerge free of the past and more able to go on than persons who have failed to grieve. This does not mean they will never think of, or feel, the loss again. Indeed, recovery from a trauma can be conceptualized as "resting in the sadness," rather than fighting or trying to escape it through some self-destructive behavior or some form of denial. (Even a constructive activity, such as working or achieving, can function as a form of denial of a significant loss.)

Once a loss has been grieved, it will no longer pose a significant barrier in the way of pursuing whatever goals or dreams clients might have for themselves. Simply put, to say good-bye to someone or something one loved deeply is excruciatingly painful. But until that good-bye is said and the loss truly mourned, the individual cannot go on to new involvements because too much psychic energy is still bound up in the lost object or person.

The Three Levels of Loss

Grieving is not simple: it involves losses on at least three levels. The first level is the loss of specific people or things or the physical, emotional, or spiritual aspects of the self that have been lost. These include tangible losses, such as the loss of a friend or relative, a home, an organ of the body, or a certain physical or intellectual ability. There are also intangible losses that can be equally important: faith in a spiritual being, loyalty to a government or institution, belief in the integrity of certain people or agencies, faith in the goodness of life and mankind. Not all trauma survivors challenge all their previous assumptions about the world, but many do. Thus, part of your role is to help clients identify the basic premises they held before the trauma that gave their lives meaning, purpose, and safety. Clients can then identify which of these have been challenged, damaged, or destroyed, by the traumatic experience and secondary wounding episodes.

For many survivors, the intangible losses are as devastating if not more devastating than tangible losses. For example, a male incest survivor who bears numerous physical scars from being abused may consider his bodily damage minor compared to the loss of his ability to truly trust others.

The second level of loss involves powerlessness. Part of the sadness of grieving stems from acknowledging that no matter what one does or did, certain losses cannot be replaced. Obviously one cannot restore certain tangible losses, yet it can be equally difficult to restore intangible losses. It is a struggle for many survivors to recreate their faith in persons or institutions that betrayed them during the trauma and, if not more important, to recreate their faith in themselves.

Many PTSD clients have lost their dignity as well as numerous vocational, social, and romantic opportunities as a result of the trauma and secondary wounding experiences. All these losses, including the loss of innocence, need to be recognized and mourned. Some clients also feel grief over the time, money, and energy spent in the healing process. "It wasn't my fault! Why do I have to be in therapy for years when my assailant doesn't?" Resentful statements such as these are often followed by grieving. This grief stems from acknowledging that one has been scarred by the trauma and that some of the scars may never go away.

Survivors of family traumas, such as child abuse, battering, suicide, and so on, need to mourn the loss of the dream of the ideal family they always desired. They may secretly hope that their mother, father, or other family member will change to finally be supportive of them. As they slowly absorb the reality that most likely their family members and the family system will never change or that they will never regain what they have lost, the grieving begins. After the grieving, however, they can go on to meet their own needs.

The third level of loss involves confronting one's mortality. When clients grieve the losses resulting from their trauma, they are also, on some level, grieving their mortality. Mortality is the ultimate expression of powerlessness. Although most people are aware that someday they will die, they do not think about this fact very much. However, this reality is forced upon one in grieving the deaths of others or the death of a part of oneself.

The Five Stages of Grief

In her landmark book, *On Death and Dying,* Elizabeth Kubler-Ross (1981) explains that the grieving process consists of five stages: denial, anger, bargaining, depression, and acceptance. Not only those who are dying, but those who suffer major losses in life, usually experience the five stages of grief. However, these "stages" do not always occur in precise order. A person can be in more than one stage at a time, and the length of time spent in each stage varies from person to person, as does the intensity of feeling. Throughout the five stages, feelings of fear, despair, disorganization, guilt, anxiety—even adrenaline surges may be experienced (Staudacher 1987, 1991).

Denial

In the first stage—denial or shock—the loss created by the trauma and its aftermath is not acknowledged. For example, an abused wife would most likely go into denial or shock the first time her husband beat her. Her disbelief that someone she loved and trusted could turn on her would probably make her unable to identify her losses. But those who have been abused have many losses: their hope for protection and care from a loved one, the physical injuries they have suffered, and so on.

Similarly, those who have seen others die as a part of their trauma —whether in a war, hurricane, car accident, or technological disaster—would be likely to go into denial regarding the deaths they observed. They might feel they were dreaming instead of living real life. Some individuals deny the reality of the deaths around them by unconsciously hoping for miraculous resurrections.

Anger

Once denial is cracked, clients can expect to be flooded with anger. They may be angry at life for giving them such hardships. If they are religious, they may be angry at their deity. If they have been abused, they may experience an intense rage at the individual who abused them. They may also be angry at themselves for seemingly accepting the abuse. They have yet to learn that perhaps they had no choice but to accept it.

Bargaining

The bargaining stage of grief is characterized by fantasies of "what if" and "if only." It is also characterized by excessive and irrational self-blame. If a client was carelessly driving a car that caused a ten-vehicle crash on the highway, killing a dozen people, then he or she has every right to hold him or herself responsible for the trauma. Similarly, if a client killed or abused others, and in the process was also abused or hurt, then he or she needs to take responsibility for his or her actions.

However, it's more likely that the client did not cause the trauma or its aftereffects. When clients continue to punish themselves for the what-if's and if-only's, they achieve no purpose other than wearing themselves out and perhaps destroying themselves.

Depression

There are many kinds of depression: the normal fluctuations in mood experienced by almost everyone, clinical depressions, and the depression associated with the grieving process. Clients experiencing this last type need to be reminded that this is a normal response. As trauma survivors, they are under severe stress. Not only are they coping with everyday feelings and needs, but they are coping with the trauma, as well as the reactions of others. They are also probably making complex arrangements for reordering their lives and obtaining medical, psychological, legal, and other help for themselves (and perhaps even for others involved in their trauma).

Depression is a natural response to these stresses and all the various losses they have suffered. Even though the depression associated with the grieving process is temporary, it can still be intense and painful. Grieving clients may also suffer some of the symptoms associated with clinical depression: difficulty con-

centrating, low self-esteem, changes in eating and sleeping habits, feelings of fu-
tility and hopelessness, or various physical problems such as backaches, headaches, vomiting, or constipation.

Extreme fatigue, and its opposite, physical agitation, are common to depression. Grieving clients may find every task an overwhelming burden, see little
hope for themselves or their situation, feel tired all the time, and receive little
or no pleasure even from people or events that normally would have pleased
them.

Review the *DSM-IV* definitions of depression if you need to ascertain whether
a client may be suffering from more than the depression associated with grief.

Acceptance

Acceptance is the final stage of grief. After clients have passed through the
other stages, they will feel less depressed and enraged about the trauma. They
will simply accept it and the emotional toll it has taken on them, their family,
and any others involved. Acceptance does not mean they are happy, but rather
that they have stopped fighting their own limitations and the reality of what
has happened to them.

They can compensate themselves somewhat for what they have lost. However, part of acceptance is realizing that whatever compensations they arrange
for themselves are only partial, at best. There is no way to restore what they
have lost. In the acceptance stage, they accept their scars and they accept that
all they can do is seek support for themselves when they go through periods of
remembering the trauma. They learn to be kind and loving to themselves but
realize that even their self-love cannot take away all the pain.

The Nonsequential Aspects of Grieving

As mentioned above, the model of the grieving process as consisting of five
stages does not mean that clients will progress neatly from stage to stage. Human emotions never come in neat packages. There are transitional states, where
one moves from one stage to the next. But one can also be in more than one
stage at a time. For example, the acceptance stage is often colored by anger, depression, and bargaining. Or a client may reach the acceptance stage only to
have the anniversary date of the trauma, another major life loss or trauma, or
some other trigger set him or her back to an earlier stage.

Because grieving is a process, it takes time. A client cannot expect to sit down
one day and decide that she or he will set aside a few hours that week to grieve
and be done with it.

There is no timetable or schedule for grieving. Some therapists talk about six
months to two years to recover from the death of a loved one and five years to
overcome the effects of a divorce. However, there are no published statistics
about how long it takes to finish grieving the losses inherent to a trauma. Much
depends on the nature of the trauma itself.

The depth and length of a client's grieving process will depend on the extent
and meaning of their losses. It will also depend on their cultural background,
their personalities, and the number of other demands that are placed on their
time and energies.

Also, because your clients have PTSD, they can expect to have recurring times
of grieving. People and situations that remind clients of the trauma or of secondary wounding experiences can trigger a renewal of both grief and anger. They

can also expect that when they have new losses, they may react more intensely than they feel is warranted. They may be correct in their assessment, in a sense. However, clients need to discard the notion that they are overreacting and instead simply acknowledge that trauma survivors are more reactive to subsequent grief and loss than are individuals who have not been traumatized. It is as if the new wounds open up the old wounds, and they feel both at once.

Consequently, for example, if a client was traumatized once, then subsequently involved in a minor car accident, he or she might react with more depression and sorrow than the others who were present. This strong reaction can be accounted for by the fact that the trauma has expanded the client's ability to feel intensely.

Obstacles to Grieving

People fear grieving because they fear suffering and the loss of control and vulnerability it implies. When the pain of loss engulfs people they feel defenseless and weak, and so they are. True grief is so consuming that, at least temporarily, grieving people cannot function as before. For this reason, in societies where grief is respected and supported, the bereaved often are not expected to perform their normal roles or meet their usual responsibilities. They are, in essence, given a prescribed period of time off from the normal work of life to complete another kind of work: grieving.

Unfortunately, in American culture, a display of strong emotion is considered a sign of weakness or even of mental instability. To grieve "too long" is considered a sign of self-pity or dwelling in the past.

The "appropriate" response to loss is usually a form of stoicism. For example, when President Kennedy was shot, Mrs. Kennedy was widely praised as a loyal wife and a brave and strong person for not shedding a tear during his funeral. However, if Jacqueline Kennedy had been living in some other society, such behavior might have been considered heartless and a disgrace to her husband. In other societies, the bereaved are permitted, if not expected, to cry openly, to moan, to scream, or even to try to jump into the casket.

Part of the stigma that attends emotionality in our culture stems from the fact that emotionality is associated with women who are presumed to be weak, hysterical, irrational, and needy partially because they are inherently "emotional." In contrast, men are endowed with the presumably superior traits of rationality, intellectuality, and emotional self-control. Men who are heavily invested in the traditional male sex role, which equates strength with emotional control, and women who need to distance themselves from the denigration attached to the traditional female role, will do their best to suppress their feelings and appear cool, calm, and collected, regardless of the situation. The irony here is, of course, that recognizing and grieving a loss is the first step toward restoring emotional control.

Clients who experienced significant losses before the trauma and were able to grieve those losses, at least in part, will be less afraid of grieving than those for whom grieving is a totally new and unknown experience. All who grieve, especially those unfamiliar with grieving, will have concerns such as the following:

> If I grieve, how long will it take? How much will it hurt? Will it change my personality?

> If I let myself grieve, can I make the grieving stop when I can't stand it anymore, or am I totally powerless?

If I grieve a loss once, for example, by crying for a while, will I be done with it, or will I have to grieve that same loss some more?

If I have to grieve the same loss more than once, how will I know when the grief will strike? Will it overpower me again the second time like the first time? Will I have the strength to go on after giving in to the sorrow?

These questions are legitimate and need to be given honest, not "Pollyanna," answers. Otherwise clients' fears about grieving can become magnified and they could run from the process even harder than they did prior to beginning therapy. You need to tell them that there is no way to predict how long or how deeply they will grieve. Undergoing the grieving process may result in their changing their priorities or lifestyle, or it may not. Although it may feel for a time as if the grief will swallow them and they will never emerge alive, these feelings do not reflect reality. Grieving may feel like dying, but one does not die.

In fact, although it seems unbelievable while one is grieving, the time of intense grief eventually passes. How long it takes for the acute grieving period to lift is unpredictable; the time needed varies from one individual to another. Yet it is certain that after the catharsis of grieving, there is renewal. The loss is always there, but there is a new energy for the present. It is also certain that without the catharsis of grieving, there can only be stagnation.

Identifying Losses

To facilitate the grieving process and to legitimize their grief, clients need to become as aware of their losses as possible. Just as clients cannot deal with their anger without knowing what they are angry about, they cannot deal with their grief until they identify their losses. This is especially the case with clients who are ashamed of grieving for fear they are only feeling sorry for themselves or feeling sad about unimportant things.

This interpretation of grief trivializes it, yet it is a natural result of the pain and death denying tenor of our society. However, when clients who so malign their grief begin to list their losses, both tangible and intangible, they often suddenly begin to realize they in fact have every right and reason to grieve, and that they have a lot of grieving to do. In some cases, however, itemizing losses (as the following exercise has clients do) gives birth not to the grief but to anger and rage. In that case you will need to help the client with those feelings, as discussed earlier in this chapter.

When clients consider their losses, they need to take into account the full range of losses: financial, emotional, medical or physical losses, philosophical, spiritual, and moral. The following handout, Identifying Your Losses, may be completed as a homework assignment or discussed in a session. Probably more than one, if not several, sessions will be required. Even more so than others, this exercise should not be rushed.

When you present this exercise to clients, emphasize how important it is. Also, warn your client that completing the exercise may involve some pain and anger—perhaps a great deal of pain and anger. However, once they identify their losses and begin to grieve them, they can then use their understanding of what they have lost to empower themselves and enrich their lives. For example, once they know what they have been cheated of, they can begin to make plans to compensate themselves as much as possible, if they choose to. They might also begin to make some adjustments in their lives so that, as much as possible, they

Identifying Your Losses

Make a written list of your financial, emotional, medical or physical losses, and your philosophical, spiritual, and moral losses. Take some time to complete this exercise. It's far more important than it may at first appear. The paragraphs below list examples of these different types of losses.

Financial Costs

Make a list of all the financial losses you have sustained as a result of the trauma or any secondary wounding experiences. Consider both direct and indirect costs.

Direct costs include money and property stolen, medical bills, relocation expenses, legal fees, babysitting, and transportation costs (to go to court, doctor's appointments, and so on), days lost from work, and the costs of mental health care to cope with the trauma. Include in your direct cost list any financial costs borne by relatives and friends.

Indirect costs include the cost of lost opportunities, for example the loss of career opportunities you were unable to pursue due to medical, psychological, or other conditions stemming from the trauma. Perhaps you had to go to court to prosecute your offender several times, and while you were busy with attorneys and the court system, you missed out on applying for a new job or working on a new project that could have led to a promotion.

Emotional Costs

From what emotional symptoms have you suffered and for how long? How have you had to limit social, vocational, and other aspects of your life because of symptoms resulting from the trauma, or secondary wounding experiences? These are all losses.

Other aspects of the emotional cost of the trauma are the costs to your family members and friends. How did the trauma affect your relationships with the significant others in your life? What emotional costs did they have to bear as a result of your trauma or secondary wounding experiences?

Medical and Physical Costs

Have any of your physical or mental abilities been negatively affected by the trauma or by secondary wounding experiences? If so, please list which ones and how they have been impaired. How have these medical or physical limitations affected other aspects of your life: your job, relationships, sex life, creative pursuits, and so on?

Philosophical, Spiritual, and Moral Costs

What cherished beliefs about yourself, specific people, people in general or about specific groups, organizations, or institutions were negatively affected by the trauma or by secondary wounding experiences? Be as specific as possible in your listing.

can prevent certain losses from recurring. Or they might use the insights they gained from identifying their losses to otherwise help themselves or others.

Coping with Grief

For those who are actively grieving, a concept such as "coping with grief" can feel like an insult or a cruel joke; the very words may engender a tirade of anger and pain. "How am I supposed to 'cope' with seeing young men split in half?" a combat veteran might say. "How do I 'cope' with losing my arm in a car accident?" says a teenager. "I'm supposed to 'cope' with being beaten and raped?" asks a mother of four. "Is it possible to 'cope' with seeing a fire destroy your home and community?" asks a severely shaken businessman. "Is there truly any way to 'cope' with feeling like an orphan in your own family?" asks a formerly abused child.

The anger and questions of these survivors are legitimate. Coping does not mean "overcoming" or "whitewashing" the very real losses trauma can create. Clients who have truly undergone trauma can never forget what happened, and they will have scars. Thus, instead of suggesting to clients that if they follow a few simple directions they will be able to cope with their intense pain, give them a new definition of coping—one that is appropriate for trauma survivors. For example, you could say something like this:

> The scars will be with you forever. However you can take
> some steps toward dealing with the trauma directly and
> constructively, rather than indirectly and destructively. You can
> make an effort to confront and try to ease your emotional,
> physical, and spiritual scars. There are steps you can take to
> make your life in the present as fulfilling and meaningful as
> possible. And, finally, when you are ready, you can begin to
> accept, rather than deny or fight, the limitations the trauma
> has imposed on your life.

In essence, coping means that the past is not allowed to totally destroy the present. Coping means that despite their extremely negative experiences, clients can preserve at least part of their heart, soul, and self-respect. Coping with grief, and with the recurring sense of loss that so often afflicts trauma survivors, means that they learn to live with the sorrow. They learn to accept the grief, without allowing the fact that they are grieving to plunge them into depression, self-hatred, or despair.

Grief is so unfamiliar to most people that when they first experience it, they feel as if something is wrong with them. However, people who have had a major loss, even a loss not of the proportion of a trauma, soon learn that grief and sadness are natural and permanent parts of life.

Expressing Grief

Expressing grief does not erase the pain, but it does help. Clients need to be encouraged to express their grief in any way that is right for them. Clients who can cry are fortunate. Encourage them to weep, scream, or wail for all they want, for as long as they want, preferably in a safe accepting environment. However, not all clients are capable of crying and, even those who can cry can gain further insight into their grief by expressing it by writing. For example, they can write letters to or about the persons they lost or to those they now feel alienated from. They can also write letters to parts of themselves they feel were lost, as well as to any agencies or institutions that failed them. Instruct your clients that they need not show their writing to anyone, although they can if they want to.

Additional suggestions on writing about grief can be found in *Beyond Grief*, by Carol Staudacher (1987).

For example, she suggests taking a sheet of paper for each emotion felt during the day. At the top of each page, one writes a word or two describing the feeling, and beneath that one writes about the thoughts and actions that feeling inspires. "You may also write about why you think you have the particular feeling," Staudacher says. If writing is a comfortable outlet for you, it could be more helpful in resolving personal issues than you would imagine." Clients who do not like writing about their feelings directly, might want to write a poem or a short story that expresses their grief indirectly.

Writing is not a helpful medium for some clients, especially (obviously) if they are illiterate or dyslexic. For such clients, you might suggest singing, drawing, painting, or making a piece of sculpture that expresses their grief. Or they might want to express their grief through movement to music.

Even gardening can be a form of expressing grief. One survivor of an airplane crash, for example, bought several new kinds of vegetable plants, one for each person who died in the crash. He tended to his plants lovingly, pretending they were the deceased, and gave away the produce to the needy in honor of the dead.

Creating a Time and a Place to Grieve

Grieving requires psychic energy and time. Clients in life situations in which they are besieged with many external demands may have little time, and no private place, to grieve. Usually the office or other places of employment, where certain amounts of emotional composure are expected, are not appropriate places for clients to weep or grieve in other ways. They may need to take time off from work, go for long walks at lunch, or find some quiet spot so that they can have the freedom to feel their feelings without being stared at, reprimanded, or considered odd.

At home, too, clients may need to create a particular space or set aside time for emotional expression. If, however, economic and other realities make such privacy nearly impossible, then their grieving process may be forestalled. It is not uncommon, for example, for trauma survivors whose circumstances involve significant economic, legal, or medical problems to—by necessity—be so involved in responding to these problems that the grieving process is postponed. Only after these other problems are resolved, is their grief free to emerge, at the point when they have the time and energy to grieve.

Giving Dignity to Grief

In many societies, people who have lost loved ones are helped by religious and other rituals that acknowledge their losses and permit them to receive the support and consolation of others. For example, certain Christian groups hold memorial services at specified intervals after a death. In Judaism, a full year after a death is recognized as a time of grief and healing, with distinct stages observed, including seven days of sitting *shivah*, a time when the bereaved gather to talk about their memories both of the death itself and the life that preceded it. "The condolence call provides the mourner with the opportunity to tell his story many different times to many different people, each of whom are enjoined to allow the mourner to speak first so that his interests are allowed to be the focus of conversation" (Gorden 1975).

Similar rituals can help clients give dignity to their own grief. Rather than seeing their sorrow as a sign of "going crazy" or "dwelling in the past," they need to remember that the people, qualities, or values they are mourning are worthy of their grief. One way clients can both express their grief and give dignity to it is to create a memorial for it. Some people set aside a corner of their home or a special drawer where they keep mementos or writings about the trauma as a form of memorial. If their grieving involves the loss of one or more people, they may want to hold a religious service, if they feel this would meet their needs. Alternatively, they may want to hold an informal service with others who understand their pain, or raise funds for a memorial contribution honoring the deceased.

Another way to think of an appropriate form of memorial is to consider what the deceased might have wanted as a commemoration. However, when clients' grief involves intangibles, such as the loss of certain qualities within themselves (their innocence, for example, or the loss of certain mental or physical abilities) they may need to create a personal memorial service for themselves. In designing such a service, clients might be helped by researching how other cultures observe and mourn death.

Chapter 10

Final Healing Stages

The title of this chapter should not be taken to suggest that healing is ever necessarily total or complete. Rather, the phrase "final healing stages" means a time in the healing process when the client becomes ready to embrace two important processes: self-empowerment and reconnection with others and society at large.

According to Herman (1992), trauma devastates people because it disempowers them and causes disconnection between them and others. Trauma can also cause a disconnection or alienation from the self. Not only the pain, fear, and loss involved in the trauma debilitate but aftereffects of the trauma and secondary wounding experiences often propel survivors into a lifestyle characterized by passivity and social isolation, which results in a sense of hopelessness and feeling of abandonment. Alternatively, as in the case of domestic violence survivors, subsequent events reinforce a previous lifestyle fraught with loneliness, self-abasement, exploitation by others. Survivors may also exhibit antisocial behavior and other forms of aggression, both of which can be understood as, in part, retaliatory responses to feeling powerless and isolated.

Some survivors, in contrast, are fortunate enough to be reintegrated into their families and communities shortly after the trauma, usually as the result of a few people's support. Often these reintegrated survivors are able to resume their pretrauma activities. Some, as a direct result of the trauma, even assume a more active, masterful stance toward life than they had prior to the trauma. However, these functional individuals are not our concern. Those survivors whose trauma has resulted in disempowerment and disconnection are the ones this chapter is designed to help you help. For this group, the "final" stages of healing involve reconnection and empowerment (Herman 1992).

To become empowered after having been traumatized means to regain strength. For some clients, this includes physical strength, but the main ways clients empower themselves lie in the areas of making healthy, independent choices for themselves—rather than allowing other people or "ghosts" from the trauma to make decisions for them. These ghosts can include negative thinking, low self-esteem, and the many fears that are the natural result of having been traumatized.

In essence, clients' empowerment means that the trauma is no longer the central organizing factor in their life. Although the trauma and its effects cannot be erased—and will remain a factor in clients' decisions, interactions with others, and inner life—they no longer dominate.

Assessing Client Progress

Survivors who are ready to embark on the final stages of empowerment and connection are able to do so only because they have made the following strides:

1. They have been able to remember and piece together enough of their traumatic histories to form a narrative. These narratives may be spotty, and there may be some confusion or ambiguity about certain aspects of what occurred. However, the trauma is no longer just fragmented memories, unrelated dreams or nightmares, and incomprehensible symptoms. It is no longer a mystery or a semi-mystery, but a coherent or semi-coherent story.

2. Because clients have a clearer picture of what transpired, and because they have learned what PTSD is, they can make some sense out of their symptoms and begin to forgive themselves for having them.

3. Due to having learned and practiced anger management techniques and ways of handling trigger situations, they have established some control over their worst symptoms.

4. They have established a trusting relationship with at least one person, you, their therapist, on whom they can rely when they feel afraid—of the past, the present, the future, of themselves or others.

As a result of these four achievements, "final-stage" clients are ready to re-engage in life: to form new relationships or to heal broken ones and to take a more active stance in other areas of life. They may even decide to seek compensation for their trauma-related injuries and insults; yet this more active stance, or empowerment, is not limited to seeking retribution or compensation. First they have to realize that they have power, which, for some survivors, is an achievement in itself. Then they have to find a means of expressing that power or control, beginning with a few self-chosen areas. This may mean learning new skills, setting new goals, or reviving old dreams, in whole or in part.

In sum, with the trauma sufficiently remembered, with some of the feelings and thought patterns generated by the trauma identified and processed, and with sufficient measures taken so that clients feel somewhat safe internally and externally, they can then begin the process of empowering themselves and reconnecting with other people. However, arrival at this stage does not mean that all clients are at the final stage of the healing process.

For some clients, especially survivors of long-term or extreme abuse, the healing process may take many years, if not decades. In fact, a client's very progress in therapy may make possible the resurrection of further traumatic memories. As clients grow in self-knowledge and self-respect, in managing and accepting their PTSD symptoms, and in creating an increasingly safer and more loving world for themselves, they become, in a sense, psychologically stronger. As a result, their inner selves will feel able to tolerate the release of any still repressed memories.

For example, a rape survivor might make good progress in dealing with the rape and then, two years after terminating therapy, begin to have flashbacks about early childhood physical or sexual abuse. Or a natural catastrophe or car accident survivor might be ready to leave counseling when memories of a prior criminal victimization, kidnapping, torture experience, or other horror emerge.

In other instances, the healing process leads not to the release of long-buried traumatic memories but to more detailed and precise memories of the trauma that brought the client to therapy in the first place. For example, a male incest survivor may remember perpetrators in addition to his uncle or may begin to recall in detail the times as a child when he asked for help from teachers, neighbors, or other family members, only to be ignored or blamed for the abuse.

In these and other instances where the process of healing from one trauma sets the stage for the emergence of further memories and feelings, the client will once again undergo the disorientation and pain of the first healing process. However, since the client has had experience with healing, she or he can probably move somewhat more quickly and easily through this second healing process.

Even if the passage of time, combined with inner growth, does not result in new traumatic memories—for eventually there may be no new memories—the individual's interpretation of the trauma and its impact may change and mature. In this sense, healing is never truly finished. However, the progress that has been made can and should be recognized and appreciated.

Reinforcing Gains

Before clients go on to explore areas of their lives in which they want to exert increased control, it is useful to buttress their confidence in their ability to do new things, to take risks and grow, by recapping the progress they have made so far. They might not consider having undergone therapy for the trauma and other concerns as an achievement worthy of consideration. Yet it is a brave act, involving time, money, and effort, and it represents a substantial investment in acquiring emotional and spiritual self-knowledge and the kind of behavioral controls over their emotions they will need to be successful in the larger world.

Emotional Growth

Clients often do not give themselves full credit for the degree to which they have attained mastery over the trauma and their secondary wounding experiences. These successes need to be pointed out to clients as specifically as possible. For example, you could say this to a client who had problems with anger:

> A year ago you were not able to wait a half hour for a friend
> without having a rage reaction, because waiting reminded you
> of waiting for help to arrive after the accident and the help
> never came. I remember how mad you were at yourself
> because you couldn't control your anger. You were so enraged
> with your friend when he'd be late, you'd lash out at him so
> viciously that it only alienated him.
>
> Then, within six months, you learned to run around the
> block until you were exhausted, tear up newspapers, and write
> your feelings down instead of cursing your friend for being
> late. Even then it was hard for you to be civil with him when
> he arrived. However, you were able to tell him that you didn't
> like being kept waiting and not unload on him all the anger
> that belonged to the people who betrayed you during the
> trauma.
>
> Today you still don't like to be kept waiting, but you realize
> that his being late doesn't have the life-or-death implications
> that being late had during the trauma. You've also worked

through enough of your anger about the trauma so that when you are kept waiting, your level of anger is almost one-tenth what it was before. And you are learning to accept that your friend isn't perfect, that he has a real problem with tardiness.

True, you can't sit calmly and wait for him; you still need to walk around the block when he's late. You still get angry with him, but you aren't plummeted into an uncontrollable fury. Today you are freer than ever from the rage that wanted to strike out at everything in sight. Remember how you hated being saddled with that anger? "It's not fun at all. How do I turn it off?" you used to ask me.

Somehow, it has lessened, through your hard emotional work, through all that talking, all that raging, all that crying you've done in this room and with others. And your reward is that today you can even manage a smile for your friend instead of wanting to attack him when he walks in the door.

Now that's progress, because you aren't letting the effects of the trauma ruin something you want to have in your life today—a beautiful friendship with someone who, although he has an annoying habit of being late, you love a great deal and who loves you too.

If there is one rule in working with PTSD clients it is to reinforce, reinforce, reinforce—any positive qualities they have that emerge and any steps, however small, they make toward progress. (This does not mean, of course, denying or ignoring the client's difficulties. After all, clients come to therapy to understand and deal with their deficiencies, conflicts, and other problem areas, not with their strengths.) Yet, in your role as "reinforcer," you can point out to clients that they have taken the risk of looking at their traumatic past, rather than running from it; have made the effort to gather additional information about what happened to them; and have taken the additional risk of sharing what happened and how they felt about it with another.

Armed with this new information and feedback, they have been able to view the trauma more objectively. Most likely, they overestimated what they could have done to mitigate the situation and underestimated their utter powerlessness or the many difficulties posed to them by the numerous double binds inherent to traumatic situations. Another bold step they have taken (and you should emphasize this) is that they took the risk of looking at and feeling their emotions. Many people never examine or get to know their emotional selves. As a result, they live "half-lives" because they are afraid to acknowledge, much less deal with, their fear, anger, grief, and other strong emotions.

Even though in our society such individuals are often viewed as strong because they seem immune to the upheavals caused by emotions, in fact they are emotionally ignorant or weak. Inevitably, some day a crisis, loss, or even a trauma will enter these people's lives, and they will be ill-prepared to cope with it, except perhaps through denial, substance abuse, or some other nonconstructive means. In a sense, such individuals can be considered to be in emotional kindergarten, whereas your clients, who have braved the storms of profound grief, paralyzing despair, and all-consuming anger or murderous rage, and have learned to recognize and cope with these emotions, can be seen as having a bachelor's, if not an advanced degree, in emotional awareness and control.

Existential and Spiritual Growth

Your clients also need to appreciate that somewhere in the healing process they took a spiritual or existential look at their trauma. Part of this perspective includes the awareness that their victimization occurred in a social and historical context as well as a psychological one. Part of your role as therapist is to educate clients on the socio-political context of the trauma, partly because it is a fact that traumatic events do not occur in historical vacuums and partly because much of the self-blame survivors typically feel is lifted when they learn that what occurred involved forces larger than themselves.

Therefore, another achievement for which your clients need to learn to take credit is their attainment of a heightened awareness of social injustices. For example, traumas involving injuries to women and children often involve the unequal power distribution by age and sex. Similarly, traumas involving ethnic, economic, and religious issues have as their setting long histories of bigotry and unequal power. Once clients became conscious of certain unpleasant sociopolitical realities, they probably felt the anger and sorrow that attend this raised consciousness. They need to take credit for facing, rather than denying or avoiding, some of the brutalities and injustices that are part of human existence, and for having the courage to feel the painful feelings associated with such an awareness.

Another of your clients' achievements is their encounter with their own mortality. This has probably led them to ask some searching questions about life in general and more specifically, about what they want to do with their lives. The knowledge that they too will die can motivate people to vigorously pursue their dreams and goals.

With the grueling processes of memory retrieval, coping with emotions, learning to control symptoms, and trigger events confronted and somewhat mastered, clients can think about the trauma from a new perspective. At this point, the process begins of evolving an ever-maturing philosophical or existential perspective on the trauma. With some of the major emotional work out of the way, the client can begin to grapple with the meaning of the trauma, and perhaps the trauma itself will point out future directions for the client's life, such as a "survivor mission."

Victor Frankl, a psychiatrist who was interned in a Nazi concentration camp and who later worked with survivors of the camps, believed that the great pain involved in certain traumas, like his own, could be turned around to give great meaning to life through "self-transcendent giving" or some form of meaningful activity. For example, Frankl documents case after case of inmates in the camps who gave up their lives for someone, or something, they considered meaningful. His theory was that people could tolerate numerous kinds of deprivations—economic, physical, sexual—as long as they felt their life had purpose (Frankl 1955, 1959, 1975).

Frankl's concepts suggest that therapists can help PTSD clients by assisting them to find ways of giving to the world in honor of their life-or-death experiences. Such actions help clients to transform their pain into prosocial constructive activities, which reduces their need to act out or repress their pain and other feelings. Frankl stresses that such giving (which can take the form of a variety of survivor missions) is not an emotional defense nor an emotional escape, except in those cases where trauma survivors "prematurely involve themselves in self-transcendent activities without regaining to consciousness their memories and feelings about the trauma." Such survivors may be using the activity surrounding survivor missions to "avoid the conscious awareness of painful feelings such as terror and rage" (Lantz 1992).

To help clients appreciate their progress, you may want to devote some sessions to taking stock. The following handout, Taking Stock of Your Progress, can be completed jointly in session or given to the client as a homework assignment.

Refinding the Self

Clients may want to find new directions in life, but not know how to commence the journey. They may make comments such as, "For so long now I've been preoccupied with what happened during the trauma. Now I'm ready to get into the present, but it's like starting all over again. Where do I begin?"

One place clients can start is where they left off. You can explore with them who they were and what they were interested in before the trauma and see if there are any interests of their pretrauma self that they could, or would want to, pursue now.

In this way, empowerment can begin with refinding the self, the person that existed before the trauma. The questions you need to ask in this regard can include the following:

What was the client like before the trauma?

Are any aspects of the pretrauma self salvageable?

Does the client want to revive any part of that self or any of his or her pretrauma goals?

The handout Rediscovering Your Pretrauma Self is designed to help clients remember and define who they were before the trauma. It can be completed as a writing assignment, or you can ask these questions in a session. You may want to suggest that clients center themselves with deep breathing exercises or muscle relaxation before beginning.

Reconnecting with Others

Relationships that are nurturing, kind, and loving—whether with people, pets, a spiritual being, or some other higher power of one's understanding—are energizing and potentially healing. In this sense, PTSD clients who counter the natural pull of their PTSD symptoms toward mistrust and fear of others with an active effort to develop and use a support system will be empowered by the human connections they make.

As Judith Lyons (1991b) points out, following trauma, survivors either move toward people or pull away. In some cases, trauma survivors retreat simply because they do not have the psychic or physical energy to relate to people or engage in social and other activities as they did before. Especially immediately following the trauma, survivors may be so involved with their feelings and with practical matters that, of necessity, they allow their human relationships to slip. Also, some survivors harbor such shame about what occurred during the trauma or about any symptoms they are experiencing that they "hide" from others, even from family members and people they know love them.

Some individuals are so severely injured physically by trauma that they have to "drop out" of normal work, social, or family activities. When trauma results in blindness, amputation, or some other major physical limitation, the trauma

Taking Stock of Your Progress

You have grown considerably as a result of the healing process—mentally, emotionally, and spiritually. To appreciate the extent of your growth, consider the following questions. Reply to them in writing; begin the first page with the heading "My Progress."

Note that these questions are not meant to imply that what you thought and felt before were distortions. Many of those thoughts and feelings were based in reality.

Mental or Cognitive Growth

1. What have you learned about how the conditions of trauma influenced your view of what occurred during the trauma, your role in causing the trauma or influencing its outcome, your self-esteem, and your view of other people?

2. What have you learned about how the victim-blaming mentality of certain people and institutions affected your view of what occurred during the trauma, your view of your role in causing the trauma or influencing its outcome, your view of yourself, and your view of other people and institutions?

3. What have you learned about reality? More specifically, what have you learned about how people react when their lives are threatened? What have you learned about how bureaucracies and other organizations operate? What have you learned about human error, human cruelty, or human indifference?

4. What have you learned about your ability to control your life? In what areas can you exert control? In what areas are you not able to exert control?

Emotional Growth

5. What have you learned about yourself emotionally?

6. Which emotions do you still struggle with?

7. What are your most trying emotional situations today?

8. Do you have any unfinished emotional work to do regarding the trauma or secondary wounding experiences? If so, what?

Existential or Spiritual Growth

9. How did the trauma change your view of the meaning of life?

10. How did the trauma change your view of human nature?

11. How did the trauma confirm or change any of your previous spiritual or moral beliefs? How did it change your views of right or wrong, of sin, or of injustice?

12. What have you learned about the personal meaning of the trauma? Did you view it as a punishment of sorts or from inside some other personal framework? Has the healing process changed your original views of the personal meaning of the trauma? If so, how?

13. Do you now see the trauma (and any secondary wounding experiences that followed) as purely random events in which you just happened to find yourself trapped for reasons having little to do with your personality, morality, or any other aspect of yourself? Or do you still attach some personal meaning to these experiences? If the trauma still has a special personal meaning for you, what is that meaning?

Rediscovering Your Pretrauma Self

Part One: Who Was I Then?

Try to recall what city you were living in at the time the trauma occurred. Who were you living with, and what were you doing? Did you have a job or were you in school or raising a family? Try also to recall your physical self. How did you wear your hair? What did you weigh? What kind of clothes did you like?

Form as vivid and detailed a picture of yourself as possible. Use photographs of yourself from that time if you have them. As you look at the photographs or concentrate on the vision of yourself in your mind, ask the person you see, "Who were you? What were you like? What would you be like and what would you be doing right now if the trauma hadn't happened?"

To further activate your memory, think about the losses you have identified and discussed in therapy. Are there aspects of your pretrauma self that you feel were killed or wounded during the trauma? These may include your faith in certain people or institutions, your innocence, your sense of humor, your illusion of invulnerability, as well as some of your intellectual, vocational, or recreational interests.

As you write about your pretrauma self, consider the following questions:

1. What did you do for fun?

2. What were your major worries and anxieties?

3. What did you like about yourself then?

4. What didn't you like about yourself?

5. Who were your friends?

6. How were you getting along with your family?

7. Did you have any religious or spiritual beliefs? If so, what were they?

8. Did you have any firm philosophical or existential convictions? If so, what were they?

9. What dreams or goals did you have for your life, and what were your interests?

10. Of the goals and interests you had prior to the trauma, which ones would you like to pursue now or in the near future?

11. Of the pretrauma goals and interests you are still drawn to, which would you realistically be able to pursue? What obstacles would stand in your way?

Part Two: Salvaging the Past

If the obstacles are insurmountable, your goals cannot be considered as possibilities. If the obstacles are not insurmountable, what stands between you and what you want? Even if you cannot achieve all of a certain goal, you may be able to achieve part of it.

For example, you may have loved dancing at parties prior to the trauma. Then the trauma occurred. Your interest in socializing diminished. You became so de- pressed you did not have the desire, nor the energy, to go to parties, much less dance at them. If you were severely injured you may no longer be able to dance as you once did. Or perhaps your body was spared, but your face was disfigured, or you may feel so scarred on the inside that you have trouble mixing with others.

As a result, you may lack the confidence to attend parties and have a good time as others do. Yet in your heart you still love music, and the part of you that enjoyed dancing is not quite dead.

What can you do? If your physical condition permits, you could simply go dancing somewhere that you need not interact with others, if you choose not to, and stay only as long as you are comfortable. If you are disabled, you can still sway or otherwise move in time to the music. Some people confined to wheelchairs dance by moving their chairs to the beat. Others take jobs as disc jockeys. Although they cannot dance, they love music and dancing so much, it brings them joy to be near it.

What if one of your pretrauma ambitions was to pursue a certain course of study? Could you go back now? If you cannot return full time, is it possible for you to attend part-time or to take one course at a time? If even that is too costly in terms of time and money, are there any local junior college or adult school classes or workshops in your field of interest? Usually such classes are low-cost.

If you cannot attempt to pursue a certain interest right away, perhaps you can plan to pursue it in the future.

The main question to keep asking yourself is, "Is there a piece of my dream that can be turned into reality?" Even if all you can salvage is a sliver of your dream, grab it and nurture it to the best of your ability.

survivor's entire lifestyle may be transformed. This usually includes some shrinkage of the survivor's relational world, at least initially, as well as a period of withdrawal to make necessary adjustments. However, when survivors' initial tendencies toward withdrawal are reinforced by rejecting or denigrating reactions from others, survivors can retreat even further, and may ultimately develop a lifestyle characterized by social withdrawal and alienation.

As discussed in chapter 2, it has been clinically documented that survivors who receive adequate support following the trauma are at less risk for developing PTSD than those survivors who had a double trauma: the trauma itself and the secondary wounding experience of being rejected or discounted by meaningful others and important social groups (van der Kolk 1990a; Courtois 1988; Lyons 1991b; Williams and Williams 1987; Catherall 1992). According to van der Kolk (1990a), the incidence of long-term PTSD can be significantly reduced if survivors receive adequate emotional validation. As long as the survivor has at least one person to turn to who can provide some assurances and emotional stability, recovery from the trauma is expedited.

However, in some circumstances, a survivor's attachment system is destroyed. For example, combat soldiers continually lose their attachment system in battle. Similarly, refugees, concentration camp survivors, torture victims, and sole survivors of vehicular accidents and natural catastrophes sometimes lose all or parts of their attachment system.

Family abuse survivors who speak out against the abuse or take other active stances sometimes have analogous experiences. They can become outcasts from their own family because they are breaking one of the unwritten rules of secrecy frequently found in violent homes: the violence is not to be talked about or significantly challenged.

Other family members may blame the fleeing survivor for the abuse or see him or her as disloyal for having abandoned the family as a whole or for having abandoned the violent family member, who may be seen by some family members as caring, emotionally needy, or victimized himself or herself. They may also resent the family member who leaves because they fear the abuser will retaliate against them for this individual's departure or will eventually victimize them instead. Even if remaining family members sympathize or support the survivor who has had the courage to flee, they may fear that the abuser will punish them if they have contact with one who left. This situation can leave the fleeing family member functionally alone.

Survivors who are rejected, to one degree or another, by the people they love the most at the time they most need these people may adopt in defense a counterdependent stance of "I don't need anyone"—utter denial of the heightened dependency needs that follow traumatization. However, all human beings have a need for their fellow creatures, and trauma survivors are in special need of support, particularly when the trauma is fresh or when they are undergoing the healing process. In addition, the more intense and prolonged the trauma they endured, and the more harmful and numerous their secondary wounding experiences, the more support the client may need.

Assessing and Expanding the Client's Support System

Your role as therapist is to, first, assess the client's current support system. If the current support system is inadequate—if, for example, you are *it*—then you need to explore with the client ways of finding further support. If a client is reluctant to turn to family members, friends, outside support groups, twelve-step programs, and so on, you need to discuss the reasons for this hesitancy.

Clients sometimes fear that sharing with certain people or groups will be destructive, and sometimes they are right. In other cases, however, your clients' fears about being rejected or restigmatized may not be realistic. For example, some clients may view the situation in black-and-white terms. If people or groups are not 100-percent supportive 100 percent of the time, your client may refuse to even consider sharing with them. You need to address such absolutist thinking in your sessions.

You need to help your clients look at their fears realistically and assist them in selecting individuals and groups would be most likely to profit from emotionally. You can help them learn how to accept and handle feedback that is basically supportive, but is not perfectly so. Conversely, you may also need to support clients in avoiding those people and organizations with whom interacting would be just another destructive secondary wounding experience.

If clients resist the idea of establishing a support system out of pride, you can speak to them as follows:

> It is critical that you get support and continue to get support as long as you need it. It is hard enough being a trauma survivor *with* support, but being without support is an unnecessary and lonely battle.
>
> If you already have a support system in family or friends, you may or may not need to be involved in counseling or with a survivors' group after you have undergone the healing process. However, if you are not so fortunate as to have an existing support system, you will probably need to be involved with a therapist or group for many years, just as you are with your family and friends.
>
> There is no need to feel ashamed of your need for support. Most people need emotional support in life. Those who claim they don't usually have serious emotional problems or are in denial of a basic human need.
>
> Think of getting support as a form of preventive medicine. Why wait until you feel so overwhelmed or depressed that you require intensive therapy or hospitalization, or develop an addiction, psychosomatic illness, or other psychological symptom, to cope with your scars and feelings? Would you berate diabetics for needing insulin all their lives? Would you ridicule heart patients if they needed to do some exercise every day for the rest of their lives? Then why begrudge yourself what you may need for your mental and physical health?

Survivor Groups

In general, some form of group therapy for trauma survivors is highly recommended. A group experience helps reduce the stigma and sense of isolation associated with being a survivor of trauma and provides invaluable peer support and interaction. In most groups—but especially in self-help groups where there is no professional leadership—participants are able to give as well as receive.

Clients' self-esteem can increase by leaps and bounds as they see the ways in which they are able to help other survivors.

Some clients may not be ready for a group experience until they have first received some individual therapy and have both intellectually and on a gut level accepted the reality of the trauma and the seriousness of its consequences. Thus, clients should not be forced into a group until they are ready. Group therapy is also not suitable for clients who are either suicidal or homicidal, extremely dependent, overly susceptible to the suggestions of others, or whose health is severely handicapped by an addiction.

Recent years have seen the growth of numerous self-help and professionally led support groups for trauma survivors. Groups for survivors of war, rape, incest, and various forms of family abuse are becoming fairly common and thus easy to find. Groups for survivors of crime, natural catastrophes, vehicular accidents, and other forms of trauma may be harder to find. To search for a survivor group appropriate for a particular client, consult agencies, hospitals, police department, and libraries and newspapers. (Survivor groups may be listed in the classified ads, in the community section, or in sections pertaining to family life and mental health.) A full range of these groups may or may not exist in your area.

You may also want to check with the local chapter of the American Psychological Association, the American Psychiatric Association, or the National Association of Social Workers to see if they can help you locate a survivor group. Other therapists with expertise in trauma may also be able to refer you to such a group. (Appendix B lists further resources.)

Clients involved in a twelve-step program such as Alcoholics Anonymous, Narcotics Anonymous, Overeaters Anonymous, Al-Anon, or Nar-A-Non, might ask at meetings whether anyone knows of a survivor group appropriate for them. Also, if your client has a physical or emotional problem related to the trauma, for example if he or she lost a limb or developed some other physical or emotional problem such as depression, you might want to inquire about survivor groups organized around the specific physical or emotional concern, rather than the type of trauma endured.

Some survivor groups are led by professionals, others by survivors only. Some have a religious basis or are identified with a certain faith or denomination. Some groups—especially those conducted by mental health professionals—may be time-limited and require regular attendance. Others are open-ended and clients can drop in. You will need to inquire about the leadership, structure, and fees for the groups that exist in your area. If you don't have any luck in finding a group that fits your client's needs or experiences, you might consider starting one yourself.

Groups charge anything from a nominal fee to the full hourly rate for a therapist. Self-help survivor groups and church-led groups that do not employ professionals are usually either free or charge only what is necessary to meet expenses. Survivor groups that are led by professionals vary in price. Some offer a sliding scale; others do not.

Twelve-Step Programs

Twelve-step programs exist for a variety of problems, from drug and alcohol addiction (Narcotics Anonymous) and Alcoholics Anonymous to eating disorders (Overeaters Anonymous), overspending (Debtor's Anonymous), gambling (Gamblers Anonymous), and compulsive sexual activity (Sex and Love Addicts Anonymous). Most twelve-step programs offer tremendous support and encouragement to those who are struggling to overcome addiction. However, clients who are abusing alcohol, drugs, or food to such an extent that they are physically ill, unable to take care of themselves or a danger to themselves or others may need hospitalization (see "The Possibility of Relapse" below).

Even though twelve-step groups are not professionally led, thousands of people have benefited from them immensely. You should be aware, however, that all groups are not the same and that there is a wide variability in the nature of the meetings, their leadership and membership. Some groups, for example, encourage forgiveness to the extent of discouraging the expression of anger. This might be inappropriate for some clients, particularly if they are crime, abuse, or torture survivors. By reading the group's literature, and talking to other members if possible, you and your client can decide whether or not a particular group is right for him or her.

The purpose of any therapy is to provide support for clients and help them regain self-esteem, confidence, and trust in themselves and others. If participation in a group experience fails to approach these goals, you and your client need to reevaluate options.

Those clients who find solid twelve-step meetings (or survivor groups) that both accept and strengthen them are especially empowered, because in these groups they not only have the opportunity to receive, but to give. Such giving is empowering, for through it clients see that their ability to give to others is based on the very aspects of themselves toward which they harbor (or used to harbor) shame and guilt. These aspects include their brokenness due to the trauma, their dysfunctional ways of coping with the trauma, their mental confusion about who they are and where they are going next, their dependency needs, their pain and their anger.

The purpose of a support group is not to cause clients to become overly dependent or to allow individuals within their support system to direct their life. Similarly, empowerment does not mean dominating or exploiting others.

A Note of Caution

Blame-the-victim attitudes and misunderstandings about the nature of trauma and abuse exist in twelve-step programs just as they do in the general public. Some sponsors and program members, just like some therapists, family members and friends, may be uncomfortable with the intensity of trauma survivors' feelings and experiences and may give them negative feedback when they speak up. Your clients need to be cautioned that not everybody will understand or feel comfortable listening to their accounts of traumatic experiences.

"Take what you want and leave the rest" is an often-heard slogan in twelve-step programs. Your clients need to remember that slogan in terms of what they hear at meetings and in terms of the people they meet. Trauma survivors should always be selective about who they talk to about their deepest feelings—because not everybody will be able to tolerate or understand them.

Another source of concern is that twelve-step programs stress critical self-examination. Members are asked to take inventories of their past mistakes and to come to acknowledge, and deal with, their character defects. The goal is spiritual progress, not spiritual perfection. This goal may be admirable; and self-awareness, even of one's defects, is valuable and necessary for psychological growth as well as spiritual growth. But it's especially important for survivors to build their self-esteem and acknowledge and deal with their rage at their abusers, victimizers, or others who might have hurt or failed them during the trauma or its aftermath. Thus, clients need a program that recognizes and honors those needs.

Participation in a twelve-step program should ultimately build clients' self-confidence and help them vent their rage outward in appropriate ways, rather than inward toward themselves or other inappropriate victims. If this is not the case—for example, if your client has an overly critical and controlling sponsor within the group—discuss your concerns with the client.

For example, Joshua N. attended a Narcotics Anonymous meeting near his home for over three months before he decided it wasn't helping him. Although there were other survivors in the meetings, they rarely shared their experiences. When Joshua shared, he felt like an outsider; his intense feelings of rage and sorrow were misinterpreted as "emotional binges" or "character defects." There were also many individuals at the meeting who were court-ordered to attend NA and who were not dedicated to recovery. Some of them acted as if the meeting were a joke: Afterwards they swapped not only drugs, but stories about how they had beaten up or raped others.

Since twelve-step meetings tend to differ in focus and membership, Joshua was advised by his therapist to try and attend other NA meetings until he found one in which he felt comfortable. As an alternative to meetings, Joshua read twelve-step literature and completed recommending writing and other assignments available in twelve-step program workbooks. He also contacted the national NA headquarters and obtained audio cassettes of NA conventions and special meetings.

Bonnie C., on the other hand, had an extremely positive experience with Overeaters Anonymous. After the first meeting she attended, she no longer felt alone. She found a sponsor, whom she telephoned every day with her food plan for that day and whom she contacted whenever she felt hungry, angry, lonely, tired, or afraid (the usual times when she tended to become obsessed with food or binge). When her sponsor was unavailable, she had the phone numbers of at least two dozen other OA members she could call and talk to.

Over time, Bonnie learned to turn to her OA sponsor and friends rather than to food for support. Although there were other abuse survivors in Bonnie's OA group, they tended not to talk about being abused in the meetings. They did, however, talk about it on the telephone, and eventually Bonnie began to attend meetings of Incest Survivors Anonymous (ISA) with some of her OA friends. At ISA meetings, Bonnie developed even more friendships. Because she had the benefit of individual counseling and some experience in OA, she was able to be helpful to quite a few incest survivors who were just beginning to look at their abuse experience or who did not have the financial means or emotional willingness to be involved in individual counseling. As her ability to make friends and give to others grew, so did Bonnie's sense of empowerment.

Considering Retribution

After being victimized or traumatized, it is possible for survivors to fall into one of two extreme modes of reacting. The one extreme is for them to continue the trauma role of being powerless, and passively allow others to abuse or take advantage of them in many current life situations. An example would be a rape victim who overworks at her job, overgives to her boyfriend, and volunteers to take care of her elderly parents and others at the expense of her own social life. Because she is giving so much to others and doing so little for herself, she finds herself depressed much of the time. She attributes her depression to the rape, which is valid. However, some of her depression is also the result of her present self-sacrificial lifestyle. If she could only remove the sense of guilt and defilement she has as a result of the rape, she might feel less obligated to cleanse herself and prove her goodness through self-denial.

At the other extreme are trauma survivors who are determined never again to be taken advantage of or exploited by anyone or any force. Determined to rid themselves of the victim role, they are unwilling to give to anyone or any cause unless they are assured of getting back at least an equal return. If they feel their rights are threatened in some manner, they will fight for those rights regardless of the cost.

A former victim who desires to shed the shackles of passivity and negativity, and makes efforts to do so, is worthy of admiration. It is truly heroic to fight for one's rights against many odds. However, in making decisions about how far to push for one's rights, one's physical, emotional, spiritual and financial well-being also need to be considered.

In some situations there comes a point where it is self-defeating for clients to stand up for themselves or seek revenge or compensation even through legal means. This is not to say that clients should give up or remain victims in their thinking. However, sometimes trauma survivors need to put themselves first, before any cause or fight for justice or anything external to themselves, however important the other issues may be.

For example, Joe L. lost one of his children and his home when, without adequate warning, a tornado hit the town he lived in. Other residents also lost property and family members. Joe, like many of the town's citizens, was justifiably enraged at the town council, since the members had known months before the tornado hit that the city's warning equipment was in need of repair. The council then procrastinated on distributing compensation. Joe started the fight for what he was due determined to win. He didn't want to be worn down by the town council's procrastination and legal maneuvers as he and his neighbors had been over the equipment-repair issue. For more than a year, Joe spent ten to fifteen hours a week on his case, and paid two lawyers' fees as well, with no real results.

Eventually, Joe decided to accept what the council was offering—even though it was only half what he felt he was due, and even though it disappointed and angered some of his neighbors. He decided it was more important to be with his wife and two surviving children and get on with his life than to continue to pursue retribution.

This story is not meant to imply that clients should not use legal channels to fight those institutions or persons who hurt them. On the contrary, it may be critically important for them personally to do so, as well as for the survivor group they represent. Indeed, if survivors of various injustices had given up pursuing their rights when they met the first obstacle, we would not have civil rights legislation, health and safety regulations, battered women's shelters, and many other protections.

As was stated in the section "Refinding the Self," above, it is up to the client which aspects of the pretrauma self will be pursued. Similarly, in considering legal or other actions aimed at receiving compensation, it is up to the client whether or not to pursue certain courses of action. Although empowerment consists of more than seeking compensation, often clients' first steps toward empowerment do begin with attempts to "get back" at least part of what was lost.

The following is a list of questions to consider with your clients when contemplating whether to pursue legal claims and compensations:

> How much time, energy, and money is the client willing to put into the fight for his or her rights? Is it more difficult and stressful for the client to fight for his or her rights against an obstinate or complicated bureaucracy or to give in and accept an unfair settlement to the case?

> In all likelihood, a large amount of paperwork and delay will be involved. To get through it, the client may need the support of many family members, friends, or other survivors. Can the client ask for and receive that support?

> Other survivors' knowledge and advice can be invaluable in pursuing the client's rights. What have those people already tried to obtain their lawful rights? Could your client possible unite with other survivors to claim his or her rights?

> Can the client in question permit himself or herself to give up the struggle to obtain what is legally his or hers if the struggle should become too costly—emotionally, socially, vocationally, or financially?

> Can the client handle defeat? Is the client prepared to acknowledge the possibility of defeat and can he or she prepare for this eventuality so that it is not devastating?

If a client, in pursuing a legal remedy, is not receiving a response to an application or other inquiry, he or she needs to try to find out why, by telephoning or writing to the proper authorities. If they are unresponsive or have frustrated the client's attempts to obtain lawful compensations, there may be a grievance board or committee to which the client can appeal.

Under such circumstances, the client may ask for your intervention in the form of a phone call, letter, or appearance. Since your actions may have legal ramifications, you need to be aware of the policies of your agency (or profession) on such matters. If you are in private practice, you may need to consult with an attorney to find out any possible legal consequences to you. You also need to decide for yourself how much time and energy you can devote to this client's legal and other formal pursuits. If you are going to charge for time spent on such matters outside of your normal sessions, you need to make your client aware of the additional expense.

If you are working with survivors in a group or with survivors who know each other from the same twelve-step program or for some other reason, then you need to be aware that survivors talk about their therapists—you—with one another. If you decide to help one survivor with a court or some other agency battle, but not to help another survivor, you may have to answer for your decision to the survivor you did not assist or to the group as a whole.

Your decisions on these matters should be well thought out. Consultation with colleagues, an attorney, or both, is advisable.

The Issue of Revenge

Most trauma survivors have revenge fantasies. Whether or not they obtain any legally mandated compensations to which they are entitled, and whether or not those who broke the law during the trauma are ever brought to justice, clients probably harbor at least a few vengeful thoughts and feelings toward whomever or whatever they feel was at fault in their trauma and secondary wounding experiences. Some clients are only dimly aware of these feelings; others are all too conscious of them and struggle against them on a daily basis.

The rage born of injustice has ignited nations into massive political and social changes. Some of that kind of rage—righteous rage—burns in your victimized clients. They are entitled to be angry at whatever injustices they suffered, either at the hands of others or from the hand of fate. And they wouldn't be human if they did not want to strike back at that which wounded them.

Although you need to stress to your clients that it is not in their best interests to strike back violently, you also need to help them become aware of their vengeful feelings and thoughts. It can be extremely therapeutic, in fact, for some clients to air their revenge fantasies. Some of their nonviolent fantasies of retribution might be worth considering as a basis for positive action.

For example, several years ago, as reported in a publication by the U.S. Commission on Civil Rights (1978), in New York City a woman was assaulted by her husband. Still carrying the knife he had cut her with, he chased her into the streets and continued to beat her, in front of a number of witnesses. The neighbors, fearing the woman would be murdered in front of their eyes, telephoned the police. The police arrived, but did nothing. They claimed there was insufficient evidence of assault, and refused to arrest the abuser. They also did not assist the woman in getting to a hospital.

The woman swore revenge. Marshalling her profound rage and hatred toward the police, she found dozens of abused wives in the area who had had similar experiences with the police. Together, they filed a class action suit against the New York City police department. It was the first such class action suit in New York's history. These women had seemingly unlimited anger at the injustices they had experienced at the hands of the police. Their anger and desire for revenge empowered them to withstand the numerous obstacles thrown in their way. Eventually they won, and the results of their victory are still benefiting women today. By directing their anger in a prosocial manner, rather than in an antisocial or self-destructive way, they were able not only to help themselves, but to change history.

A Note of Caution

The following exercise asks clients to describe their vengeful fantasies. It is important that your asking the client to share such thoughts not be construed by the client as suggesting that you support her or his acting on these fantasies. You need to clearly state, more than once, that there is a vast difference between talking about vengeful acts and committing them.

In fact, you should ask clients if they feel that they can complete the exercise without being triggered into harming other people, property, animals, or themselves. In my experience, some clients have shuddered at the prospect of talking about their desire for revenge. They were afraid, or even certain, that such an exercise would lead to out-of-control behavior or predispose them to later violence.

If a client falls into one of the following categories, do not attempt the revenge fantasy exercise unless you are extremely certain it will not provoke aggression or defenses against aggression (such as self-mutilation) *and* you have had considerable experience conducting therapy with such clients:

- Combat veterans or police officers

- Those who have formal or informal training in fighting, killing, sabotage, or another form of destruction

- Those who have beaten or otherwise physically abused, or have sexually abused, others

- Those who like to torture animals

- Those who have killed people

- Those who are currently or have frequently been suicidal, homicidal, or both

- Those who suffer from severe depression, hallucinations, a psychosis, or psychotic episodes

- Those who enjoy watching others suffer or property being destroyed

- Those who are afraid that if they dare to think about their revenge fantasies, they will act on them

Not talking about the revenge fantasies won't make them go away. However, you do not want to trigger a violent response in individuals who, almost automatically, due to training, mental suffering, or history, may react with violence.

The following handout, Revenge Fantasies, can be completed as a homework assignment by those clients you feel are stable enough and have enough control over their aggression or self-destructiveness to attempt the exercise without harming themselves or others. It can also be completed in your office, in writing or orally.

The Question of Compensation

Just as clients might secretly (or not so secretly) have revenge fantasies, they probably have some notions about what they think they deserve as compensation for all the hardship and heartache they have suffered. As part of their therapy, clients can identify all that they feel entitled to as compensation for having suffered the trauma and the secondary wounding experiences that followed.

Compensations fall into three categories: those to which the client is entitled by law; those that the client feels he or she should receive, but which are not legally mandated; and those that lie in the realm of fantasy—the client would like to have these compensations, but they are simply not available in the real world.

The following handout, Pursuing Compensations, can be completed as a homework assignment or in session. The second part of the exercise concerns the issue of self-compensation. These questions are designed to help clients identify those material objects and lifestyle changes they can give themselves.

Self-Care as Compensation

When clients do not include the following means of self-compensation on their list, be sure to remind them of these important means of giving to themselves. If they seem unable to accept that they deserve such self-care, their reluctance in this area needs to be discussed. It may reflect residues of self-blame or self-hate from the trauma.

Revenge Fantasies

Use the following statement as a beginning for a list of your revenge fantasies. List those fantasies you have on a recurring basis first, then go on to those you think about less frequently. You can even go ahead and make up some new ones if you like.

> I am still angry at _____ and _____.
> Sometimes when I become really angry, I fantasize that I
> _____ or _____.

Your fantasies need not be realistic, nor do they necessarily have to be particularly "vengeful." They might simply be dreams of yourself becoming successful and admired, while those who have hurt you do not. Be sure to write down as many fantasies as you can think of.

Now review your list of fantasies. First, go through and put a check mark by those that, if you acted on them, would cause physical harm to someone or something. Put a second check mark by those that, if acted on, would harm you or people you love. Under no circumstances act out those fantasies. Now, review your list again. Be sure that those fantasies you have left unchecked are in fact nonviolent.

Of those nonviolent fantasies you have listed, put a star by those that could promote your well-being or might spare others from suffering what you suffered. Then think about which of these might you consider pursuing. Make a list of the pros and cons of pursuing each of those you have selected.

For example, suppose one of your revenge fantasies is writing a letter to an organization that failed to respond to your needs as a trauma survivor. You would want to find out how the organization handles such grievances and follow their established procedures. If you have evidence to support the idea or strongly suspect that the organization might retaliate against you for writing such a letter, you might decide not to pursue that course of action—or to postpone acting until a later time when there would be less risk. Similarly, if your revenge fantasy is to publicly expose an official of the organization who was particularly demeaning to you, weigh the consequences in terms of your self-interest, as well as in terms of what you feel compelled to do out of a sense of justice.

Depending on the organization in question, following established procedures for filing grievances may or may not bring about quick results, or any results at all. However, such procedures are available and should be used as a starting point.

Pursuing Compensations

This exercise has two parts: The first is to identify the compensations you deserve or would like to have. The second is to think of ways to compensate yourself.

Part One: Listing Compensations

Take three sheets of paper (and have some more in reserve). At the top of the first page write "Compensations I am entitled to by law," on the second page write "Compensations I should be entitled to by law but am not promised," and on the third page write "Compensation fantasies: what I would receive in the best of all possible worlds."

Then, on the first page list all the compensations you are entitled to by law. For example, combat veterans are entitled to certain benefits by law. Survivors of natural catastrophes in this country are also legally entitled to certain types of assistance. Crime victims have certain legal rights as well. You may need to do some research to find out what your legal rights are. Many communities have free or sliding-scale legal aid services.

On the second page, list all the compensations you feel should be provided to you but are not. For example, you may feel you should be entitled to free or low-cost therapy to help overcome the trauma, or that your spouse, children, or other affected family members should have access to such help.

On the third page, list all the compensations you would like to have, but at this point you feel are simply not available in the real world. As you complete this part, do not let reality inhibit you. Pretend you can have anything you want, and don't limit yourself to material objects. For example, you may wish you could have back parts of your youth or certain mental faculties, such as the ability to concentrate. Would you like a parade in your honor or the apology of your abuser? How happy would it make you to receive a proclamation from the head of some institution that you were right and the organization was wrong?

Let your imagination run free. From your compensation fantasy you can evolve a more realistic list of experiences, attitudes, and objects that can serve as forms of compensation for your sufferings.

Before you begin writing, you may want to review your losses you have explored in therapy. Reviewing your losses may spark your imagination about what you would like in return.

Part Two: Self-Compensations

You may or may not receive the compensations you are entitled to by law. However, you can make efforts to compensate yourself. Using what you wrote above about the compensations you deserve and dream about, what can you realistically give yourself as a form of compensation? Although you can certainly include material items such as clothing, a home, or a new car, and experiences such as vacations and entertainment, these things may be beyond your means.

Many trauma survivors find that, although it is important to give themselves material goods and pleasurable experiences, it is also important to treat themselves with loving kindness on a daily basis. It has also proven important to them to respect the impact of the trauma on their personalities and habits, as the following stories indicate.

> Loretta, an incest survivor, allowed herself six years to go through college rather than the regular four years. "I was so pressured during my childhood," she says, "I didn't want to repeat that experience in college. Also I wanted to make time for both individual and group incest therapy. If I carry the regular workload, I'll never take the time necessary to heal myself."

> Mike, also a family abuse survivor, compensates himself by trying to retrieve what he can of his childhood. He describes it like this: "My father left my mother when I was six. After that, my childhood ended. My mother became an alcoholic and began to beat me. I was so busy recovering from the physical abuse and taking care of younger brothers and sisters, I hardly ever played.

> "Today I am trying to compensate myself for my lost childhood by being on a baseball team. I also play games with my sons, vicariously enjoying being a kid by being with kids. Last week I bought myself a train set and I'm considering taking swimming lessons. I realize I could be making money, going to night school, or doing good works instead of playing so much. But the good works I'm doing now are for myself. At least for the present, I need to make up for the past any way I can."

> Joanne, a hurricane survivor, compensates herself by taking the anniversary day of the hurricane off from work every year and holding a small memorial service for her friends who died in the storm. She also makes a point of not pressuring herself at work. "I'm a trauma survivor. I can't handle as much stress as others. Maybe I'll achieve less than others in life. But I simply cannot, or refuse to, recreate the trauma by exhausting myself as if some catastrophe was going on."

You can also compensate yourself emotionally by trying not to punish yourself for the reemergence of symptoms in the presence of trigger events or at anniversary times. "Each time, the stick I beat myself with gets smaller and smaller. And I use it for a shorter period of time," says one survivor.

Another way of taking emotional care of yourself is to keep a daily journal of your feelings and allow yourself time to talk to others about your problems and concerns. You can carry the load alone if you want to, but why suffer needlessly? If help is available, take it.

Spiritually, you may want to give yourself the time to meditate, pray, or engage in other activities you find rewarding.

The preceding ideas are only suggestions. Only you know what will help you feel compensated. Over time, the experiences and objects you desire as forms of compensation may change. That's fine. Just be sure to continue to compensate yourself.

Safety

One way clients can compensate themselves is to make their lives as safe as possible on a very basic physical level. This is particularly important in the case of crime or family abuse victims. They need to be sure they have done all they can to protect themselves from further crime and abuse. For example, they need to be aware of various forms of legal and police protection available and consider ways of installing home-protection devices with which they feel comfortable.

Self-defense courses are also useful. Even if the tactics are never used against an attacker, it is empowering for clients to have these techniques at their command.

Some therapists and therapy programs for trauma survivors include time in the wilderness or outdoors as an exercise in facing danger in moderate doses. The philosophy of such programs is that trauma survivors can increase their life options if, instead of avoiding all dangerous situations, they learn to modulate their responses to danger. These programs hope to teach, for example, that there are levels of danger, that one can survive the initial anxiety reaction to danger, and that one can even learn to control some of the anxiety or panic reactions to threatening situations. Clients might want to consider one of these programs if they truly want to and you feel it is safe for them to do so.

However, they may not be ready to face the anxiety and fears that can arise in such programs. Also, any program being considered needs to be carefully researched to be sure there are adequate safeguards for the participants and adequate help should a participant suffer a severe psychological reaction. Programs that push participants to go beyond what they feel are their limits, that do not curb any competitiveness that may arise among the participants, or that offer "fast fixes," are to be avoided.

Clients who are not family abuse or crime survivors, as well as those who are, may want to secure their homes, automobiles, and other property as much as possible. For example, are their parking areas and entryways well lit and windows secure against break-ins? Do they have a fire extinguisher and smoke detector? Are there hazards in their homes that could be avoided, for instance, piles of newspaper or other flammable materials? Is the electrical wiring in good condition? Are stairs and banisters sturdy? Do they check the tires, brakes, and otherwise maintain their cars so that they have the assurance their cars are in good running order?

The list of precautions clients can take is endless, but you need to stress that they owe it to themselves to take the time to make sure their immediate environment is safe, including their work environment. Clients may want to ask others, for example, safety inspectors at work, car mechanics, and home inspectors and safety officials, for specific ways in which they can make their world as safe as possible. They can also talk to their neighbors. Neighborhood crime watch and other community efforts have proven to be one of the best ways to ensure a safe environment.

Physical Health

Critical to empowerment is taking care of physical and medical needs. Survivors who struggle with survivor guilt, low self-esteem, or even extreme self-hatred sometimes unconsciously neglect their bodies as a form of self-punishment. Because they feel responsible for others' deaths or injuries in the trauma, or because their self-esteem was crushed, they often do not feel they deserve to take the time or spend the money on their medical and physical needs.

Even if this does not feel comfortable, natural, or necessary to clients, they need to check out any medical concerns. They also need to permit themselves adequate sleep and take the time necessary to exercise and eat properly. These suggestions may sound elementary, but it is common for individuals with PTSD, depression, or addiction problems to neglect their body because they experience anxiety in taking care of themselves medically or physically.

Emotional Self-Care

In order to feel safe with their emotions, clients need to understand their symptoms and other responses to the trauma and, for as long as necessary, avail themselves of the help of mental health professionals, family members, and friends. Another way clients can take care of themselves emotionally is to ask for help with tasks that overwhelm them, either at work or at home. Regardless of their occupation, they will at some point or another be given tasks that cause them intense internal pressure. "It's too much for me," they feel, yet they may hesitate to share that feeling with coworkers. However, that feeling is the same feeling they had during the trauma.

Perhaps no help was available during the trauma. But clients can ask for help now. Depending on the circumstances, they may be able to share with coworkers that a particular assignment is creating confusion or stress and ask them for suggestions in handling the task. This does not mean clients are asking others to do their work for them, but rather that the coworkers probably have insights that could lighten the client's task.

The Possibility of Relapse

Even clients with considerable recovery can relapse. In fact, "relapse is part of recovery" is a slogan often heard at twelve-step meetings. A relapse can be a minor slip or a major setback. In cases where the clients have relapsed into abusing alcohol, drugs, or food to such an extent that they cannot take care of themselves or pose a danger to themselves or others, hospitalization or intensive care may be needed.

Such relapses occur for three major reasons. First, there may be fear at embarking on a new, more positive life or in accepting a more positive identity. The client may revert to the addiction to avoid coping with the very progress that has been so hard won. In such cases, the specific fears need to be identified, as well as the bases for the fear. What does the client feel will occur due to his or her progress? Will there be social ostracism, jealousy from a family member, physical attack, death, or some other negative consequence? On some level, many trauma survivors internalize their abuser or the abusive aspects of their past experiences. It is these that punish the survivor for his or her progress.

Second, relapse may signify the emergence of yet another aspect of the trauma—or another trauma. In this case, the relapse is positive, and clients need to be told that the relapse signifies that they are moving along in recovery, not failing in their efforts. In such cases, clients need to be assisted with the healing process for the new traumatic material.

Third, relapses occur because addiction is addiction—something that is managed, never conquered. Perhaps the relapse was triggered by the presence of the addictive substance or an addicted friend or family member. Whatever the cause, acknowledging the possibility of relapse, yet working to avoid it, is an important aspect of self-care.

A Special Note About Family Abuse Survivors

In violent homes, typically one individual is singled out as the victim. (This is not always the case, however. In some homes, almost all the children or family members are beaten by the abuser.) In homes where one individual is the prime victim, that person, whether a child or an adult, is often mistreated by other family members as well. The others may not hit or sexually molest the victim, but they frequently demean or exploit him or her emotionally, financially, or in other ways.

Even after the victim has left the original site of the abuse, other family members may perpetuate the exploitation of the victim through verbal abuse or other means. Some of the subtler forms of mistreatment include treating the abuse survivor as the black sheep of the family or assuming that the abuse survivor will always be available to do favors for the family.

In working with family abuse survivors, then, be sure to closely examine ways in which family members or caretakers other than the abuser might be exploiting the client. These people may not be aware of their behavior because it was or is a part of a family system that they perpetuate unconsciously or semiconsciously. An added complication is that these family members may also be sources of kindness and love toward the client. Yet at the same time they automatically treat her or him like a second-class citizen. These complex factors make it that much more difficult for your client to demand respect and receive emotional support.

Limits to Healing

Making generalities about the limitations of healing is difficult because trauma survivors vary not only in their individual personalities but in the severity and duration of the traumas they endured. Yet it can be said that both you and your clients may be disappointed when therapy does not heal the scars of the trauma as rapidly or as thoroughly as might be desired. In some cases, the process of healing can be painfully slow. In others, it is not only slow but some of the scars may be permanent.

If your client is truly a trauma survivor with PTSD, not a trauma survivor without PTSD or simply an unhappy person or a person who needs to learn more functional ways of viewing him- or herself or of coping with life, then it is almost axiomatic that some of the aftereffects of the trauma cannot be thought, compensated, or wished away.

These negative effects, whether psychological, social, economic, or physical, cannot be talked or intellectualized out of existence either. They may not be in the forefront of the client's mind every minute of the day, but they persist. Therapy can help restore clients to normal or pretrauma levels of functioning. Therapy can even help clients grow beyond their pretrauma levels of functioning. But both you and your client need to be aware that no amount or kind of therapy can remove the trauma from the client's memory.

Indeed, amnesia is not the goal of the healing process. Recovery for trauma survivors lies not in "feeling better all the time," nor in never thinking about the trauma again, but rather in being able to find comfort in interpersonal relationships—especially intimate ones—and being able to be involved with, function in, and contribute to society. Recovery also entails being able to focus on the positives in life and to experience a wider range of feelings than fear, anger, and self-hatred.

Regardless of how hard clients work in therapy, as trauma survivors, they will be subject to unwanted, recurring thoughts of the trauma, to nightmares, and perhaps even to flashbacks. Even years after the trauma has been dealt with in counseling, clients may have times of rage, emotional pain, numbing, anxiety attacks, physical pain, and other symptoms related to the trauma. Therapy cannot take away all the pain, rage, or numbness, but it can bring these emotions under clients' control by increasing their emotional connectedness to others and their sense of purpose in life.

In addition, therapy does not have any answers to existential or spiritual questions, such as "Why me?" or "Why is there injustice, brutality, and hatred in the world?" The healing process can encourage clients to think about these questions and draw their own conclusions, but for some clients, such questions may never be answered satisfactorily—no matter how long they sit in your office.

There are some areas that therapy cannot heal or can only begin to heal. Survivors of extended torture; survivors of wars or community upheavals that devastate not only the survivor's family but the very fabric of his or her society and culture (such as the conflicts in Cambodia, Somalia, El Salvador, Iraq, the former Yugoslavia), and survivors whose traumas involved the loss of most or all of their family members, have losses that are so great and so irreplaceable that often the most a mental health professional can do is to keep the survivor from becoming psychotic or committing suicide. Lofty notions, such as "finding meaning in the trauma" or evolving a "survivor mission," in these cases are best saved for a select few who are particularly gifted, spiritual, and psychologically and physically intact.

Therapy also has limits for individuals who suffer from profound moral pain resulting from having committed actions during the trauma that violated their personal code of ethics or societal codes of ethics. Combat veterans can fall into this category. Although not all war veterans suffer from moral pain—in the form of guilt about having killed—conflicting feelings about the role of warrior can be an important issue in therapy with some veterans.

For some, the moral pain comes from having killed any human being at all, even a clearly identifiable enemy. For others, killing enemy troops was justifiable, but killing others, either by accident or deliberately, is an ongoing source of remorse. Still others went beyond killing to committing atrocities, such as mutilating the dead, torturing unarmed civilians, raping children, having intercourse with corpses, or even eating body parts of the enemy.

It is very difficult for some combat veterans to forgive themselves for such behavior solely by learning to reframe their actions in terms of the pressures of the trauma—even though the pressures of war are responsible, to a great extent, for the unleashing of such barbarism. Veterans who struggle with understanding how they ever committed such acts or who find that a part of them is still capable of, if not desirous of, committing such acts in the present, often search for help beyond therapy in some form of spiritual or religious counseling.

Similarly, abused women and children who are forced by their perpetrator or circumstances to hurt other family members or to commit illegal acts (such as stealing), or acts they feel are immoral (such as prostitution, having sex with strangers, or posing or dancing nude) can feel shame and guilt about these survivor behaviors that is so deep and profound that psychological help is of little or no assistance. Often these people seek spiritual help or the help of the arts. There are also instances where captives have been forced to injure, sexually abuse, torture, or even kill family members and friends in order to save their lives or the lives of other family members. To say that such individuals can get over their experiences by simply undergoing a therapeutic process would be to mock their pain and torment.

On the other hand, the healing offered as part of the therapeutic process can ameliorate even the most tragic of traumatic situations. At the very minimum, it can begin to arrest self-destructive or violent tendencies in the suffering individual (which only add new pain and destruction onto that generated by the trauma).

Although therapeutic interventions have their limitations, healing can result in reduced frequency of and fear of symptoms, reduced fear of insanity, rechanneling of anger and grief into positive directions, and a change of the client's self-perceived status from victim to survivor. Healing can also promote a change of outlook from rigid to flexible and spontaneous, and can foster an increased appreciation of life, a sense of humor, and a profound empathy for others who suffer.

Case Example

Roger M., a combat veteran, sought counseling because his alcoholism had led to a blackout during which he was involved in a serious car accident and because his wife was threatening to leave him due to his numerous absences from home, his verbal abuse toward her and their two children, and the financial drain his drinking imposed on the family budget.

In the first stages of counseling, Roger felt he could solve his problems if he simply stopped drinking, "shut his mouth," and stayed home more. He soon learned that much more was involved.

Alcoholics Anonymous meetings proved unhelpful for Roger until he found a meeting that combat vets as well as civilians attended. After the alcohol abuse was arrested, Roger experienced more anger at everyone—including himself and his family—and he wanted to leave home and withdraw from people by going camping even more frequently.

The feelings of grief and anger associated with his war experiences eventually emerged and were identified as such, and Roger began to be able to differentiate the past from the present. As part of his growing self-mastery, he was able to speak to himself as follows: "I'm angry that so many of my friends died so pointlessly, but I will not take out my anger on my family as I have in the past by yelling at them, and I will not take it out on myself, by drinking." Now when Roger becomes angry at a family member, but feels he will overreact and become verbally abusive because his present aggravation taps into his storehouse of rage from the war, he simply leaves the room to go for a walk or to pray.

Roger has learned to exert self-control in a way he never knew possible. He hopes someday not to overreact at all, but in the meantime he has less fear about being with his family because he knows that he has coping techniques available to help manage his anger. Similarly, when Roger has the urge to leave home and go camping, he's learned to ask himself what is he feeling that makes him want to run away. He's been able to call members of his support group and his therapist at these times to help him figure out what he is feeling. He can now also share some of his emotions with his family, instead of disappearing without giving them a clue as to when he'll return, as he did in the past.

Yet still he cannot participate in many family functions, and he still feels like an outsider in his own family because he so often is riddled with intrusive memories of war, and the rage and sadness that leave him feeling confused, disoriented, and alienated from others.

However, part of the culmination of his therapy was learning to accept his feelings, rather than fight them, and learning that he can continue in a present-day activity—for a limited time at least—while having trauma-related feelings. At times he must excuse himself, and some activities he cannot participate in at all. For example, football and other contact sports remain powerful triggers, so he cannot attend his son's games. But, in the past he used to denigrate his son for playing football, calling him a "war monger" and "stupid" for playing football instead of developing his academic skills. Roger no longer does this, though he still sometimes wishes he had chosen to go to college rather than join the military. He still feels football is a warlike sport, but he realizes that if he is to have a relationship with his son, he will have to refrain from making derogatory comments and make the effort to explain to his son that watching football stimulates thoughts—even flashbacks—of men's wounded bodies flying through the air and landing dead on the ground. Although he can't go to his son's games, he has identified other activities the two of them can enjoy together.

In addition, Roger has made great strides in the grieving process. In the initial stage of therapy, he denied his grief and all grieving was expressed as anger, inertia, or self-hatred. As he began to feel, he wrote poems about his dead buddies. Now, in the empowerment stage, he has begun to share the poems with others and will self-publish them. He has also built a small shrine-like monument in part of his backyard to honor his dead friends, and to honor his own grief. He can now go to his own backyard, instead of to the streets, when the emotional pain becomes overwhelming. Sometimes his wife or one of the children will silently join him. They no longer have a father and husband who leaves home at unpredictable times. He can now grieve without alienating the people he loves and needs and who love and need him.

He also has identified anniversary dates. He marks them on the calendar and expects to be angrier, more depressed, and more desirous of drinking at these times. He has committed to trying to call his therapist and friends more at these times, and he has learned to remind himself that he's not losing his mind, rather he's having an anniversary reaction. This cognitive restructuring does not lessen the unwanted emotional states that come with anniversaries, but it does temper his self-disparagement. It also assures Roger that there will be an end, that after the anniversary time passes, he will be less tormented. This hope helps him to endure more positively, so that now, after several years, his anniversary reactions are less intense, because he has worked through some of the feelings associated with them and is thus less afraid.

Chapter 11

Other Professional and Therapeutic Concerns

Challenges inherent to working with trauma survivors include the distinct possibility of clients becoming suicidal or homicidal. You have a greater risk of experiencing the death of a client (either by suicide or as the result of addiction or other escapist behavior) in working with trauma survivors than in working with the general population.

Other professionals—social workers, psychologists, psychiatrists, and paraprofessionals such as addiction counselors—may not know about PTSD. Even worse, they may not want to know about it, may see it as an excuse, or may consider you a "softie" or a "pushover" for giving the trauma any weight at all. Colleagues might insist that one of your clients has a character disorder, when your assessment indicates PTSD with no secondary diagnosis. The client may not meet even half of the *DSM-IV* criteria for personality or character disorder, yet your colleagues insist on this diagnosis.

At this point, you realize you have touched something irrational in your colleagues: the same irrational hostility and disbelief that some trauma survivors have confronted over and over again, not only in mental health but in other areas as well. Suddenly you understand secondary wounding on a gut level.

If and when this happens, seek support from others in your field or related fields who are knowledgeable about PTSD and trauma. Including PTSD as a possible diagnosis for clients who qualify may mean you are "rocking the boat" in your particular agency. Like anyone who introduces change in a profession, you can expect resistance and hostility, but such is the price of making history.

What follows is a by-no-means-complete list of some of the personal and professional obstacles you may encounter in working with trauma survivors. If you sometimes experience frustration in working with trauma survivors, try not to chastise yourself. If you have made a serious attempt to educate yourself and to truly listen to your clients, you are probably helping them more than you realize. Never forget that the mental health field is still in the infancy regarding knowledge and treatment of PTSD.

Special Difficulties in the Therapist-Client Relationship

When you are the first person the trauma survivor turns to for help, your responses and guidance are especially significant. This is especially true if the trauma is recent and the client's memory receptors are consequently still on alert. In these cases what you say and do will be imprinted in the client's memory more vividly and in a more lasting manner than if you encountered the client some time after the trauma had occurred. On the other hand, you may be the fourth or fifth therapist the client has turned to. In this case, you may have to cope with emotional scars and secondary wounding experiences inflicted by previous therapists or mental health programs that were uninformed about PTSD.

Whether you are the client's first therapist or one of a series, there are many areas in which you will need to display exquisite sensitivity and great caution. As stressed in earlier chapters, in addition to the regular dynamics of therapy you will need to attend carefully to both verbal and nonverbal cues about how many memories and how much emotion the client can tolerate. You want to respect the clients' true limits in getting in touch with the trauma, but you are also there to encourage and support them as they take the risk of looking at the past. At times, you may "nudge" a client too hard, whereas at other times you miss an opportunity to help a client explore another aspect of the past because of your fear of pushing. Consequently, you need knowledge and training in order to respond as beneficially as possible (see appendix B).

In addition, it is wise for you to read about the specific kinds of trauma endured by your clients. Understanding the particulars of the stresses of combat, the dynamics of family violence and incest, and the psychological, social, and economic aftermaths of community disasters (natural catastrophes, technological disasters) is necessary for two reasons. First, you need this information to help educate your clients; often PTSD clients come to therapy thinking they are the only ones who have endured the traumas they experienced or that they are the only ones who have reacted as they have (with PTSD and other symptoms). Your knowledge of trauma in general and their kind of trauma in particular can help assure them that they are not alone in their experience. Second, your familiarity with the kind of trauma endured by your client will communicate to your client that you are competent and will enable you to be more sensitive to their particular needs and problems. Appendix B lists suggested reading in a number of categories.

When You Can't Be There

Counseling trauma survivors is hard work. In the first place, you need to practice therapy somewhat differently than you have learned thus far in your career, and you need to be especially considerate of your clients' sensitivities, given that their central nervous systems and emotional capacities may be especially reactive. Second, the therapeutic relationship is a critical variable in treatment outcome, regardless of client diagnosis or the kinds of therapy you practice. However, your relationship with a client assumes special importance when that client is a trauma survivor.

All forms of trauma tend to break, or at least severely damage, many of the survivor's connections to other people and social institutions, even those forms of trauma caused primarily by natural forces rather than human beings. Consequently, establishing a working relationship with the client is crucial in reestablishing the survivor's personal relationships and preventing the development of chronic PTSD, with its devastating long-term side effects. These include problems in holding down a job or forming close personal ties due to mistrust of others, low frustration level, memory problems, anxiety attacks, and depression. In cases where the trauma was inflicted by a trusted loved one, your relationship with the client is even more important in that it can be a major step toward enabling the client to trust and be emotionally intimate with other people.

For example, Janice K., like many abused girls, functioned as the emotional caretaker of her abusive parent. Also like many abused girls, she ran away from home at a young age and married an abusive man, toward whom she again assumed the role of emotional caretaker. Eventually Janice divorced her abusive husband, but she continued to assume the caretaker role with her children, with her coworkers, and even with members of her support group, to the neglect of her own needs.

After several months of therapy, Janice was finally able to differentiate her needs from those of people she felt obligated to and those of her loved ones. She had just begun to take steps toward meeting her needs, when a crisis hit her home. Since it was a particularly stressful period in Janice's life, her therapist invited her to telephone the office if necessary, until the crisis was over. The therapist agreed to talk to Janice for up to ten minutes at no charge.

One day, Janice in desperation, did telephone. The therapist, however, was about to leave work and could not give Janice the promised ten minutes. However, instead of having the receptionist tell Janice that she was too busy to take the call, the therapist took the phone call herself and stated, "I know you are calling for a very important reason, because for you to ask for something, you must really need it. I also know how sensitive you are about reaching out for help and then being put off. All your life when you reached out for help, people were too busy or not interested enough to stop what they were doing to help you.

"Now here I am in the position of needing to leave work when you call. We can talk for about five minutes now, but not for the full ten minutes I had promised. If this feels as if I am abandoning you or putting you off, we can discuss it in our next session. I am giving you a clear communication, however, that I am glad you called and I want you to call again during this time of crisis. The best times to call are ... "

In handling the phone call in this manner, the therapist acknowledged Janice's difficulties with reaching out. While it may not be necessary to provide such explanations for all clients, those survivors with issues revolving around caretaking or abandonment need to be given extra special consideration in the scheduling of appointments and telephone calls.

Transference and Countertransference

The classical definition of transference is an incorrect or false association between a current relationship and a past relationship (Kluft 1992b). The person experiencing such transference is, usually unknowingly, viewing a present relationship as a repetition of one that occurred in the past. In some cases, the person may even subtly or overtly try to recreate the past relationship in the present.

Transference occurs in therapeutic relationship when a client imposes upon the therapist qualities and expectations that belong to individuals in her or his past. Hence the client may act and react to the therapist as she or he did to certain significant others—not only parents and caretakers from childhood, but individuals involved in the trauma. Transference is not bad or undesirable; once it occurs, it can be understood and examined and the client can grow in self-awareness.

Countertransference refers to the therapist's transferring onto the client qualities belonging to individuals in the therapist's past. In essence, countertransference refers to the therapist's having a distorted or neurotic perception of the client (Kluft 1992b) or to the therapist's having exceptionally strong feelings toward the client because some aspect of the client reminds the therapist of someone toward whom he or she had strong feelings or of issues that are emotionally charged for the therapist.

In dealing with trauma survivors, you will encounter not only normal transference issues but quite possibly what Richard Kluft (1992b) has labeled "traumatic transference" or the client's "constant expectation of harm." He asks those who would work with trauma survivors, especially survivors of long-term or severe trauma, to consider the following question: "Do you want to work with clients who see you, or have the potential of seeing you, as the 'bad guy,' as someone who you aren't . . . for years perhaps?"

As therapy progresses, the problem of being seen as the "bad guy" only escalates. For example, as you succeed in helping clients retrieve memories, they will eventually come to feel the pain, anger, and other emotional turmoil associated with those memories. In fact, if you are doing PTSD therapy correctly you will inevitably retraumatize your clients with their own trauma, to one degree or another. Although you can make many efforts to minimize retraumatization, you cannot spare them the upheaval of the remembering and reliving experiences necessary for healing. Consequently, some clients may learn to associate you with emotional pain, as well as with the shattering of the comfort of denial and their preferred or illusory view of their lives.

On the other hand, other trauma survivors may want you to be their double, to think and act as they do (Kluft 1992b); may treat you as their "magic helper" or, in the case of some abused children and battered wives, may make you a substitute for the idealized caretaker or husband they never had. When you fail to measure up to their expectations, you may have to contend with their hostility, disappointment, and feelings of betrayal.

In examining your own countertransference, honesty is required. If you are sexually attracted to, morally repelled by, inordinately fond of, or otherwise have some strong feeling toward the client, this does not automatically mean you should stop working with the client or that you are an inadequate therapist. You first need to be aware of your reaction and then decide whether your reaction hinders the therapy. If necessary, you can seek professional consultation on the matter. Excellent discussions of countertransference issues can also be found in Courtois 1988; Herman 1992; Sonnenberg, Blank, and Talbott 1985; and Williams 1987a. (See the references listed at the end of the book or the "Further Reading" section of appendix B.)

Keeping the Proper Perspective

Kluft points out that therapists working with trauma survivors tend to adopt one of the following roles: detective, savior, advocate, or balanced therapist. You might want to consider which of these stances you might be assuming toward a given client.

In the detective role, the therapist functions as a "private eye," who searches not only for the client's symptoms, but for the client's lies and deceptions. The "detective" therapist operates from a position of mistrust and disbelief of the client, rather than from the required position of trust and belief. According to Kluft (1992b), the detective role serves to distance the therapist from the client's pain and victimization. The empathic connection is lost and subsequently few therapeutic advances can be made. (There are, however, instances where such a role is appropriate, as is discussed in the section on assessing PTSD for nonclinical purposes, below.)

In the savior position, the therapist assumes that his or her love and concern can "save" the client. Concern for the client is an important ingredient in therapy, but concern alone is not enough, and, when extended in an inappropriate manner, may cause the client to become overdependent on the therapist. Since one of the principal goals of PTSD therapy is to empower the client, the client must learn to see power emanating from the self, not the therapist. Although the therapist is supportive, clients need to know that it is they themselves who are tolerating the emotional intensity of traumatic recall and who are taking risks to change their lives. The therapist needs to know this as well.

In addition, if the therapist, even out of loving concern for the client, comes to idealize the client as a victim, the client is robbed of the therapist's objective evaluation of his or her reality testing and interpersonal skills (Kluft 1992c).

An advocacy position in which the therapist supports (or perhaps even initiates) the client's pursuing his or her rights or compensations in the real world, is not an unhealthy position. In fact, it can be an energizing stance vis-à-vis the client. However advocacy, like love, is not enough. The client needs to process the trauma cognitively and emotionally in order to heal. A large financial compensation for injuries sustained during the trauma may create temporary elation, but unless the client has made strides in the inner healing process, she or he may become even more depressed on realizing that the material compensation does not stop the nightmares, the fear, the hyperreactivity to trigger situations, and other symptoms of PTSD.

The most balanced therapist position combines enough of the detective approach that the therapist can question the client on certain distortions in attempting to clarify the client's thinking about the trauma; enough love or concern that the client feels supported and important; and enough advocacy that the client knows he or she is justified and will be supported in any attempt to obtain legally mandated compensations for some of the injuries and losses sustained during the trauma.

If You Have Experienced Trauma

If you have PTSD, your reactions to your PTSD clients may be problematic and conflictual. On the one hand, you may overidentify with your clients. On the other hand, you may find yourself distancing yourself from them. Or you may vacillate between the two extremes.

Giving such mixed messages to clients can wreak havoc in the therapeutic relationship, especially with clients who are family violence survivors. Abused children, battered women, and others who have been physically assaulted by a caretaker or loved one usually receive double messages from the abuser, such as

"Come close/Go away" or "I love you/I hate you." If, because of unresolved or unacknowledged PTSD, you are ambivalent toward your clients and vacillate in your responses to them, you are to some extent recreating the emotional climate of the trauma in your sessions. Consequently, if you are a trauma survivor with PTSD or other trauma-related symptoms, and you do not plan to seek help, then you need to stop seeing trauma survivors and work with other kinds of clients.

If you have experienced a trauma and you have only begun to work through your experience, you might want to consider waiting to work with trauma survivors until you and your therapist decide you have made sufficient gains in your own healing process. For example, seeing traumatized clients when you are still in the emergency stage of your healing process is ill advised. You cannot be of maximum assistance to other trauma survivors until you have been strengthened by increased understanding of your own pain.

Furthermore, you need to be aware of the possible benefits and disadvantages of survivors treating survivors. Some of these are outlined in "Warrior Therapist: Vets Treating Vets" (Catherall and Lane 1992). The authors of that article point out that some of the advantages to clients in having a survivor for a therapist include an increased ability to trust, increased possibility of being understood, a greater tolerance on the therapist's part for horror stories and intense emotions, and increased insight. Therapists who have had or continue to have some degree of PTSD "are privy to insights about PTSD that cannot be found in any textbook. This can contribute to the sensitivity with which the therapist conducts the treatment and approaches key issues."

On the other hand, Catherall and Lane also state that survivor therapists working with fellow survivors may struggle with more intense transference and countertransference issues than in the average therapeutic relationship. Also, in working with PTSD clients, the survivor therapist reexposes him- or herself to trauma, which may stimulate PTSD symptoms. Other possible disadvantages for the therapist, the authors point out, are "overidentification with the client ... the exacerbation of survivor guilt ... [and a] shift from emphasis on therapy to victim advocacy."

When Skepticism Is Appropriate: Assessing PTSD for Nonclinical Purposes

Since PTSD became an official diagnosis in 1980, there have been increasing numbers of clients seeking a diagnosis of PTSD for purposes of compensation or litigation, rather than healing. A related problem is that many individuals who have suffered legitimate traumatic experiences exhibit symptoms that do not fall into the DSM criteria for PTSD. For example, people who have suffered on-the-job accidents and other forms of trauma are sometimes refused compensation because they "only" develop partial PTSD or because their reaction to the trauma takes the form of psychosomatic problems or a psychiatric problem other than PTSD. These individuals feel cheated, and rightly so. Thus, to obtain the benefits they feel they deserve, they might feign PTSD.

In such situations, you are no longer a therapist but an assessor, and it is legitimate for you to wonder if a particular client is exaggerating or fabricating symptoms for financial or other self-serving purposes (which is not to say you should show your suspicion openly). If you are to function as an assessor for legal or other purposes, then you should read Judith Lyon's "Issues to Consider in Assessing the Effects of Trauma: Introduction" (1991a). In this article, Lyons outlines some of the issues and dilemmas facing assessors of PTSD, such as that assessors must be cognizant that PTSD can present in a variety of ways, can coexist with other disorders, and can change over time. She stresses that, during the interview, the therapist should "be alert to the possibility of deception or exaggeration without adopting a suspicious stance which would be detrimental to the development of trust and respect for the individual being assessed."

She also suggests that assessors use as many indicators of PTSD and truthfulness as possible. For example, you can examine prior medical and other records and use some of the recent objective measures of PTSD, such as the PK scale of the Minnesota Multiphasic Personality Inventory (MMPI) developed by Terence Keane, Paul Malloy, and John Fairbank (1984). (These are covered in more detail in appendix B.) You can also use some of the other clinical interviews and objective measures discussed in appendix B.

Bear in mind, however, that these objective measures are still relatively new and may not adequately cover every kind of trauma reaction. Consequently, in most cases the assessment of PTSD depends on the interview. Yet there is no uniform presentation in PTSD clients. Some are in numbing and evidence no emotional reactivity while describing the trauma. Others are emotionally effusive, teary-eyed if not hysterical. Some PTSD clients can remember every detail of their experiences; others suffer from partial or almost total amnesia. Some clients present with almost pure PTSD, others with dual diagnoses. Sometimes the presentation of PTSD is masked by other problems. When severe early childhood trauma has resulted in the development of a character disorder or a multiple personality disorder, the problem of assessment becomes even more problematic.

There are no rules for assessing PTSD, save for the *DSM-IV* criteria, which will probably continue to be revised over time due to new research findings on PTSD. There are, however, a few specific questions that can be asked to separate truth-tellers from fabricators. You can ask them, for example, to give as many details as possible about their nightmares, flashbacks, and other reliving experiences. In these detailed accounts, you may be able to separate fabrication from authenticity. Even this can be tricky, however, since PTSD sufferers often have only partial recall of their dreams and reliving experiences.

Clients may also avoid talking about the trauma or their symptoms in order to ward off the painful aftereffects of thinking about events that irrevocably changed his or her life—even into clinical interviews, creating the appearance that the client either was not traumatized or suffered few ill effects from the trauma. However, this pattern of minimizing or discounting both the trauma and effects are part of PTSD. Social isolation and other forms of withdrawal from others are more certain signs of PTSD. Some individuals with PTSD usually find emotionally close relationships painful or conflictual. However, if the client is also a substance abuser, his or her discomfort with interpersonal relationships may not be evident, in that the substance may ameliorate the stresses of interpersonal relationships.

Even more important is the individual's affect or emotional state. Can you sense that he or she is in genuine pain or suffering from hopelessness? Do you get the sense that the client feels out of control mentally or emotionally due to flashbacks and mood swings? In my experience, clients who truly suffer from

PTSD are rarely happy or excited about it. If clients seem overly enthusiastic about their symptoms, you may begin to wonder about their sincerity.[1]

You can also interview family members and friends for verification purposes. However, this too can be unreliable, in that a PTSD sufferer may have learned to hide his or her symptoms from others in order to fit in socially or maintain a job.

Issues in Working with Self-Mutilating Clients

Since self-mutilation has not been researched much, literature on self-mutilation (other than substance abuse or eating disorders) is limited. Furthermore, there are few professional guidelines for handling clients who injure themselves. Such a situation leaves mental health professionals with difficult decisions to make about, for example, which self-mutilating behaviors are potentially life threatening and according to what standards: medical, legal, or professional? How does a mental health professional decide at what point a seemingly not-too-dangerous self-mutilating behavior might become a suicide attempt? If a relatively minor self-mutilating behavior, such as excessive scratching, suddenly mushrooms into a more dangerous behavior, such as cutting to the point of bleeding, will the mental health professional be considered liable?

When self-mutilation looks like a suicide attempt or as if it might lead to a suicide attempt, it is generally suggested that the therapist recommend, if not insist, upon hospitalization. However, clients are not always compliant with therapists' suggestions, and, if the therapist is dealing with a dysfunctional family, family members may be of little help. Usually one or more family members are in denial of the family's problems, including the self-mutilation, and may minimize or discount it. The client's life may have to be in imminent danger for the client or family member to take responsible action. By this time, the client may already have suffered significant injury, and members of the family can easily project their guilt about the situation onto the therapist and accuse the therapist of not doing his or her job.

Lawsuits can follow. Therefore, it is of utmost importance that the therapist be aware of any self-mutilating behavior on the part of the client, address the issue with the client, and monitor not only the behavior, but his or her efforts to alleviate this extremely distressing and potentially dangerous behavior. However, these tasks may be easier described than done. The first steps—determining the existence of self-mutilation and monitoring it—require that you create an atmosphere in which the client feels free to share about self-abuse. (Chapters 4 and 6 discuss assessing for and interventions for self-mutilating behavior, respectively.)

As you track and document the self-mutilating behavior, notice if it increases drastically in frequency or in severity. If so, family members and other authorities

---

1. On the other hand, Jordan, Nunley, and Cook (1992) point out that overreporting of symptoms may be the norm among some traumatized groups. In a rather unique study, these researchers found that PTSD symptoms were overreported among both combat veterans who were already receiving compensation and those who were seeking to be compensated. The latter group did not overreport any more than those who were already receiving financial compensation. The authors conclude that overreporting of symptoms among combat veterans exists. However, the motivation does not appear to be financial gain, but a desire to be heard. Referring to those veterans who overreported their symptoms, the authors write, "Thus their high F scores [on the MMPI] may be more accurately viewed as a 'cry for help' from someone who has not been heard in the past rather than mere exaggeration of symptoms for the sake of getting compensation."

need to be marshalled to urge the client to seek increased help and hospitalization. If the client is a minor, parents or other responsible parties need to be informed immediately of the self-mutilation practices and the possibility of suicide attempts.

For less serious forms of self-mutilation, some therapists adopt the suicide-prevention model and try to effect a contract with the client, in which the client agrees orally or in writing to stop the self-mutilation. However, this approach is not recommended; in many cases, such a contract may be entirely counterproductive and lead to an escalation in self-mutilation or to an actual suicide attempt.

For example, Calof (1992) gives the example of a female client who would clutch her neck and squeeze it so tightly that he feared for her life. On the surface, the client's behavior seemed to be suicidal or a reenactment of what was done to her in her abusive family of origin. However, it was later revealed that her behavior reflected an "unconscious identification" with a relative who died by hanging. In clutching her neck, the client was attempting to save her relative's life. For the therapist to have insisted on a contract with this client to stop her behavior would have been disastrous.

Had this client agreed to such a contract, she would most likely have suffered from intense guilt at not having attempted to save her relative. This guilt might have led her to punish herself through some other form of self-abuse or even suicide. On the other hand, had the client refused to make the contract with the therapist, or had made the contract and then broken it because of her unresolved need to try to save her dying relative, she would have feared being abandoned by the therapist and would consequently have lost another caring relationship in addition to those lost with her parents (when they began to abuse her) and with the hanged relative who had been kind to her. To lose yet another positive relationship could have had a devastating effect on the client.

Given the confusion and the lack of research and professional guidance in this area, it can be easy for mental health professionals to view self-mutilating clients as nuisances, immature individuals whose self-injuries are primarily bids for attention. As Calof stresses, when we therapists see clients repeat self-injurious behavior for the dozenth time, rarely do most of us think that "Oh, this person is a victim, a survivor of great sufferings that have brought him or her to this point." Instead, we tend to become annoyed, if not angered, at victims for their acting-out behavior.

In the first place, as stated, their behavior leaves us with a myriad of professional questions for which we do not have easy answers or guidelines. As a result, we may be left vulnerable professionally. Secondly, because their behavior can disturb our schedules and tax us more than other clients, it may ignite in us a moral rage that is all too easily directed at the client. Calof stresses that this rage properly belongs to the perpetrator. However, because the victim is available (whereas the perpetrator is not) or because we are not familiar with the client's story, the rage is displaced.

It is important to keep in mind that healing is a process, often a slow one. Just as we must respect the defenses of our clients, while at the same time trying to help them understand what might be behind those defenses, we must also respect self-mutilating behavior. Regardless of how destructive, frightening, and perhaps personally repulsive the client's behavior might be, it serves an important purpose—it tells the world that "something is wrong, something horrible happened to me." The behavior will need to remain until the client finds other ways to communicate the pain and anger to the world. A simple contract where the client commits to not self-mutilate is rarely enough. In order for the self-mutilation to come to an end, clients need to develop other ways of modulating feelings and telling their story (Calof 1992).

The Issue of False Memories

Lately there has been growing concern in the legal and mental health communities, as well as among the general public, about the extent to which therapists can create "false memories" of trauma, either through suggesting to clients that they were traumatized on the basis of their presenting symptoms or through interpreting clients' dreams and fantasies as evidence that trauma occurred. To date, most of the false memory concerns have focused on early childhood sexual trauma rather than on other forms of trauma. Experts in the field of early childhood sexual abuse interpret the rise of the false memory accusation as a form of societal resistance against acknowledging that child sexual abuse exists and is so extensive (Herman 1992; Courtois 1988; Briere and Conte 1993).

However, if a therapist strongly suggests to a client that she or he was sexually abused as a child, or if a vulnerable or highly impressionable individual becomes overwhelmed from listening to the stories of abuse survivors in a group and overidentifies with the survivors, false memories could arise. Such instances are, however, relatively rare (Schwartz 1993).

The rise in reported childhood sexual abuse cannot be attributed to false memories induced by irresponsible or untrained therapists, although such individuals do exist. Rather the rise in recall of early trauma can be attributed to the fact that at no time in history has there been greater cultural awareness of childhood sexual trauma and greater cultural permission to talk about it. In addition, our society is full of triggers, in the form of media presentations on the subject, both fictional and factual.

Personal Challenges

In addition to the compassion, tolerance, objectivity, study, and other hard work you need to devote to working with PTSD clients, you may find these cases affecting your personal experiences and outlook. They may even revive fears and traumas you believed were buried.

Listening to Horror Stories

No matter how wise in the ways of the world you think you are, listening to your clients talk about their traumas can be extremely exhausting and even harrowing. By definition, trauma is shocking, so you should expect to feel shocked sometimes. Your adrenaline may begin to pump as you listen to your clients' horror stories or their far-from-neutral feelings. Don't be surprised if you start having nightmares about some of your client's episodes. After hearing or reading about traumatic episodes you can also expect to feel emotionally numb or dead. You are not emotionally dead however; you are simply recuperating from the intense emotionality involved in truly listening and responding to your trauma survivors' stories.

It is also possible that you will find yourself "enjoying" or being inordinately interested in some of the more sexual, more violent, or more sadistic aspects of your clients' stories. You may, for instance, find yourself becoming sexually aroused in listening to accounts of rape, incest, or physical abuse or find yourself identifying with the aggressor in situations of combat, domestic violence, or stranger crime. It may come as a shock to you that you, like some of your clients, have a darker side that is not buried as deeply in your psyche as you had thought. You may respond with guilt to encountering this dark side, or you may find that you don't feel guilty at all. Then you might feel guilty about not feeling guilty.

Remember all these feelings: the shock, the adrenaline, the numbing, and the guilt. This is the cycle of feelings that constitute PTSD. Multiply those feelings of yours twenty or thirty times, and imagine them appearing unpredictably, for no apparent reason. Picture others viewing you as crazy for having these feelings. Add a few memory problems, flashbacks, anxiety attacks, and perhaps a few physical injuries caused by the trauma, and you begin to understand what it feels like to have PTSD—and why your support and empathy are essential to your clients' healing.

Confronting Fears of Victimization

Working with trauma survivors challenges all your defenses that say you and your loved ones are immune to tragedy. Your conviction that you and your family will be spared criminal victimization would likely be shattered when your well-dressed, respectable, middle-class client who is compulsive about everything, including home security, walks into your office with a bandage where his eye used to be. "The alarm system didn't work," he says. He was beaten and robbed at seven o'clock on a Sunday morning.

Similarly, your belief that your wife, daughter, and sister (not to mention yourself, if you are a woman) are immune from sexual assault can no longer be sustained as more and more of your women clients reveal that they were victims of incest or rape. For so long you thought, "It only happens among the lower classes. It could never happen in my family, to my friends." Suddenly the statistics on rape and sexual abuse become real and believable to you, and your illusions about the society you live in shatter. Observing the deep scars sexual assault leaves on its victims, you can no longer distance yourself from the personal tragedies behind these statistics.

As a therapist and as a human being, when you confront a trauma survivor you have a choice. Either you bear the anxiety of knowing that the next victim could be you, or someone you love, or else you build defenses against the client and what that person represents: the many losses and injustices inherent to random victimization. Unfortunately, such defenses usually entail somehow blaming the victim for what he or she has experienced. If you find that you are stymied in your ability to be supportive of the client, are having difficulties viewing the client objectively and making appropriate interventions, or are constantly fighting negative or critical attitudes toward the client, it is time for you to let go of the case.

It may also be time for you to seek assistance in dealing with your fears of victimization. Perhaps a consultation with a trauma expert or a few individual therapy sessions might be helpful. Regardless of which you choose, your fears need to be addressed and dealt with for you to be of use to trauma survivors.

Appendix A

A Brief History of Traumatology

Post-traumatic stress disorder is a new name for an old problem. Under different names, PTSD has been documented by doctors, historians, and poets as far back as the days of the ancient Greeks. For example, the historian Herodotus wrote that during the battle of Marathon in 490 B.C., an Athenian soldier who suffered no wounds became permanently blind after witnessing the death of the soldier standing next to him (Bentley 1991). Achilles and Agamemnon, military heroes in Homer's *Illiad*, suffered from classic symptoms of PTSD (Shay 1991). In fact, today, their rage reactions and other symptoms are being studied in hopes of shedding light on combat-related PTSD and associated problems such as combat addiction (Shay 1991; Solursh 1989)

In the 1600s, Samuel Pepys wrote of the panic and distress of those who survived the great fire of London during that era: "A most horrid, malicious, blood fire ... So great was our fear ... it was enough to put us out of our wits." For weeks after the fire, Pepys, like many other survivors of the fire, suffered insomnia, anger, and depression—all common forms of acute PTSD (Bentley 1991).

In the late nineteenth century, Jean-Martin Charcot, a neurologist living in France, observed individuals confined in mental institutions who were suffering from physical symptoms—convulsions, amnesia, paralysis, intense physical pains, and other such maladies—that had no medical or neurological basis (Herman 1992). At the time, such persons, primarily women, were deemed to be suffering from "hysteria." In an effort to determine the cause of these nonmedical symptoms, Charcot put these individuals into trance states using hypnosis. When people spoke, they related histories of severe physical and sexual abuse as children that were followed by their running away from their childhood abusers, only to be revictimized on the streets or in their new homes. Ultimately, they sought refuge in state mental institutions.

Charcot concluded that childhood and other traumas were one of the causes of hysteria and other symptoms in these individuals, symptoms that are now characterized as belonging to the PTSD diagnosis. Charcot's discovery attracted much attention, including that of other reknowned doctors such as Freud, Janet, and Breuer (van der Kolk, Brown, and van der Hart 1989; Herman 1992).

Freud, Janet, and Breuer eventually joined Charcot in his work and conducted in-depth interviews with traumatized persons. These interviews confirmed Charcot's observation of trauma as the origin of hysteria and other symptoms of PTSD. When Freud returned to Vienna, however, he changed his perspective.

According to his critics he did so for economic and political reasons. For example, had Freud maintained the thesis that the hysterical and other symptoms of the many upperclass women he had as clients were due to childhood sexual and other abuse, he would have been condemning the men who paid the bills for his treatment sessions with these women and the men with whom he associated professionally. Even in professional, medical, and intellectual circles, the society of Freud's Vienna was not ready to acknowledge or accept that wealthy, highly respected members of society were sexually abusing their children. Thus, had Freud continued to support this unpopular and unacceptable thesis, he would have severely endangered his livelihood and his standing in the professional community. Ultimately, Freud abandoned what he had learned from Charcot's work in France and stated that hysteria among women was due to childhood fantasies and conflicts, not actual childhood trauma. Freud's position essentially blames the victim and has been the object of considerable feminist criticism (Herman 1992; Chesler 1972; Millett 1969).[1]

Janet, however, did not abandon his empathic stance toward "hysterical" women. Although his writings were rejected by many of his contemporary colleagues, today his works on dissociation and on healing from childhood trauma are of great interest to mental health professionals who seek to understand the long-term effects of child abuse and domestic violence (van der Kolk, Brown, and Hart 1989).

The effects of trauma became issues of public concern and professional interest in World War I, during which large numbers of soldiers suffered psychiatric breakdowns in response to the prolonged and vicious nature of trench warfare. During World War I, PTSD and PTSD-like symptoms incapacitated and caused the evacuation of some 10 percent of American enlisted men (Goodwin n.d.; Grinker and Spiegel 1983). According to one source, "Shell shock," "battle fatigue," or "war neurosis"—the names given to combat-related trauma during and immediately after World War I—also resulted in almost 40 percent of British battle casualties (Showalter 1985).

Evacuated men who could no longer fight because they couldn't stop crying, because their memory and ability to concentrate were impaired, or because they were so emotionally and physically numb they could barely move or respond to commands, were not only a military "embarrassment," but a severe drain in terms of morale and money. Consequently, the military began to formally consider the problem of combat stress and work on means of preventing the loss of men to war trauma or in current language acute PTSD. During World War II, for example, elaborate screening devices were employed. Designed to weed out those who could not withstand combat, the screening devices were evident failures. At various points during World War II, over 300 percent more men suffered from PTSD symptoms than during World War I (Goodwin n.d.; Grinker and Spiegel 1983).

After World War II, military experts concluded that it was not the personal or moral strength of the soldier, but the length of his exposure to combat that caused him to "break." Armed with the knowledge that the trauma of war was often enough to impair even the strongest and toughest of men (Goodwin n.d.; Grinker and Spiegel 1983), the tour of duty during the Vietnam conflict was set to thirteen months. It was assumed (or hoped) that this relatively short exposure

---

1. For a more detailed discussion of Freud's changed perspective on female hysteria see Kate Millett's *Sexual Politics* (New York: Doubleday, 1969) and Phyllis Chesler's *Women and Madness* (New York: Avon Books, 1972).

to combat would lessen psychological problems. Unfortunately, this approach also proved ineffective: PTSD or PTSD-like symptoms have been recorded in well over one third of combat soldiers who returned from Vietnam. These symptoms persist today (Weiss et al. 1992).

Likewise, numerous World War II and Korean War veterans still suffer from nightmares and other symptoms of PTSD—a fact that has recently been brought to the attention of the United States Congress as part of a movement to open Vietnam Veterans Outreach Centers to older veterans who have never received help for their PTSD (*Congressional Record* 15 July 1987).

Today there is ongoing interest in the reactions to combat and in preventing combat stress—both in the United States military and in other military establishments, notably, that of Israel. The reasons for this interest are both practical and humanitarian (Soloman et al. 1992; Avraham et al. 1992; Cooper 1992).

One of the offshoots the political efforts of Vietnam veterans to gain attention for their mental health needs was the validation of what women's rights advocates had been saying for years: that many of the "mental health" and other problems of women were not due to their inferiority, mental and emotional weakness, or other defects, but were due to victimization and exploitation. Previously, the PTSD symptoms of rape victims, battered women, and abused children had been called "rape crisis syndrome" (Burgess and Holmstrom 1974a,b; Russell 1975), "battered women syndrome" (Walker 1979; Hilberman and Munson 1977–78), and "child abuse accommodation syndrome" (Summit 1983). Today these are recognized as forms of post-traumatic stress disorder.

When PTSD was recognized by the American Psychiatric Association in 1980, the definition of trauma included not only combat, but all of the varieties of domestic violence, rape, and other forms of assault. In many ways, the recognition of combat trauma as a form of PTSD helped to legitimize and remove stigma from female and child survivor of domestic and street violence. The most recent studies of psychological effects of trauma confirm the prevalence of PTSD among victims of incest and childhood sexual and physical abuse (Herman 1992; Courtois 1988; Finkelhor 1979; Brown and Finkelhor 1986; Herman, Russell, and Trocki 1986; Gorcey, Santiago, and McCall-Perez 1986; Russell 1975; Eth and Pynoos 1985).

Today increasing numbers of traditional mental health professionals and organizations are recognizing the need to address the problems of abused children (as well as the sexual abuse of clients by mental health professionals). One possible reason for this increased interest shown in the professional literature "may be associated with social and political events outside the scientific community (publicized attacks, attention from popular media, heightened public awareness from judicial rulings)" (Blake, Albano, and Keane 1992).

Since the inclusion of PTSD in the *DSM-III* in 1980, the field of traumatology has come into its own. Efforts are now under way to create formal credentialing for PTSD therapy and research on reactions to trauma are at an all-time high. A recent study of psychological abstracts from 1970 to 1990 revealed a dramatic increase in the number of trauma-related studies (Blake, Albano, and Keane 1992). However, the increased interest in trauma and its effects were not uniform across categories of trauma. Most of the research concerns war-related trauma and sexual abuse. Research on natural catastrophes, technological disasters, Holocaust survivors, refugees, torture survivors, vehicular accidents, and other kinds of trauma remains minimal.

Appendix B

Professional Education and Resources

The guidelines and therapeutic interventions presented in this book are a beginning, but you will need to attend workshops and read materials pertaining to the specific kinds of trauma your clients have endured in order to provide them with the best of care. Unfortunately, this may be easier said than done, for a number of reasons.

For example, until recently, there have been very few workshops or seminars on PTSD. Since 1990, and especially since the Persian Gulf War, there has been increased interest in PTSD, with a parallel rise in the number of PTSD workshops and presentations. But, these workshops are still not widespread, and they provide only an introduction to the subject. A great number of these workshops concern child sexual abuse; relatively few workshops exist regarding the treatment of crime victims, physical abuse survivors, and those who have lived though serious accidents and natural catastrophes.

The literature and outcome studies available parallel this problem. The few outcome studies that have been completed deal with select populations, usually rape victims, child sexual abuse survivors, and occasionally war veterans. Professional materials are likewise available on the subjects of incest and other forms of child sexual abuse, rape, physical abuse, and war veterans. (Some of these resources are listed below.)

In contrast, there are relatively few professional articles or books on how to help survivors of vehicular accidents, technological or occupational disasters, and natural catastrophes. In such cases, you will have to rely on your general knowledge of trauma and PTSD counseling, adapting your approach to the specifics of the trauma and the individual clients involved.

However, the increased interest in trauma and treating trauma survivors is gradually making traumatology a field of its own within the various mental health professions. If you persevere in your search for workshops and reading material that promise to be of assistance to you in your work, you will be increasingly able to find such training. The following are a few places to begin your search (see also "Curricula," below):

- Local and state psychological, social work, and psychiatric associations may offer PTSD seminars at their meetings and conventions.

- A newsletter that lists PTSD workshops is published by the International Society for Traumatic Stress Studies, 435 N. Michigan Avenue, Suite 1717, Chicago, IL 60611-4067.

- Local Veterans Administration Medical Centers or Readjustment Counseling Centers offer PTSD inservice programs, which often are open to nongovernment professionals and may be free of charge.

Resources

Alternative Means of Assessment for PTSD

Since PTSD became an official diagnosis, numerous researchers have tackled the problem of assessment (Keane, Weathers, and Kloupek 1992). In 1991, for example, a special section of the journal *Psychological Assessment* reviewed current thought and research on assessing PTSD in a variety of populations including rape victims, refugees, children, and natural catastrophe survivors. Structured interviews based on the *DSM* criteria have also been developed.

These means of assessment vary in reliability and validity, and some suffer from certain limitations. Therefore, interested practitioners would need to examine the current state of research for each instrument before using it to determine its usefulness for their purposes. Presented below are some alternative means of assessing PTSD that have some promise of reliability and validity. These include both objective, or psychometric, measures and structured interviews.

Objective Measures:

The PK scale of the Minnesota Multiphasic Personality Inventory (MMPI) (Keane, Malloy, and Fairbank 1984) is based on items of the MMPI that have been shown to distinguish PTSD clients from non-PTSD clients. It is most useful in assessing combat veterans.

The Mississippi Scale (Keane, Cadell, and Taylor 1988) comes in two versions: one for combat veterans, the other for civilians.

The Penn Inventory (Hammarberg 1992) is based on both combat and civilian survivors.

Clinical Interviews:

In addition, several structured clinical interviews are available. These include:

The structured clinical interview for the *DSM-III-R* (SCID) by Spitzer et al. (1991).

The PTSD interview by Watson et al. (1991).

The clinician administered PTSD scale by Blake et al. (1990). "A clinician rating scale for assessing current and lifetime PTSD: The CAPS-1." *Behavior Therapist* 18.

Audiotapes and Videotapes

Videotapes (as well as books) on PTSD and its aftermath are available from Varied Directions International, 69 Elm Street, Camden, ME 04843; 207-236-8506 (phone), 207-236-4512 (fax). Write for a free catalogue.

Videotapes on sexual trauma are available from Hazelden Educational Materials, P.O. Box 176, Pleasant Valley Road, Center City, MN 55012; 800-328-9000.

All audiotapes cited in the text from the Fourth Conference on Abuse and Multiple Personality, Training in Treatment are available from Audio Transcripts Ltd., 335 South Patrick Street, Suite 220, Alexandria, VA 22314; 800-338-2111.

Bibliographies

"Child Sexual Abuse: A Bibliography of Journal Studies, 1978–1982." Journal of Child Care 1, 1983.

"Forcible rape: An updated bibliography," by B. M. Pawliski. *Journal of Criminal Law and Criminology* 74, 1983.

"Post Traumatic Stress Disorders in Vietnam Veterans: An Addendum to Fairbank, et al," by S. M. Silver. *Professional Psychology* 13, 1982.

"PTSD in Vietnam Veterans: Selected Bibliographic Addendum to Fairbank, et al. Silver and Arnold," by L. Kolmar. *Professional Psychology: Research and Practice* 20, 1989.

"A selected bibliography of post-traumatic stress disorders in Vietnam veterans," by John Fairbank, Keith Langley, G. J. Jarvis, and Terence Keane. *Professional Psychology* 12, 1981.

Curricula

A curriculum for professionals who want to work with PTSD clients, "The Initial Report from the Presidential Task Force on Curriculum, Education, and Training," by Y. Danieli and J. H. Krystal (1989), is available from the International Society for Traumatic Stress Studies, 435 N. Michigan Ave., Suite 171, Chicago, IL 60611, 312-644-0828 (phone), 312-644-8557 (fax).

Support Groups

The following names and addresses provide a place to begin looking for client support groups.

AA World Services (Alcoholics Anonymous), Check local listings as well. 475 Riverside Drive, NY 10015; 212-870-3400.

Adult Children of Alcoholics, Central Service, P.O. Box 35623, Los Angeles, CA 90035; 213-464-4423.

Al-Anon Family Group Headquarters and Alateen (both for the families of alcoholics), World Service Office, P.O. Box 862, Midtown Station, New York, NY 10018; 212-302-7240. Check local listings as well.

Incest Survivors Anonymous, P.O. Box 5613, Long Beach, CA 90805; 213-428-5599.

National Association for Children of Alcoholics, 31706 Coast Highway #201B, South Laguna, CA 92677; 714-770-2189.

National Child Abuse Hotline, Childhelp USA; 800-4-A-CHILD.

National Coalition Against Domestic Violence, P.O. Box 34103, Washington, D.C. 20043; 202-638-6388.

National Organization for Victims Assistance (NOVA), 1757 Park Road NW, Washington, D.C. 20010; 202-232-6682.

National Self-Help Clearinghouse, 25 West 43rd St., Room 620, New York, NY 10036; 212-642-2944.

Further Reading

The Brunner/Mazel Psychosocial Stress Series of books and the *Journal of Traumatic Stress* are good places to start reading. The following listings provide information and guidelines on the treatment of trauma survivors.

General Information on PTSD

A Clinical Guide to the Treatment of Human Stress Response, by George S. Everly, New York: Plenum Publishing, 1992.

"The Compulsion to Repeat the Trauma: Re-enactment, Revictimization, and Masochism," by Bessel van der Kolk. *Psychiatric Clinics of North America* 12:2 (June 1989).

Handbook of Post-Traumatic Therapy, edited by Mary Beth Williams, Westport, Conn.: Greenwood Publishing Group, 1994.

International Handbook of Traumatic Stress Syndromes, edited by John P. Wilson and Beverly Raphail. New York: Plenum Publishing, 1992.

Journal of Traumatic Stress, available from Plenum Press, 223 Spring Street, New York, NY 10013.

Massive Psychic Trauma by H. Krystal. New York: International University Press, 1968.

Post Traumatic Therapy and Victims of Violence, edited by Frank M. Ochberg. New York: Brunner/Mazel, 1988. (Also contains information specific to domestic violence, sexual abuse, crime, and family counseling.)

Post-Traumatic Stress Disorder Therapy: A Clinician's Guide, by Kirkland C. Peterson, Maurice F. Prout, and Robert A. Schwartz. New York: Plenum Press, 1990.

Posttraumatic Stress Disorder: DSM-IV and Beyond, edited by Jonathan R. T. Davidson and Edna B. Foa, Washington D.C.: American Psychiatric Press, 1992.

Posttraumatic Stress Disorder: Etiology, Phenomenology, and Treatment, edited by Marian E. Wolf and Aron D. Mosaim, Washington D.C.: American Psychiatric Press, 1990.

Psychological Trauma, by Bessel van der Kolk. Washington, D.C.: American Psychiatric Press, 1986.

Shattered Assumptions: Towards a New Psychology of Trauma, by Ronnie Janoff-Bulman. New York: The Free Press, 1991.

Stress Response Syndromes, by M. J. Horowitz. New York: Jason Aronson, 1976.

Trauma and Its Wake (2 volumes), edited by Charles R. Figley. New York: Brunner/Mazel, 1985.

Trauma and Recovery: The Aftermath of Violence—from Domestic Abuse to Political Terror, by Judith Herman. New York: Basic Books, 1992.

Trauma, Transformation, and Healing: An Integrative Approach to Theory, Research, and Post-Traumatic Therapy, by John P. Wilson. New York: Brunner/Mazel, 1989.

Biological Aspects

Biological Assessment and Treatment of PTSD, edited by Earl L. Giller, Jr., Washington, D.C.: American Psychiatric Press, 1990.

"Current Advances in the Psychobiology of PTSD" (audiotape 921STSS-82). International Society of Traumatic Stress Studies, Eighth Annual Meeting, Los Angeles, 1992.

"Inescapable Shock, Neurotransmitters, and Addiction to Trauma: Toward a Psychobiology of Posttraumatic Stress" by B. van der Kolk, M. Greenberg, H. Boyd, and J. Krystal. *Biological Psychiatry* 20:3, March 1985.

"A Key to Posttraumatic Stress Lies in Brain Chemistry, Scientists Find." *New York Times*, June 12, 1990.

Manual of Clinical Psychopharmacology, by Allan F. Schatzberg and Jonathan O. Cole. Washington, D.C.: American Psychiatric Press, 1991.

"Posttraumatic Stress Disorder, Conditioning and Network Theory," by R. Pitman. *Psychiatric Annals* 18:3, March 1989.

"Posttraumatic Stress Disorder, Hormones and Memory," by R. Pitman. *Biological Psychiatry* 26:3, July 1989.

"Posttraumatic Stress Disorder: The Stressor Criterion," by Naomi Breslau and Glenn Davis. *Journal of Nervous and Mental Disease* 175:5, May 1987.

"Psychophysiologic Responses to Combat Imagery of Vietnam Veterans with Posttraumatic Stress Disorder Versus other Anxiety Disorders," by R. Pitman, S. Orr, D. Forgue, B. Altman, et al. *Journal of Abnormal Psychology* 99:1, Feb. 1990.

"Structural and Functional Correlates of Brain Systems Involved in Memory in PTSD," (audiotape 921STSS-75). International Society of Traumatic Stress Studies, Eighth Annual Meeting, Los Angeles, 1992.

"The Structure of Organization of Memory," (audiotape 921STSS-85). International Society of Traumatic Stress Studies, Eighth Annual Meeting, Los Angeles, 1992.

Children

See also "Domestic Violence."

"The Child Abuse Accommodation Syndrome," by Roland Summit. *Child Abuse and Neglect* 7, 1983.

Child Abuse: A Practical Guide for Those Who Help Others, by E. Clay Jorgensen. New York: Continuum, 1990.

Juvenile Homicide, edited by Elissa P. Benedek, and Dewey G. Cornel. Washington D.C.: American Psychiatric Press, 1989.

Post-Traumatic Stress Disorder in Children, by Spencer Eth and Robert S. Pynoos. Washington, D.C.: American Psychiatric Press, 1985.

Psychological Trauma and the Adult Survivor: Theory, Therapy and Transformation, by I. Lisa McCann and Laurie Anne Pearlman. New York: Brunner/Mazel, 1991.

Rediscovering Childhood Trauma: Historical Casebook and Clinical Applications, edited by Jean M. Goodwin. Washington D.C.: American Psychiatric Press, 1993.

"Trauma in Pediatric Populations," by Melanie Suhr. *Advanced Psychosomatic Medicine* 16, 1986.

Treating Abused Adolescents: A Program for Providing Individual and Group Therapy, by Darlene Anderson Merchant. Holmes Beach, FL: Learning Publications, 1990.

Treating Abuse Today: An International Journal of Abuse Survivorship and Therapy, available from Clinical Training Publications, 2722 Eastlake Ave. East, Suite 300, Seattle, WA 98102.

Incest and Other Child Sexual Abuse

See also "Rape and Sexual Assault."

The Courage to Heal: A Guide for Women Survivors of Child Sexual Abuse, by Ellen Bass and Laura Davis. New York: Harper and Row, 1988.

Healing the Incest Wound: Adult Survivors in Therapy, by Christine Courtois. New York: W. W. Norton and Co., 1988.

Incest-Related Syndromes of Adult Psychopathology, edited by Richard P. Kluft, Washington D.C.: American Psychiatric Press, 1990.

Moving Forward: A News Journal for Survivors of Sexual Child Abuse and Those Who Care for Them, available from P.O. Box 4426, Arlington, VA 22204.

Resolving Sexual Abuse, by Yvonne Dolan. New York: W. W. Norton and Co., 1991.

The Sexually Abused Male: Prevalence, Impact and Treatment, vols. 1 and 2, edited by Mic Hunter. Lexington, Mass.: Lexington Books, D. C. Heath and Company, 1990.

Treatment of the Adult Survivor of Childhood Abuse, by Eliana Gil. Walnut Grove, Colo.: Launch Press, 1988.

Treatment of Adult Survivors of Incest, edited by Patricia L. Paddison, Washington D.C.: American Psychiatric Press, 1993.

Victims No Longer: Men Recovering from Incest and Other Child Sexual Abuse, by Mike Lew. New York: Nevramont Publishing, 1988.

When the Bough Breaks: A Guide for Parents of Sexually Abused Children, by Aphrodite Matsakis. Oakland, Calif.: New Harbinger Publications, 1991.

Disaster

Disasters and Mental Health: Contemporary Perspectives and Innovations of Services to Disaster Victims, by the National Institute of Mental Health. Washington D.C.: American Psychiatric Press, 1986.

Responding to Disaster: A Guide for Mental Health Professionals, edited by Linda S. Austin. Washington D.C.: American Psychiatric Press, 1992.

Dissociative and Personality Disorders

Borderline Personality Disorder, by John G. Gunderson. Washington D.C.: American Psychiatric Press, 1984.

Borderline Personality Disorder: Etiology and Treatment, edited by Joel Paris. Washington D.C.: American Psychiatric Press, 1992.

Childhood Antecedents of Multiple Personality, edited by Richard P. Kluft. Washington D.C.: American Psychiatric Press, 1985.

Clinical Perspectives on Multiple Personality Disorder, edited by Richard P. Kluft and Catherine G. Fine. Washington D.C.: American Psychiatric Press, 1993.

Dissociative Disorders: A Clinical Review, edited by David Spiegel. Lutherville, Md.: Sidran Press, 1993.

Effective Psychotherapy With Borderline Patients: Case Studies, by Robert J. Waldinger and John G. Gunderson. Washington D.C.: American Psychiatric Press, 1989.

Family Environment and Borderline Personality Disorder, edited by Paul S. Links. Washington D.C.: American Psychiatric Press, 1990.

Interviewer's Guide to the SCID-D, by Marlene Steinberg. Washington D.C.: American Psychiatric Press, 1993.

Multiple Personality from the Inside Out, edited by Barry M. Cohen, Esther Giller, and Lynn W. Lutherville, Md.: Sidran Press, 1991.

Personality Disorders: New Perspectives on Diagnostic Validity, edited by John M. Oldham. Washington D.C.: American Psychiatric Press, 1990.

Structured Clinical Interview for DSM-IV Dissociative Disorders (SCID-D), by Marlene Steinberg. Washington D.C.: American Psychiatric Press, 1993.

Trauma and Survival: Post-Traumatic and Dissociative Disorders in Women, by Elizabeth A. Waites. New York: W. W. Norton, 1993.

Treatment of Multiple Personality Disorder, edited by Bennett G. Braun. Washington D.C.: American Psychiatric Press, 1989.

Domestic Violence

See also "Children" and "Rape and Sexual Assault."

The Battered Woman, by Lenore Walker. New York: Harper & Row, 1979.

Battered Women as Survivors: An Alternative to Treating Learned Helplessness, by Edward W. Gondolf with Ellen R. Fisher. Lexington, Mass.: Lexington Books, 1988.

Behind Closed Doors: Violence in the American Family, by M. A. Strauss, R. J. Gelles and S. K. Steinmetz. Garden City, N.Y.: Anchor, 1980.

Family Violence: Emerging Issues of a National Crisis, edited by Leah J. Dickstein and Carol C. Nadelson. Washington D.C.: American Psychiatric Press, 1988.

Policing "Domestic" Violence: Women, the Law and the State, by Susan S. M. Edwards. Newbury Park, Calif.: Sage, 1989.

"PTSD in Battered Women: A Shelter Sample," by Anita Kemp, Edna Rawlings, and Bonnie Green. *Journal of Traumatic Stress* 4:1, 1991.

Treatment of Family Violence: A Sourcebook, edited by Robert T. Ammerman and Michel Hersen. New York: John Wiley & Sons, 1990. (Also relevant to child abuse and family counseling.)

Family Counseling

Back From the Brink: A Family Guide to Overcoming Traumatic Stress, by Don R. Catherall. New York: Bantam, 1992.

Helping Traumatized Families, by Charles R. Figley. San Francisco: Jossey Bass, 1989.

Recovering From the War: A Woman's Guide to Helping Your Vietnam Veteran, Your Family and Yourself, by Patience H. Mason. New York: Viking Penguin, 1990.

Survivors and Partners: Healing and Relationships of Sexual Abuse Survivors, by Paul A. Hansen. Longmont, Colo.: Heron Hill Publishing, 1991.

Vietnam Wives: Women and Children Living with Veterans with PTSD, by Aphrodite Matsakis. Kensington, Md.: Woodbine House, 1988.

Feelings, Symptoms, and Concurrent Problems

Anxiety and Phobia Workbook, by Edmund J. Bourne. Oakland, Calif.: New Harbinger Publications, 1990.

Beyond Grief: A Guide for Recovering from the Death of a Loved One, by Carol Staudacher. Oakland, Calif.: New Harbinger Publications, 1987.

"The Cognitive Regulation of Anger and Stress," in *Cognitive Behavioral Interventions: Theory, Research and Procedures* by R. Novaco. San Diego: Academic Press, 1979.

I Can't Get Over It: A Handbook for Trauma Survivors, by Aphrodite Matsakis. Oakland, Calif.: New Harbinger Publications, 1992.

Men and Grief: A Guide for Men Surviving the Death of a Loved One, by Carol Staudacher. Oakland, Calif.: New Harbinger Publications, 1991.

Phobia: A Comprehensive Summary of Modern Treatments, edited by R. L. Du Pont. New York: Brunner/Mazel, 1982.

The Relaxation and Stress Reduction Workbook, 3d ed., by Martha Davis, Elizabeth Eshelman, and Matthew McKay. Oakland, Calif.: New Harbinger Publications, 1988.

Resolving Traumatic Memories: Competency Based Training for Mental Health Professionals, by David Groves. Munster, Ind.: David Groves Seminars, 1987.

"Stress Innoculation—a Preventive Approach," by D. Meichenbaum and R. Novaco. *Stress and Anxiety,* vol. 5, edited by C. Speilberger and I. Sarason. New York: Halstead Press, 1978.

Stress Management: An Integrated Approach to Therapy, edited by Lenore Walker. New York: Brunner/Mazel, 1991.

Thoughts and Feelings: The Art of Cognitive Stress Intervention, by Matthew McKay, Martha Davis, and Patrick A. Fanning. Oakland, Calif.: New Harbinger Publications, 1981.

Uncommon Therapy, by Jay Haley. New York: W. W. Norton. (Presents techniques for self-mastery. However, these would need to be adapted to the needs of the particular client and may not be suitable for everyone.)

When Anger Hurts: Quieting the Storm Within, by Matthew McKay and Patrick Fanning. Oakland, Calif.: New Harbinger Publications, 1989.

History of Traumatology

Post Traumatic Stress Disorder: DSM-IV and Beyond, by Jonathan R. T. Davidson and Edna B. Foa. Washington D.C.: American Psychiatric Press, 1993.

Trauma and Recovery: The Aftermath of Violence—from Domestic Abuse to Political Terror, by Judith Herman. New York: Basic Books, 1992.

Rape and Sexual Assault

See also "Child Sexual Abuse" and "Domestic Violence."

"The Group Treatment of Sexual Assault Survivors," by Judith Sprei and R. Goodwin. *Journal for Specialists in Group Work* 8, 1983.

"The Process of Coping with Sexual Trauma," by Susan Roth and Elana Newman. *Journal of Traumatic Stress* 4:2, April 1991.

The Second Rape: Society's Continued Betrayal of the Victim, by Lee Madigan and Nancy Gamble. New York: Lexington Books, 1991.

"Stress Management for Rape Victims," by Lois Veronen and D. Kilpatrick, in *Stress Reduction and Prevention*, edited by Donald Meichenbaum and M. E. Jaremko. New York: Plenum Press, 1983.

Simulated PTSD

"Civilian Related Post-Traumatic Stress Disorder: Assessment Related Issues, " by R. J. McCaffrey, E. J. Hickling, and M. J. Marrazo. *Journal of Clinical Psychology* 45, 1989.

"Inpatient Diagnosis of Post-traumatic Stress Disorder," by L. Hyer et al. *Journal of Consulting and Clinical Psychology* 54, 1986.

"Psychometric Detection of Fabricated Symptoms of Post-Traumatic Stress Disorder," by J. Fairbank, R. J. McCaffrey, and T. M. Keane. *American Journal of Psychiatry* 142, 1983.

Torture

International Handbook of Traumatic Stress Syndromes, edited by John Wilson and Beverly Raphael. New York: Plenum Publishing, 1992.

You can also write for annual reports and list of publications to the Rehabilitation and Research Center for Torture Victims (RCT); International Rehabilitation Council for Torture Victims (IRCT), c/o Juliane Maries, 34, DK-2100 Copenhagen O, Denmark. Texts from the center include: *Psychotherapeutic Guidelines for Treatment of Torture Survivors*, a manual in English. *Torture Survivors*, (a textbook in English and Arabic). *Publications by Staff of the RCT*, revised 1992, a bibliography.

War and Combat

"Combat Addiction: Overview of Implications in Symptoms Maintenance and Treatment Planning," by L. P. Solursh. *Journal of Traumatic Stress* 4:2, 1989.

"Learning About Combat Stress from Homer's *Iliad*," by J. Shay. *Journal of Traumatic Stress* 4:4, 1991.

Post Traumatic Stress Disorders: A Handbook for Clinicians, edited by Tom Williams. Cincinnati: Disabled American Veterans, 1987.

Stress and Coping in Time of War: Generalizations from Israeli Experience, edited by Norman A. Milgram. New York: Brunner/Mazel, 1986.

The Trauma of War: Stress and Recovery in Vietnam Veterans, edited by Stephen M. Sonnenberg, Arthur S. Blank, and John A. Talbott. Washington, D.C.: American Psychiatric Press, 1985.

References

Adler, Tina, 1990. "PTSD Linked to Stress Rather Than Character." *The APA Monitor* 21:3 (May).

Alford, J. D., C. Malhone, and E. Fielstein, 1988. "Cognitive and Behavioral Sequelae of Combat: Conceptualization and Implication for Treatment." *Journal of Traumatic Stress* 1:4.

American Psychological Association, 1984. *APA Task Force on the Victims of Crime and Violence.* Washington, D.C.: American Psychological Association.

Anixter, William, 1990. "Managing Difficult Cases: Anxiety Disorders, Alcoholism, and Substance Abuse." Paper presented at the Anxiety Disorders Association of America, Tenth National Conference, Bethesda, Md., March.

Arnold, Arthur, 1985. "Inpatient Treatment of Vietnam Veterans with Post-Traumatic Stress Disorder," in *The Trauma of War: Stress and Recovery in Vietnam Veterans*, edited by Stephen M. Sonnenberg, Arthur S. Blank, and John A. Talbott. Washington, D.C.: American Psychiatric Press.

Avraham, Yair, Mario Mikulincer, Chen Nardi, and Shlomo Shoman, 1992. "The Use of Individual Goal Setting and Ongoing Evaluation in the Treatment of Combat Related Chronic PTSD." *Journal of Traumatic Stress* 5:2 (April).

Baker, Bob, and Mary Dale Salston, 1992. "Clinical Management of PTSD Related Intrusion and Arousal Symptoms," audiotape. International Society of Traumatic Stress Studies, Eighth Annual Meeting, Los Angeles, Calif.

Bard, Morton, and Dawn Sangrey, 1986. *The Crime Victim's Book*, 2d ed. New York: Harper and Row.

Barocas, Harvey, and Carol Barocas, 1973. "Manifestations of Concentration Camp Effects on the Second Generation." *American Journal of Psychiatry* 130:7 (July).

Barrett, David, 1990. "The Use of Medication in the Treatment of PTSD." Presentation at Readjustment Counseling Program Training Seminar, Baltimore, Md., May.

Beck, Aaron T., 1973. *The Diagnosis and Management of Depression.* Philadelphia: University of Pennsylvania Press.

Bentley, Steven, 1991. "A Short History of PTSD: From Thermopylae to Hue." *The Veteran* (January).

Bigham, Denise, and Patricia Resick, 1990. "Victimization in a Chemically Dependent Population." Paper presented at the Society for Traumatic Stress, National Convention, New Orleans, La., October.

Blake, D. D., F. W. Weathers, L. N. Nagy, D. G. Kaloupek, G. Kaluminzer, D. S. Charney, and T. M. Keane, 1990. "A clinician rating scale for assessing current and lifetime PTSD: The CAPS-1." *Behavior Therapist* 18.

Blake, Dudley D., Anne M. Albano, and Terence M. Keane, 1992. "Twenty Years of Trauma: Psychological Abstracts 1970 Through 1989." *Journal of Traumatic Stress* 5:3 (July).

Blake, J. D., 1986. "Treatment of Acute Posttraumatic Stress Disorder with Tricylic Antidepressants." *Southern Medical Journal* 79:2.

Blank, Arthur S., 1985. "The Unconscious Flashback to the War in Vietnam Veterans: Clinical Mystery, Legal Defense, and Community Problem," in *The Trauma of War: Stress and Recovery in Vietnam Veterans*, edited by Stephen M. Sonnenberg, Arthur S. Blank, Jr., and John A. Talbott. Washington, D.C.: American Psychiatric Press.

Blank, Arthur, 1989. "PTSD," presentation. Veterans Administration Medical Center, Washington, D.C.

Bourne, Edmund J., 1990. *The Anxiety and Phobia Workbook*. Oakland, Calif.: New Harbinger Publications.

Briere, J., and J. Conte, 1993. "Self Reported Amnesia for Abuse in Adults Molested as Children." *Journal of Traumatic Stress* 6:1.

Briere, John, and Christine Courtois, 1992. "The Return of the Repressed: Memory Retrieval," audiotape. Fourth Annual Eastern Regional Conference on Abuse and Multiple Personality: Training in Treatment, Alexandria, Va., June 25–29.

Briere, John, Robin Grant-Hall, Lauri Anne Pearlman, and Dori Laub, 1992. "The Impact of Severe Trauma on the Self," audiotape. International Society of Traumatic Stress Studies, Eighth Annual Meeting, Los Angeles, Calif.

Brown, Angela, and David Finkelhor, 1986. "Impact of Child Sexual Abuse: A Review of the Research." *Psychological Bulletin* 99:1.

Brown, George, and Bradley Anderson, 1991. "Psychiatric Morbidity in Adult Inpatients With Childhood Histories of Sexual and Physical Abuse." *American Journal of Psychiatry* 148.

Burgess, Ann W., and Lynda L. Holmstrom, 1974a. *Rape: Victims of Crisis*. Bowie, Md.: R. J. Brady.

Burgess, Ann W., and Lynda L. Holmstrom, 1974b. "Rape Trauma Syndrome." *American Journal of Psychiatry* 131:9.

Janoff Bulman, Ronnie, and Irene Frieze, 1983. "A Theoretical Perspective for Understanding Reactions to Victimization." *Journal of Social Issues* 39:2 (May).

Burns, David D., 1980. *Feeling Good: The New Mood Therapy*. New York: Signet Books.

Calof, David L., 1992. "Self Injurious Behavior: Treatment Strategies," audiotape. Fourth Annual Eastern Regional Conference on Abuse and Multiple Personality: Training in Treatment, Alexandria, Va., June 25–29.

Carmen, Elaine, 1989. "Family Violence and the Victim-to-Patient Process," in *Family Violence: Emerging Issues of a National Crisis*, edited by Leah Dickstein and Carol Nadelson. Washington, D.C.: American Psychiatric Press.

Cassiday, Karen, and Judith Lyons, 1992. "Recall of Traumatic Memories Following Cerebral Vascular Accident." *Journal of Traumatic Stress* 5:4 (Oct.).

Catherall, Donald, and Christopher Lane, 1992. "Warrior Therapist: Vets Treating Vets." *Journal of Traumatic Stress* 5:1.

Catherall, Don R., 1992. *Back from the Brink: A Family Guide to Overcoming Traumatic Stress*. New York: Bantam Books.

Chambless, Dick, Dean Kilpatrick, and Bessel van der Kolk, 1990. "Symposium on Post-Traumatic Stress Disorder," presentation. Anxiety Disorders Association of America, Tenth National Conference, Bethesda, Md., March.

Chesler, Phyllis, 1972. *Women and Madness*. New York: Avon Books.

Chu, James A., 1992. "Working Through Impasses in the Therapy of Multiple Personality Disorder," audiotape. Fourth Annual Eastern Regional Conference on Abuse and Multiple Personality: Training in Treatment, Alexandria, Va., June 25–29.

Cohen, Barry, 1992. "The Expressive Therapies Continuum: Structure and Process," audiotape. Fourth Annual Eastern Regional Conference on Abuse and Multiple Personality: Training in Treatment, Alexandria, Va., June 25–29.

Cong. Record., 100th Cong., 1st Sess., 1987, 133, 10062-72.

Cooper, Samuel, 1992. "Anthropological Impression of Koach: Participant Observations." *Journal of Traumatic Stress* 5:2 (April).

Courtois, Christine, 1988. *Healing the Incest Wound: Adult Survivors in Therapy*. New York: W.W. Norton and Company.

Deschner, J. P., 1984. *The Hitting Habit: Anger Control for Battering Couples*. New York: MacMillan.

DSM-III-R, 1987. *(Diagnostic and Statistical Manual of Mental Disorders*, 3rd ed., revised. Washington, D.C.: American Psychiatric Association.

DSM-IV Draft Criteria (March 1) 1993. Washington, D.C.: American Psychiatric Association.

Fine, Catherine, 1991. "Cognitive Therapy," audiotape. Conference on Multiple Personality Disorder—Diagnosis and Treatment, Sheppard Pratt Hospital, Townson, Md., Sept. 27–28.

Finkelhor, David, 1979. *Sexually Abused Children*. New York: Free Press.

Frankl, Victor, 1955. *The Doctor and the Soul*. New York: Alfred Knopf.

Frankl, Victor, 1959. *Man's Search for Meaning*. New York: Simon and Schuster.

Frankl, Victor, 1975. *The Unconscious God*. New York: Simon and Schuster.

Freedy, John R., Darlene L. Shaw, Mark P. Jarrell, and Cheryl Masters, 1992. "Towards an Understanding of the Psychological Impact of Natural Disasters: An Application of the Conservation Resources Stress Model." *Journal of Traumatic Stress* 5:3 (July).

Frye, Stephen, and Rex Stockton, 1982. "Discriminant Analysis of PTSD Among a Group of Vietnam Veterans." *The American Journal of Psychiatry* 139:1.

Giller, Earl J., Jr., editor, 1990. *Biological Assessment of Post-traumatic Stress Disorder.* Washington D.C.: American Psychiatric Press.

Glover, J., 1988. "Four Syndromes of PTSD: Stressors and Conflicts of the Traumatized with Special Focus on the Vietnam Combat Vet." *Journal of Traumatic Stress* 1:4.

Goderez, Bruce, 1986. "The Many Faces of Post-Traumatic Stress Disorder." *The Veteran's Guide* (March).

Goodwin, Jim (n.d.) *Continuing Readjustment Problems Among Vietnam Veterans: The Etiology of Combat Related Post-Traumatic Stress Disorders.* Cincinnati: Disabled American Veterans.

Gorcey, M., J. Santiago, and McCall-Perez, 1986. "Psychological Consequences for Women Sexually Abused in Childhood." *Social Psychiatry* 21.

Gorden, Audrey, 1975. "The Jewish View of Death: Guidelines for Mourning," in *Death: The Final Stage of Growth*, by Elizabeth Kubler-Ross. Englewood Cliffs, N.J.: Prentice-Hall.

Grinker, R. P., and J. P. Spiegel, 1983. *Men Under Stress.* New York: McGraw-Hill.

Haley, Sarah, 1984. "I Feel a Little Sad: The Application of Object Relations Theory to Hypnotherapy of Post-Traumatic Stress Disorder in Vietnam Veterans." Paper presented at Society for Clinical and Experimental Hypnosis, San Antonio, Tex., October.

Hall, Calvin S., and Gardner Lindzey, 1970. *Theories of Personality*, 2d ed. New York: John Wiley and Sons.

Hammarberg, M., 1992. "Penn Inventory for Posttraumatic Stress Disorder: Psychometric Properties." *Psychological Assessment: A Journal of Consulting and Clinical Psychology* 4.

Hansen, Paul, 1992. *Survivors and Partners: Healing the Relationships of Sexual Abuse Survivors.* Longmont, Colo: Heron Hill Publishing.

Herman, Judith, 1989. "Recognition and Treatment of Incestuous Families," in *Family Violence: Emerging Issues of a National Crisis*, edited by Leah Dickstein and Carol Nadelson. Washington, D.C.: American Psychiatric Press.

Herman, Judith, 1992. *Trauma and Recovery: The Aftermath of Violence—from Domestic Abuse to Political Terror.* New York: Basic Books.

Herman, Judith, Diane Russell, and Karen Trocki, 1986. "Long Term Effects of Incestuous Abuse in Childhood." *American Journal of Psychiatry* 143:10.

Hilberman, Elizabeth, and M. Munson, 1977-78. "Sixty Battered Women." *Victimology: An International Journal* 2.

Jelinek, J., and T. Williams, 1984. "PTSD and Substance Abuse in Vietnam Veterans: Treatment Problems, Strategies and Recommendations." *Journal of Substance Abuse Treatment* 1.

Jordan, Randall G., Thomas V. Nunley, and Roy R. Cook, 1992. "Symptom Exaggeration in a PTSD Inpatient Population: Response Set or Claim for Compensation." *Journal of Traumatic Stress* 5:4 (Oct.).

Kardiner, Abraham, 1941. *The Traumatic Neuroses of War*. New York: Paul B. Hoeber.

Keane, Terence, 1990. "The Epidemiology of Post-Traumatic Stress Disorder: Some Comments and Concerns." *The National Center for Post-Traumatic Stress Disorder* 1:3 (Fall).

Keane, T., J. M. Caddell, B. Martin, R. T. Zimering, and J. A. Fairbank, 1983. "Substance Abuse Among Vietnam Veterans with PTSD." *Bulletin of the Society of Psychologists in Addictive Behavior* 2.

Keane, T. M., J. M. Caddell, K. L. Taylor, 1988. "Mississippi Scale for Combat Related Posttraumatic Stress Disorder: Three Studies in Reliability and Validity." *Journal of Consulting and Clinical Psychology* 56.

Keane, Terence M., Paul F. Malloy, and John A. Fairbank, 1984. "Empirical Development of an MMPI Subscale for the Assessment of Combat Related Posttraumatic Stress Disorder." *Journal of Consulting and Clinical Psychology* 52:5.

Keane, Terence, Frank Weathers, and Dan Kloupek, 1992. "Psychological Assessment of Post-Traumatic Stress Disorder." *PTSD Research Quarterly* 3:4 (Fall).

Kinzie, David J., 1989. "Therapeutic Approaches to Traumatized Cambodian Refugees." *Journal of Traumatic Stress* 2:1.

Kluft, Richard, 1991. "Natural History of MPD," audiotape. Conference on Multiple Personality Disorder—Diagnosis and Treatment, Sheppard Pratt Hospital, Townson, Md., Sept 27–28.

Kluft, Richard P., 1992a. "Revictimization," audiotape. Fourth Annual Eastern Regional Conference on Abuse and Multiple Personality: Training in Treatment, Alexandria, Va., June 25-29.

Kluft, Richard P., 1992b. "Transference and Countertransference Phenomenon with Multiple Personality Disorder," audiotape. Fourth Annual Eastern Regional Conference on Abuse and Multiple Personality: Training in Treatment, Alexandria, Va., June 25–29.

Kluft, Richard, 1992c. "Finding the Person Within: Making the Initial Assessment," audiotape. Fourth Annual Eastern Regional Conference on Abuse and Multiple Personality: Training in Treatment, Alexandria, Va., June 25-29.

Kolb, Lawrence C., Cullen Burrin, and Susan Griffiths, 1984. "Propranolol and Clonidine in Treatment of Chronic Post Traumatic Stress Disorders of War," in *Post Traumatic Stress Disorder: Psychological and Biological Sequelae*, edited by Bessel van der Kolk. Washington, D.C.: American Psychiatric Press.

Kosten, Thomas, John Krystal, Earl Giller, Julia Frank, and Dan Elsheva, 1992. "Alexithymia as Predictor of Treatment Response in Post Traumatic Stress Disorder." *Journal of Traumatic Stress* 5:4 (Oct.).

Krystal, H., 1978. "Trauma and Affects." *Psychoanalytic Study of the Child* 31.

Kubler-Ross, Elizabeth, 1981. *On Death and Dying*. New York: Alfred Knopf.

Kunzman, Kristin A., 1990a. *Healing from Childhood Sexual Abuse: A Recovering Woman's Guide*. Center City, Minn.: Hazelden Educational Materials.

Kunzman, Kristin A., 1990b. *The Healing Way: Adult Recovery from Childhood Sexual Abuse*. Center City, Minn.: Hazelden Educational Materials.

Lacoursiere. R. B., K. E. Godfrey, and L. M. Ruby, 1980. "Traumatic Neurosis in the Etiology of Alcoholism: Vietnam Combat and Other Trauma." *American Journal of Psychiatry* 137.

Langer, Ron, 1987. "Post Traumatic Stress Disorder in Former POW's," in *Post Traumatic Stress Disorders: A Handbook for Clinicians*, edited by Tom Williams. Cincinnati: Disabled American Veterans.

Lantz, Jim, 1992. "Using Frankl's Concept with PTSD Clients." *Journal of Traumatic Stress* 5:3 (July).

Lee, Evelyn, and Francis Lu, 1989. "Assessment and Treatment of Asian-American Survivors of Mass Violence." *Journal of Traumatic Stress* 2:1.

Lee, N., John Richards, and James Mitchell, 1985. "Bulimia and Depression." *Journal of Affective Disorders* 9.

Lew, Mike, 1988. *Victims No Longer: Men Recovering From Incest and Other Sexual Child Abuse*. New York: Nevramont Publishing.

Liberman, Harris, Judith Wurtman, and Beverly Chew, 1986. "Changes in Mood After Carbohydrate Consumption Among Obese Individuals." *American Journal of Clinical Nutrition* 44.

Lindy, Jacob, 1985. "The Trauma Membrane and Other Clinical Concepts Derived from Psychotherapeutic Work with Survivors of Natural Disasters." *Psychiatric Annals* 15:3 (March).

Lyons, Judith A., 1991a. "Issues to Consider in Assessing the Effects of Trauma: Introduction." *Journal of Traumatic Stress* 4:1 (January).

Lyons, Judith A., 1991b. "Strategies for Assessing the Potential for Positive Adjustment Following Trauma." *Journal of Traumatic Stress*. 4:1 (January).

McCarthy, Barry, 1986. "A Cognitive Behavioral Approach to Understanding and Treating Sexual Trauma." *Journal of Sex and Marital Therapy* 12:4 (Winter).

McKay, Matthew, Martha Davis, and Patrick Fanning, 1981. *Thoughts and Feelings: The Art of Cognitive Stress Intervention*. Oakland, Calif.: New Harbinger Publications.

McKay, Matthew, and Patrick Fanning, 1987. *Self-Esteem: A Proven Program of Cognitive Techniques for Assessing, Improving, and Maintaining Your Self-Esteem*. Oakland, Calif: New Harbinger Publications.

McKay, Matthew, Peter D. Rogers, and Judith McKay, 1989. *When Anger Hurts: Quieting the Storm Within*. Oakland, Calif: New Harbinger Publications.

Matsakis, Aphrodite, 1988.. *Vietnam Wives: Women and Children Surviving Life with Veterans with Post-Traumatic Stress Disorder*. Kensington, Md: Woodbine House.

Matsakis, Aphrodite, 1992. *I Can't Get Over It: A Handbook for Trauma Survivors*. Oakland, Calif.: New Harbinger Publications.

Millett, Kate, 1969. *Sexual Politics*. New York: Doubleday.

Mollica, Richard F., 1988. "The Trauma Story: The Psychiatric Care of Refugee Survivors of Violence and Torture," in *Post-Traumatic Therapy and Victims of Violence*, edited by Frank Ochberg. New York: Brunner/Mazel.

Nathanson, Donald, and Joan Turkus, 1992. "Shame and Self Esteem in Sexual Abuse Survivors," audiotape. Fourth Annual Eastern Regional Conference on Abuse and Multiple Personality: Training in Treatment: Alexandria, Va., June 25–29.

New York Times, 12 June 1990. "A Key to PTSD Lies in Brain Chemistry, Scientists Find."

Newman, James, 1987. "Differential Diagnosis in Post Traumatic Stress Disorder: Implications for Treatment," in *Post Traumatic Stress Disorders: A Handbook for Clinicians*, edited by Tom Williams. Cincinnati: Disabled American Veterans.

Oboler, Steven, 1987. "American Prisoners of War—An Overview," in *Post Traumatic Stress Disorders: A Handbook for Clinicians*, edited by Tom Williams. Cincinnati: Disabled American Veterans.

Ochberg, Frank, 1988. "PTSD Therapy and Victims of Violence," in *Post Traumatic Therapy and Victims of Violence*, edited by Frank M. Ochberg. New York: Brunner/Mazel.

Parsons, Erwin, 1985. "The Intercultural Setting: Encountering Black Vietnam Veterans," in *The Trauma of War: Stress and Recovery in Vietnam Veterans*, edited by Stephen M. Sonnenberg, Arthur S. Blank, and John A. Talbott. Washington, D.C.: American Psychiatric Press.

Peterson, Judith A., 1992. "Managing Abreactions in the Treatment of Multiple Personality Disorder," audiotape. Fourth Annual Eastern Regional Conference on Abuse and Multiple Personality: Training in Treatment, Alexandria, Va., June 25–29.

Pynoos, Robert S., and Spencer Eth, 1985. *Post Traumatic Stress Disorder in Children*. Washington D.C.: American Psychiatric Press.

Quinna-Holland, Kathryne, 1979. "Long Term Psychological Consequences of Sexual Assault," in *Concepts of Human Sexuality for Health Professionals*, edited by F. E. Schmitt, K. Kerfoot, and P. Grinager. New York: Appleton-Century-Crofts.

Ritter, Rick, 1984. "Bringing the War Home: Vets Who Have Battered," paper. Vet Center, Fort Wayne, Ind.

Rose, Stephen, 1991. "Acknowledging Abuse Backgrounds of Intensive Case Management Clients." *Community Mental Health Journal* 27:4 (August).

Rosenheck, Robert, 1986. "Impact of Posttraumatic Stress Disorder of World War II on the Next Generation." *The Journal of Nervous and Mental Disease* 174:6 (June).

Rossi, Ernest Lawrence, 1986. *The Psychobiology of Mind-Body Healing: New Concepts of Therapeutic Hypnosis*. New York: W. W. Norton and Company.

Roth, Walton T., 1988. "The Role of Medication in Post-Traumatic Therapy," in *Post Traumatic Therapy and Victims of Violence*, edited by Frank M. Ochberg. New York: Brunner/Mazel.

Rovner, Sandy, 1991. "Depressing Facts." *The Washington Post*, Health Section, December 17 and 24.

Russell, Diane, 1975. *The Politics of Rape: The Victim's Perspective*. New York: Stein and Day Publishers.

Rynearson, Edward K., 1988. "The Homicide of a Child," in *Post-Traumatic Therapy and Victims of Violence*, edited by Frank M. Ochberg. New York: Brunner/Mazel.

Savina, Lydia, 1987. *Help for the Battered Woman*. South Plainfield, N.J.: Bridge Publishing.

Schwartz, Mark F., 1992. "Sexual Compulsivity and Dissociation in Adult Survivors," audiotape. Fourth Annual Eastern Regional Conference on Abuse and Multiple Personality: Training in Treatment, Alexandria, Va., June 25-29.

Schwartz, Mark, 1993. "False Memory Blues." *The Masters and Johnson Report* 2:1 (Summer).

Seligman, Martin, 1975. *Helplessness: On Depression Development and Death*. San Francisco: W. H. Freeman.

Shay, J., 1992. "Reclaiming Homer's Gods," paper. Veterans Administration Medical Center, Boston, Mass.

Showalter, E., 1985. *The Female Malady: Women, Madness, and English Culture, 1830–1980*. New York: Pantheon.

Sifneos, P. E., 1975. "Problems of Psychotherapy of Patients With Alexithymic Characteristics and Physical Disease." *Psychotherapy and Psychosomatics* 26.

Sifneos, P. E., R. Apfel-Savitz, and F. Frankel, 1977. "The Phenomenon 'Alexithymia' Observations in Neurotic and Psychosomatic Patients." *Psychotherapy and Psychosomatics* 28.

Sigal, John J., 1976. "Effects of Paternal Exposure to Prolonged Stress on the Mental Health of the Spouse and Children." *Canadian Psychiatric Association Journal* 21.

Sigal, John, and Vivian Rakoff, 1971. "Concentration Camp Survival: A Pilot Study of Effects on the Second Generation." *Canadian Psychiatric Association Journal* 16.

Sigal, John, and Morton Weinfeld, 1985. "Control of Aggression in Adult Children of Survivors of the Nazi Persecution." *Journal of Abnormal Psychology* 94:4.

Silver, Steve, 1991. "PTSD." Presentation at Readjustment Counseling Program Training Seminar, Region 5, Atlantic City, N.J., April.

Silverman, Joel J., 1986. "Post-Traumatic Stress Disorder." *Advanced Psychosomatic Medicine* 16.

Slogan, G., and P. Leichner, 1986. "Is There a Relationship Between Sexual Abuse and Eating Disorders?" *Canadian Journal of Psychiatry* 31.

Solursh, L. P., 1989. "Combat Addiction: Overview of Implications in Symptoms Maintenance and Treatment Planning." *Journal of Traumatic Stress* 4:2.

Smith, John Russell, 1985a. "Individual Psychotherapy with Vietnam Veterans," in *The Trauma of War: Stress and Recovery in Vietnam Veterans*, edited by Stephen M. Sonnenberg, Arthur S. Blank, and John A. Talbott. Washington, D.C.: American Psychiatric Press.

Smith, John Russell, 1985b. "Rap Groups and Group Therapy for Vietnam Veterans," in *The Trauma of War: Stress and Recovery in Vietnam Veterans*, edited by Stephen M. Sonnenberg, Arthur S. Blank, and John A. Talbott. Washington, D.C.: American Psychiatric Press.

Solomon, Zahava, Avi Bleich, Shlomo Shoham, Chen Nardi, and Moskeh Kotler, 1992. "The 'Koach' Project for Treatment of Combat Related PTSD: Rationale, Aims, and Methodology." *Journal of Traumatic Stress* 5:2 (April).

Sonnenberg, Stephen M., Arthur S. Blank, and John A. Talbott, editors, 1985. *The Trauma of War: Stress and Recovery in Vietnam Veterans*. Washington, D.C.: American Psychiatric Press.

Spiegel, David, editor, 1993. *Dissociative Disorders: A Clinical Review*. Lutherville, Md.: Sidran Press.

Spitzer, R. L., J. B. Williams, M. Gibbon, and M. B. First, 1990. *Structured Clinical Interview for the DSM-III-R*. Washington, D.C.: American Psychiatric Press.

Staudacher, Carol, 1987. *Beyond Grief: A Guide for Recovering from the Death of a Loved One*. Oakland, Calif.: New Harbinger Publications.

Staudacher, Carol, 1991. *Men and Grief: A Guide for Men Surviving the Death of a Loved One*. Oakland, Calif.: New Harbinger Publications.

Summit, Roland, 1983. "The Child Abuse Accommodation Syndrome." *Child Abuse and Neglect* 7.

Taber, J. I., R. A. McCormick, and L. F. Ramirez, 1987. "The Prevalence and Impact of Major Life Stressors Among Pathological Gamblers." *The International Journal of Addictions* 22.

Taylor, Shelley E., Joanne Wood, and Rosemary Lichtman, 1983. "It Could Be Worse: A Selective Evaluation as a Response to Victimization." *Journal of Social Issues* 39:2.

Terr, L., 1983. "Chowchilla Revisited: The Effects of Psychic Trauma Four Years After a School Bus Kidnapping." *American Journal of Psychiatry* 140.

Terr, Lenore, 1991. "Childhood Traumas: An Outline and Overview." *American Journal of Psychiatry* 148.

Trossman, Bernard, 1968. "Adolescent Children of Concentration Camp Survivors." *Canadian Psychiatric Association Journal* 13:2 (April).

U.S. Commission on Civil Rights, 1978. *Battered Women: Issues of Public Policy: A Consultation Sponsored by the United States Commission on Civil Rights*. Washington D.C.: U.S. Commission on Civil Rights.

van der Kolk, Bessel, 1983. "Psychopharmacological Issues in Post-Traumatic Stress Disorder." *Hospital and Community Psychiatry* 34.

van der Kolk, Bessel, 1984. "Introduction" in *Post Traumatic Stress Disorder: Psychological and Biological Sequelae*, edited by Bessel van der Kolk. Washington, D.C.: American Psychiatric Press.

van der Kolk, B. A., 1986. *Psychological Trauma. Washington, D.C.: American Psychiatric Press.*

van der Kolk, Bessel, 1987. "The drug treatment of PTSD." *Journal of Affective Disorders.* 13.

van der Kolk, Bessel, 1988a. "The Biological Response to Psychic Trauma," in *Post-Traumatic Therapy and Victims of Violence*, edited by Frank M. Ochberg. New York: Brunner/Mazel.

van der Kolk, Bessel, 1988b. "The Trauma Spectrum: The Interaction of Biological and Social Events in the Genesis of the Trauma Response." *Journal of Traumatic Stress* 1:3.

van der Kolk, Bessel, 1989. "The Compulsion to Repeat the Trauma: Re-enactment, Revictimization, and Masochism." *Psychiatric Clinics of North America* 12:2, (June).

van der Kolk, Bessel, 1990a. "Symposium on PTSD." Presentation at the Anxiety Disorders Association of America, Tenth National Conference, Bethesda, Md., March.

van der Kolk, Bessel, 1990b. "Psychological Processing of PTSD: Implications for Treatment." Paper presented at the Anxiety Disorders Association of the America, Tenth National Conference, Bethesda, Md., March.

van der Kolk, B. A., H. Boyd, J. Krystal, et al., 1984. "Post-Traumatic Stress Disorder as a Biologically Based Disorder: Implications of the Animal Model of Inescapable Shock," in *Post Traumatic Stress Disorder: Psychological and Biological Sequelae.*, edited by B. A. van der Kolk. Washington, D.C.: American Psychiatric Press.

van der Kolk, Bessel A., Paul Brown, and Onno van der Hart, 1989. "Pierre Janet on Post-Traumatic Stress." *Journal of Traumatic Stress* 2:4 (April).

van der Kolk, Bessel A., Christopher Perry, and Judith Lewis Herman, 1991. "Childhood Origins of Self-Destructive Behavior." *American Journal of Psychiatry* 148:12 (December).

Veronen, Louis, and Dean G. Kilpatrick, 1983. "Stress Management for Rape Victims," in *Stress Reduction and Prevention*, edited by Donald Meichenbaum and Matat Jaremko. New York: Plenum Press.

Wadden, Thomas A., Albert J. Stunkard, and Jordan W. Smoller, 1986. "Dieting and Depression: A Methodological Study." *Journal of Consulting and Clinical Psychology* 54:6.

Walker, Lenore, 1979. *The Battered Woman.* New York: Harper and Row.

Washington Post, 30 April 1991. "Tornado Siren Failed to Work, Officials in Hard-Hit Town Say."

Washington Post, 2 Nov. 1991. "Germany's Gypsy Question: Haunting Echoes as a Hated Minority Gets 'Retransferred'."

Washington Post, 20 April 1992. "Survey Shows a Surge in Violent Crime: Sexual Assaults Rose Dramatically."

Washington Post, 4 Sept. 1992. "An Ill Wind Descends on Storm Survivors: Venting of Anger and Frustration—Part of Toll on Mind and Body."

Washington Post, 29 Sept. 1992. "For Children, Not the Cutting Room Floor."

Washington Post, 3 Oct. 1992. "Panel Cites Attacks on Women To Back Domestic Violence Bill."

Washington Post, 8 Nov. 1992. "Life as a Death Sentence."

Watson, C. B., M. P. Juba, V. Manifold, T. Kucala, and P. E. D. Anderson, 1991. "The PTSD Interview: Rationale, Description, Reliability and Concurrent Validity of a DSM-III Based Technique." *Journal of Clinical Psychology* 47.

Weiss, Daniel, Charles Marmar, William Schlenger, John Fairbank, Kathleen Jordan, Richard Hough, and Richard Kulka, 1992. "The Prevalence of Lifetime and Partial PTSD in Vietnam Theater Veterans." *Journal of Traumatic Stress* 5:3.

Williams, S. L., 1990. "Models of Treatment." Paper presented at the Anxiety Disorders Association of America, Tenth National Conference, Bethesda, Md., March.

Williams, Tom, editor, 1987a. *Post-Traumatic Stress Disorders: A Handbook for Clinicians.* Cincinnati: Disabled American Veterans.

Williams, Tom, 1987b. "Diagnosis and Treatment of Survivor Guilt," in *Post-Traumatic Stress Disorders: A Handbook for Clinicians,* edited by Tom Williams. Cincinnati: Disabled American Veterans.

Williams, Candis M., and Tom Williams, 1987. "Family Therapy for Vietnam Veterans," in *Post-Traumatic Stress Disorders: A Handbook for Clinicians,* edited by Tom Williams. Cincinnati: Disabled American Veterans.

Wilson, R. R., 1987. *Breaking the Panic Cycle: For People with Phobias.* The Phobia Society of America.

Wolfe, Barry, (chair), 1989. "New Research," audiotape of panel discussion. Rockville, Md.: Phobia Society of America.

Wong, Martin R., and David Cook, 1992. "Shame and Its Contribution to PTSD." *Journal of Traumatic Stress* 5:4 (Oct.).

Wurtman, Richard J., and Judith Wurtman, 1989. "Carbohydrates and Depression." *Scientific American* (January).

Young, Mitchell, and Cassandra Erickson, 1988. "Cultural Impediment to Recovery: PTSD in Contemporary America." *Journal of Traumatic Stress* 1:4.

Zweben, Jon, 1987. "Eating Disorders and Substance Abuse." *Journal of Psychoactive Drugs* 19:2.

Index

Note: Page numbers in *italics* refer to client handouts.

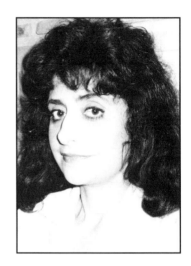

Aphrodite Matsakis, Ph.D. is clinical coordinator for the Vietnam Veterans' Outreach Center in Silver Springs, Maryland. She also conducts a private psychotherapy practice, specializing in post-traumatic stress disorder and child sexual abuse. Her previous books include *Vietnam Wives*, *When the Bough Breaks: A Helping Guide for Parents of Sexually Abused Children*, and *I Can't Get Over It: A Handbook for Trauma Survivors*.

Some Other New Harbinger Self-Help Titles

Scarred Soul, $13.95
The Angry Heart, $13.95
Don't Take It Personally, $12.95
Becoming a Wise Parent For Your Grown Child, $12.95
Clear Your Past, Change Your Future, $12.95
Preparing for Surgery, $17.95
Coming Out Everyday, $13.95
Ten Things Every Parent Needs to Know, $12.95
The Power of Two, $12.95
It's Not OK Anymore, $13.95
The Daily Relaxer, $12.95
The Body Image Workbook, $17.95
Living with ADD, $17.95
Taking the Anxiety Out of Taking Tests, $12.95
The Taking Charge of Menopause Workbook, $17.95
Living with Angina, $12.95
PMS: Women Tell Women How to Control Premenstrual Syndrome, $13.95
Five Weeks to Healing Stress: The Wellness Option, $17.95
Choosing to Live: How to Defeat Suicide Through Cognitive Therapy, $12.95
Why Children Misbehave and What to Do About It, $14.95
Illuminating the Heart, $13.95
When Anger Hurts Your Kids, $12.95
The Addiction Workbook, $17.95
The Mother's Survival Guide to Recovery, $12.95
The Chronic Pain Control Workbook, Second Edition, $17.95
Fibromyalgia & Chronic Myofascial Pain Syndrome, $19.95
Diagnosis and Treatment of Sociopaths, $44.95
Flying Without Fear, $12.95
Kid Cooperation: How to Stop Yelling, Nagging & Pleading and Get Kids to Cooperate, $12.95
The Stop Smoking Workbook: Your Guide to Healthy Quitting, $17.95
Conquering Carpal Tunnel Syndrome and Other Repetitive Strain Injuries, $17.95
The Tao of Conversation, $12.95
Wellness at Work: Building Resilience for Job Stress, $17.95
What Your Doctor Can't Tell You About Cosmetic Surgery, $13.95
An End to Panic: Breakthrough Techniques for Overcoming Panic Disorder, $17.95
Living Without Procrastination: How to Stop Postponing Your Life, $12.95
Goodbye Mother, Hello Woman: Reweaving the Daughter Mother Relationship, $14.95
Letting Go of Anger: The 10 Most Common Anger Styles and What to Do About Them, $12.95
Messages: The Communication Skills Workbook, Second Edition, $13.95
Coping With Chronic Fatigue Syndrome: Nine Things You Can Do, $12.95
The Anxiety & Phobia Workbook, Second Edition, $17.95
Thueson's Guide to Over-the-Counter Drugs, $13.95
Natural Women's Health: A Guide to Healthy Living for Women of Any Age, $13.95
I'd Rather Be Married: Finding Your Future Spouse, $13.95
The Relaxation & Stress Reduction Workbook, Fourth Edition, $17.95
Living Without Depression & Manic Depression: A Workbook for Maintaining Mood Stability, $17.95
Coping With Schizophrenia: A Guide For Families, $13.95
Visualization for Change, Second Edition, $13.95
Postpartum Survival Guide, $13.95
Angry All the Time: An Emergency Guide to Anger Control, $12.95
Couple Skills: Making Your Relationship Work, $13.95
Stepfamily Realities: How to Overcome Difficulties and Have a Happy Family, $13.95
The Chemotherapy Survival Guide, $11.95
The Deadly Diet, Second Edition: Recovering from Anorexia & Bulimia, $13.95
Last Touch: Preparing for a Parent's Death, $11.95
Self-Esteem, Second Edition, $13.95
I Can't Get Over It, A Handbook for Trauma Survivors, Second Edition, $15.95
Dying of Embarrassment: Help for Social Anxiety and Social Phobia, $12.95
The Depression Workbook: Living With Depression and Manic Depression, $17.95
Prisoners of Belief: Exposing & Changing Beliefs that Control Your Life, $12.95
Men & Grief: A Guide for Men Surviving the Death of a Loved One, $13.95
When the Bough Breaks: A Helping Guide for Parents of Sexually Abused Children, $11.95
When Once Is Not Enough: Help for Obsessive Compulsives, $13.95
The Three Minute Meditator, Third Edition, $12.95
Beyond Grief: A Guide for Recovering from the Death of a Loved One, $13.95
Leader's Guide to the Relaxation & Stress Reduction Workbook, Fourth Edition, $19.95
The Divorce Book, $13.95
Hypnosis for Change: A Manual of Proven Techniques, Third Edition, $13.95
When Anger Hurts, $13.95
Lifetime Weight Control, $12.95

Call **toll free, 1-800-748-6273,** to order. Have your Visa or Mastercard number ready. Or send a check for the titles you want to New Harbinger Publications, Inc., 5674 Shattuck Ave., Oakland, CA 94609. Include $3.80 for the first book and 75¢ for each additional book, to cover shipping and handling. (California residents please include appropriate sales tax.) Allow four to six weeks for delivery.

Prices subject to change without notice.